Brain Metastasis

Metastasis:
A Monograph Series

Volume One
Pulmonary Metastasis 1978
Volume Two
Brain Metastasis 1980
Volume Three
Lymphatic System Metastasis
(in preparation)

Brain
Metastasis

EDITED BY

Leonard Weiss, Sc.D., M.D., Ph.D.

Department of Experimental Pathology
Roswell Park Memorial Institute
Buffalo, New York

Harvey A. Gilbert, M.D.

Department of Radiation Therapy
Southern California Permanente Medical Group
Los Angeles, California

Jerome B. Posner, M.D.

Department of Neurology
Memorial Sloan-Kettering Cancer Center
New York, New York

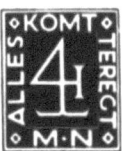

Martinus Nijhoff Publishers
The Hague/Boston/London

Published by:
G. K. Hall & Co.
70 Lincoln Street
Boston, Massachusetts 02111

Sole distributor outside the USA, its dependencies, the
Philippine Islands, and Canada:
Martinus Nijhoff Publishers
P.O.B. 566
2501 CN The Hague, The Netherlands

ISBN-13: 978-94-009-8801-9   e-ISBN-13:978-94-009-8799-9
DOI: 10.1007/978-94-009-8799-9

Contributors

Deepchand Bajpai, M.D.
Department of Radiation Therapy
Hahnemann Medical College
230 North Broad Street
Philadelphia, Pennsylvania 19102

Richard S. Benua, M.D.
Nuclear Medicine Service
Memorial Sloan-Kettering Cancer
Center
1275 York Avenue
New York, New York 10021

Ronald Blasberg, M.D.
Laboratory of Chemical
Pharmacology
Division of Cancer Treatment
National Cancer Institute
Building 37, Room 5C21
Bethesda, Maryland 20014

Luther W. Brady, M.D.
Department of Radiation Therapy
Hahnemann Medical College
230 North Broad Street
Philadelphia, Pennsylvania 19102

Irwin D. J. Bross, Ph.D.
Department of Biometrics
Roswell Park Memorial Institute
666 Elm Street
Buffalo, New York 14263

Kenneth W. Brunson, M.D.
Department of Developmental
and Cell Biology
School of Biological Sciences
University of California
Irvine, California 92718

John E. Byfield, M.D., Ph.D.
Radiation Therapy Department
Southern California Permanente
Medical Group
1510 North Edgemont
Los Angeles, California 90027

Thomas Campbell, M.D.
Department of Internal Medicine
Southern California Permanente
Medical Group
1510 North Edgemont
Los Angeles, California 90027

Paul Y. M. Chan, M.D.
Department of Radiation Therapy
Southern California Permanente
Medical Group
1510 North Edgemont
Los Angeles, California 90027

N. L. Chernik
Memorial Sloan-Kettering Cancer
Center
1275 York Avenue
New York, New York 10021

Florence Chu, M.D.
Department of Radiation Therapy
Memorial Sloan-Kettering Cancer
Center
1275 York Avenue
New York, New York 10021

Michael D. F. Deck, M.D.
Department of Radiology
(Neuroradiology)
Memorial Sloan-Kettering Cancer
Center
1275 York Avenue
New York, New York 10021

Joel R. L. Ehrenkranz, M.D.
Department of Neurology
Memorial Sloan-Kettering Cancer
Center
1275 York Avenue
New York, New York 10021

Peter J. Fitzpatrick, M.D.
Department of Radiology
Princess Margaret Hospital
500 Sherbourne Street
Toronto, Ontario M4X 1K9
Canada

Kaspar Fuchs, M.D.
Department of Neurosurgery
Southern California Kaiser
Permanente Medical Group
1510 North Edgemont
Los Angeles, California 90027

Joseph H. Galicich, M.D.
Neurosurgical Service
Memorial Sloan-Kettering Cancer
Center
1275 York Avenue
New York, New York 10021

Francis W. Gamache, Jr., M.D.
Department of Neurology
Memorial Sloan-Kettering Cancer
Center
1275 York Avenue
New York, New York 10021

Harvey A. Gilbert, M.D.
Radiation Therapy Department
Southern California Permanente
Medical Group
1510 North Edgemont
Los Angeles, California 90027

Frank R. Hendrickson, M.D.
Department of Radiation Therapy
Rush Presbyterian St. Luke's
Medical Center
1725 Harrison
Chicago, Illinois 60612

A. Robert Kagan, M.D.
Radiation Therapy Department
Southern California Permanente
Medical Group
1510 North Edgemont
Los Angeles, California 90027

Colin W. Keen, M.D.
Department of Radiology
Princess Margaret Hospital
500 Shelbourne Street
Toronto, Ontario M4X 1K9
Canada

L. B. McDowell
Memorial Sloan-Kettering Cancer
Center
1275 York Avenue
New York, New York 10021

Garth L. Nicolson, Ph.D.
Department of Developmental
and Cell Biology
University of California
Irvine, California 92717

Herman Nussbaum, M.D.
Department of Radiotherapy
Southern California Permanente
Medical Group
1510 North Edgemont
Los Angeles, California 90027

Herbert F. Oettgen, M.D.
Department of Immunology
Memorial Sloan-Kettering Cancer
Center
1275 York Avenue
New York, New York 10021

Lloyd J. Old, M.D.
Department of Immunology
Memorial Sloan-Kettering Cancer
Center
1275 York Avenue
New York, New York 10021

Stanley E. Order, M.D.
Department of Radiation
Oncology
Johns Hopkins Hospital
601 North Broadway
Baltimore, Maryland 21205

Russel H. Patterson, Jr., M.D.
Department of Neurosurgery
The New York Hospital-Cornell
Medical Center
525 East 68 Street
New York, New York 10021

Michael Pfreundschuh, M.D.
Department of Immunology
Memorial Sloan-Kettering Cancer
Center
1275 York Avenue
New York, New York 10021

Jerome B. Posner, M.D.
Department of Neurology
Memorial Sloan-Kettering Cancer
Center
1275 York Avenue
New York, New York 10021

Marcus E. Raichle, M.D.
Department of Neurology
Washington University School of
Medicine
660 South Euclid
St. Louis, Missouri 63110

Joseph Ransohoff, M.D.
Department of Neurosurgery
New York University School of
Medicine
550 First Avenue
New York, New York 10016

Aroor R. Rao, M.D.
Department of Radiation Therapy
Southern California Permanente
Medical Group
1510 North Edgemont
Los Angeles, California 90027

Stanley T. Rapoport, M.D.
Laboratory of Neurophysiology
National Institute of Mental
Health
Building 36, Room 2D-10
9000 Rockville Pike
Bethesda, Maryland 20014

Leorard Sadoff, M.D.
Radiation Therapy Department
Southern California Permanente
Medical Group
1510 North Edgemont
Los Angeles, California 90027

William R. Shapiro, M.D.
Department of Neurology and
Cotzias Laboratory of Neuro-
Oncology
Memorial Sloan-Kettering Cancer
Center
1275 York Avenue
New York, New York 10021

Hiroshi Shiku, M.D.
Department of Immunology
Memorial Sloan-Kettering Cancer
Center
1275 York Avenue
New York, New York 10021

Toshitada Takahashi, M.D.
Department of Immunology
Memorial Sloan-Kettering Cancer
Center
1275 York Avenue
New York, New York 10021

Ryuzo Veda, M.D.
Department of Immunology
Memorial Sloan-Kettering Cancer
Center
1275 York Avenue
New York, New York 10021

Nicholas Vick, M.D.
Department of Neurology
Evanston Hospital
2650 Ridge Avenue
Evanston, Illinois 60201

John Wagner, M.D.
Department of Neurology
Southern California Permanente
Medical Group
1510 North Edgemont
Los Angeles, California 90027

William M. Wara, M.D.
Division of Radiation Oncology
University of California Medical
Center
330 Moffitt
San Francisco, California 94143

Bruce A. Warren, M.D.
Department of Pathology
The University of Western Ontario
Health Sciences Centre
London, Ontario N6A 5C1
Canada

Leonard Weiss, M.D.
Roswell Park Memorial Institute
666 Elm Street
Buffalo, New York 14263

Myron Wollin, M.S.
Department of Radiation Therapy
Southern California Permanente
Medical Group
1510 North Edgemont
Los Angeles, California 90027

Preface

Of those people dying with cancer, many die as a result of metastases. In spite of this, a surprisingly small number of texts have been devoted to this clinically important topic.

The present series of monographs originated in discussions, which convinced us of the need for texts on metasasis which would contain not only basic and clinical observations on human beings and where necessary, on experimental animals but also discussions of the state of the art in diagnosis and therapy. In order to achieve this in-depth approach, for which publication was preceded by small workshops, it was necessary to impose limitations on the scope of the topic. Metastasis is therefore discussed by site, and the series is organized accordingly. The first volume in the series, *Pulmonary Metastasis*, was an expanded version of a Workshop held at Roswell Park Memorial Institute in 1977. This, the second volume, is based on a similar workshop on metastasis to the brain, held at the Memorial Sloan-Kettering Cancer Center in September, 1978. In organizing both the workshop and in editing this volume, we have been exceptionally fortunate to receive the generous cooperation of Dr. Jerome B. Posner, a practicing neurologic oncologist who has given freely of his expertise in this specialized field.

We have not attempted to include in each volume of this series a complete study of the basic sciences, as this would lead to a great deal of repetition. Some general areas which are relevant to brain metastasis have already been discussed in the first volume, and others will appear in future volumes. In this book, however, we have attemped to cover those basic topics of specific interest to brain metastasis.

Leonard Weiss
Harvey A. Gilbert
Jerome B. Posner

Contents

Contributors

Preface

Acknowledgments

Introduction

PART 1

BASIC ASPECTS OF BRAIN METASTASIS

Chapter 1	Brain Metastases: A Clinician's View Jerome B. Posner	2
Chapter 2	The Cell Periphery and Metastasis Leonard Weiss	30
Chapter 3	Experimental Brain Metastasis Kenneth W. Brunson and Garth L. Nicolson	50
Chapter 4	The Role of Brain Metastases in Cascade Processes: Implications for Research and Clinical Management Irwin D. J. Bross	66
Chapter 5	Arrest and Extravasation of Cancer Cells with Special Reference to Brain Metastases and the Microinjury Hypothesis B. A. Warren	81
Chapter 6	Quantitative Aspects of Osmotic Opening of the Blood-Brain Barrier Stanley L. Rapoport	100
Chapter 7	Brain Tumor Microvasculature Nicholas A. Vick	115
Chapter 8	A Model for Brain Metastasis William R. Shapiro	134

Chapter 9   Pharmacokinetics and Metastatic Brain Tumor
Chemotherapy   **146**
Ronald G. Blasberg

Chapter 10   Human Cancer Immunology   **165**
Herbert F. Oettgen, Hiroshi Shiku,
Toshitada Takahishi, Thomas Carey,
Lois Resnick, and Lloyd J. Old

PART 2

THE DIAGNOSIS OF BRAIN METASTASES

Chapter 11   Clinical Manifestations of Brain Metastasis   **189**
Jerome B. Posner

Chapter 12   Computed Tomography of Metastatic Disease
of the Brain   **208**
Michael D. F. Deck

Chapter 13   Radionuclide Imaging of Cancer Metastases in
the Brain   **242**
Richard S. Benua

Chapter 14   Positron-Emission Tomography   **246**
M. E. Raichle

PART 3

THE TREATMENT OF BRAIN METASTASIS

Chapter 15   Analysis of the Benefit of Palliation of Brain
Metastases   **257**
Stanley E. Order

Chapter 16   The Memorial Hospital Experience   **265**
Florence Chu

Chapter 17   The Hahnemann Experience   **269**
L. W. Brady and D. Bajpai

Chapter 18   RTOG Experience and New Concepts   **279**
William M. Wara and Frank R. Hendrickson

Chapter 19   The Princess Margaret and Ontario Cancer
                 Foundation Experience   **286**
                 P. J. Fitzpatrick and C. W. Keen

Chapter 20   The Southern California Permanente Medical
                 Group Experience: Functional Results   **303**
                 Harvey Gilbert, A. Robert Kagan,
                 John Wagner, Kaspar Fuchs,
                 Herman Nussbaum, and Aroor R. Rao

Chapter 21   Clinical Effects of Radiation on the Adult
                 Nervous System   **314**
                 M. Wollin, A. Robert Kagan, Harvey Gilbert,
                 Herman Nussbaum, Paul Y. M. Chan, and
                 Aroor R. Rao

Chapter 22   Chemotherapy of Metastatic Central Nervous
                 System Carcinoma   **328**
                 William R. Shapiro

Chapter 23   Adrenocorticosteroid Hormones   **340**
                 Joel R. L. Ehrenkrantz

Chapter 24   Combined Chemotherapy and Irradiation in
                 the Treatment of Brain Metastases from
                 Lung Cancer   **364**
                 Paul Y. M. Chan, John E. Byfield,
                 Thomas Campbell, Leonard Sadoff, and
                 Aroor R. Rao

Chapter 25   Surgical Therapy of Brain Metastases   **384**
                 Joseph Ransohoff

Chapter 26   Treatment of Brain Metastases by Surgical
                 Extirpation   **394**

Appendix   Neuropathology Work Book   **421**

Acknowledgments

Chapter 3
These studies were supported by U.S.P.H.S.-National Cancer Institute grant CA-15122 and National Cancer Institute contract CB-74153 from the Tumor Immunology Program to Dr. Nicolson. We thank A. Brodginski, G. Beattie, and S. Rosan for technical assistance.

Chapter 4
This work was supported by U.S.P.H.S.-National Cancer Institute grant CA-11531.

Chapter 5
The authors gratefully acknowledge the support of grants from the National Cancer Institute of Canada.

Chapter 9
The helpful suggestions and criticisms of Dr. Joseph D. Fenstermacher and Dr. Clifford Patlak are gratefully acknowledged.

Chapter 10
This work was supported in part by U.S.P.H.S. grants CA-19765, CA-08748, CA-19267 and contracts CB-64162 and CB-74145 from the National Cancer Institute, by a grant from the J. M. Foundation, and by a grant from the Studienstiftung des Neutschenwolkes.

Chapter 14
This work was supported in part by U.S.P.H.S. grants HL-13851 and NS-06833.

Chapter 16
This work was supported in part by U.S.P.H.S. grants CA-06973 and CA-17970 from the National Cancer Institute.

Chapter 19
These patients were cared for by many of the staff of the Princess Margaret Hospital, and we are grateful to them for allowing us to review their cases. Mrs. Shaheen Khan performed the computer and statistical analyses, and Miss Lois Reid provided the secretarial skills.

Introduction

Cancer is the disease most dreaded by people in western society. Although not the major killer—heart disease kills more people than cancer—or the most painful or mutilating of illnesses as compared with the pain and mutilation of major trauma and burns, cancer evokes more fear and dread in our population than any other illness. There are a variety of reasons for the fear that cancer evokes; some are rational, and some not so rational. At least one reason is that of the major illnesses, cancer alone has the capacity to begin at a single focus and spread in what appears to be a capricious fashion and to involve almost any organ of the body. While the spread may not be as capricious as many believe (see Chapter 4), metastasis of the brain is probably the cancer that evokes the most fear. There are good reasons for fear of brain metastasis, for brain metastases are common, severely disabling, and exceedingly difficult to treat successfully.

This monograph is devoted to brain metastases arising from any source. It is a record of the proceedings of a workshop on brain metastasis held at Memorial Sloan-Kettering Cancer Center on September 25–26, 1978. The purpose of that workshop was to bring together a widely diversified group of clinicians and scientists, each of whom has an interest and expertise in some area related to brain metastasis. The hope was that by exchange of information we would improve our understanding of those problems faced by our colleagues and in the long run, would enhance the quality of our own work. The 24 participants in this small workshop believe that we met our goals and that the exchange of information in both the formal and informal sessions was valuable. We, the editors of this monograph, hope that by supplying the medical and scientific public with the formal proceedings of the workshop we will be able to bring our readers up to date on the current knowledge about this most vexing problem.

This monograph is divided into three parts: Basic Science, Diagnosis, and Treatment. In the first part we have brought together two kinds of scientists, those interested in metastatic cancer in brain or elsewhere and those interested in the structure and function of the brain whether or not it is affected by tumor. We begin with a general overview of the problem of brain metastasis by indicating some reasons why brain metastases represent a serious and significant clinical problem. We then proceed to a general consideration of metastasis and to a consideration of the unique aspects of the brain as a recipient of metastatic tumor. The second part concerns diagnosis, and in it we attempt to bring the reader up to date on the clinical and laboratory diagnosis of brain metastasis. The third part discusses treatment in general and reviews recent experiences with surgery, radiation therapy, chemotherapy, and immunotherapy. Our comments concerning each of these aspects of brain metastasis and its corresponding part in this monograph are found in the Introduction. Our comments are here to tie the chapters of the monograph together and to indicate to our readers the present state of our knowledge of both scientific and clinical problems associated with brain metastasis.

We hope these introductory paragraphs will guide readers as they consider each of the chapters in this monograph.

The essential assumptions regarding metastasis to any organ are that cancer cells must be detached from the primary tumor, must disseminate to distant sites, must be arrested and retained at these sites, and then must grow into metastases. These steps are extremely complex and involve a number of sequential interactions between cancer cells and their environments at the cell periphery. It therefore follows that unique features which can account for metastasis have been sought in the peripheries of malignant cells. With the exception of tumor rejection antigens, which in human beings are weak, these studies have identified no absolute quantitative or qualitative differences between *all* normal and *all* malignant cells. Weiss argues in Chapter 2 that it would be much more to the point to compare nonmetastasizing cancers, such as basal cell carcinoma, with metastasizing cancers in order to focus on features related to metastasis. Possibly the present obsession in the literature with differences among a few types of so-called normal cells and their transformants, has less value in the present context than the properties of cancer cells and their interactions with hosts. This approach is less global but possibly more potentially productive than the important but distinct problem of how cancer cells differ from their normal counterparts.

Animal experiments show that approximately 10^4–10^6 cancer cells are released every 24 hours from each gram of solid tumor. In comparison, the number of "clinical" metastases developing in tumor-bearing animals is small, and it is likely that fewer than 0.1% of cancer cells escaping into the circulation survive the trauma of the metastatic cascade. Is this de facto selection evidence of preexisting metastatic subpopulations in tumors, as perhaps indicated by the work of Brunson and Nicolson (Chapter 3) on subpopulations of B16 cells? B16 cells grown in the brains of mice in passage experiments, selectively grow in the brains of other animals after intravenous injection but seldom form tumors in other organs such as the lung. The peripheral chemistry of these cells differs from lines not exhibiting a preference for brain. Are such differences related to reported differences in response to chemotherapy between various primary cancers and their metastases? Brunson and Nicolson report differences in sensitivity of the different lines to retinoic acid, but the direct relationship of this work to the human situation is not at all clear.

If some subpopulations of cells within solid tumors prefer brain, we might reasonably expect brain metastases to develop at about the same time as those in other well-vascularized organs. This is not the case: brain metastases seldom occur in the absence of metastases elsewhere and are a terminal event (see Chapter 4). Weiss presents evidence for modulation of cancer cell surfaces at the metastatic site and suggests that site-associated modifications may be the result of metastasis rather than its cause. In addition, cells may exhibit temporal metastatic preference as a result of local proliferation and/or degeneration in their mitotic or metabolic states. These and other nonexclusive explanations for differences between the cancer cells of primary tumors and their metastases are discussed in Section I.

The peripheral properties of cancer cells are also emphasized by Warren in Chapter 5. He describes the ultrastructural changes associated with intravasation of malignant cells by active movement through ruptured basement membranes and the extravasation of cancer cells from arrested tumor emboli through local injured areas. Data is presented to support the microinjury hypothesis of tumor cell arrest, in which the proportion of the blood which flows through so-called microcirculatory modules causing blockage and injury or which flows directly into venules causing comparatively less injury is determined by the tone of autonomous precapillary sphincters, which are subject to feed-back control. This widens the discussion of mechanisms of metastatic patterns into usually overlooked areas of physiology and pharmacology.

Discussion of chemotherapy for brain metastases usually involves the terms *blood-brain barrier* and *sanctuaries*. Realities of the blood-brain barrier in the normal brain are discussed in depth by Rapoport in Chapter 6. There is absolutely no question that structural and functional studies have verified the barrier's existence in *medium* brain tissue. In Chapter 7, however, Vick presents parallel studies of the barrier in and close to brain tumors and provides compelling evidence that endothelial fenestrations and discontinuities in these regions present no detectable barrier to movement of molecules as large as peroxidase (M.W. 40,200 daltons). Tumors are heterogeneous structures, and many of their interactions with noncancerous tissues, including invasion and growth, occur in their peripheral regions. It is therefore interesting that Shapiro in Chapter 8 notes that barriers exist in the peripheral regions of at least some tumors. In view of these discordant findings generalizations about the presence of blood-brain barriers in relation to brain metastases are probably out of place, since both the type of tumor and the region of tumor examined must be considered.

Discrimination also must be made between the two basic types of blood channels seen in tumors. Neovasculature derived from host capillary sprouts in response to angiogenic factors is expected, initially at least, to constitute a barrier. Wherever and whenever the vascular endothelium of this type becomes fenestrated, the barrier will disappear on a regional basis. Vascular clefts, which act as channels in some parts of some tumors, are lined with cancer cells which exfoliate into them and do not form barriers. On present evidence, failure in effective chemotherapy of brain metastases could be due to one or more factors: failure of drugs to reach all regions of the cancer, failure to enter cancer cells, or inactivation of drugs within the cells. Shapiro's observation in Chapter 8 that the blood-brain barrier is apparently intact in micrometastases adds to the chances that prophyllactic chemotherapy will fail to prevent brain metastases. In this connection, Rapoport's observation that the blood-brain barrier in rats can be reversibly opened by infusion of hypertonic solutions of arabinose or mannitol into the carotid artery may have therapeutic significance: these studies show that such osmotic treatment can increase cerebrovascular permeability to poorly diffusing agents by 10–20 fold.

Many problems of apparent drug resistance in cancer cells in other organs and experimental animals can be overcome by changes in dose, timing, or route of administration. For these reasons, Blasberg's comments in Chapter 9 on the pharmacokinetics of brain tumors have considerable interest. This author develops models which take into account the 20 m² of capillary surface in the brain in relation to the compartmentalization of blood-brain transport and considers factors which optimize the concentration of drugs in brain tumors. In analyzing time-dependent effects of drugs, Blasberg considers the effects of controlling the rate and duration of drug administration, the inhibition of drug clearance and inactivation, and the use of rescue techniques. These considerations confirm the general impression that lack of success in cancer chemotherapy may not be due to ineffectiveness of the available anticancer drugs but rather to the manner in which they are administered.

Throughout the meeting individual patients who survived for some years after treatment for brain metastases were discussed, but the majority of patients who received treatment only survived without neurologic symptoms long enough to succumb to extracranial disease. Although it has been well-known for years that brain metastases are a comparatively late event in the natural history of many cancers, particularly those of the bronchus and breast, we are indebted to Bross (Chapter 4) for a systematic attempt to uncover the dynamic sequence of metastatic patterns by analysis of autopsy data. The resulting cascade hypothesis interprets the data to show that breast cancer first metastasizes to the vertebrae or lungs and from these generalizing sites disseminates to the brain and other organs. In contrast, primary bronchogenic cancer diffuses metastases directly to the brain and other organs without intermediate generalizing sites. The fact that patients with brain metastases from both primary bronchogenic and mammary cancers do equally poorly may well reflect the later diagnosis of the bronchogenic cancers, which currently respond poorly to therapy within the thorax. In either case, only comparatively rarely will the brain be the only metastatic site in disseminated cancer, a fact which has determined current therapeutic approaches.

DIAGNOSIS

Accurate diagnosis is essential not only for the appropriate treatment of the individual patient but also to allow clinical investigators to collect reliable data and compare the effects of different treatment modalities. The first chapter in this section, by Posner, considers the clinical manifestations of brain metastasis. Chapter 11 emphasizes that patients suffering from brain metastasis can present with a wide variety of clinical symptoms and that the course of these symptoms is not always the classical gradual onset and inexorable progression. Not all patients with cancer suffering from neurological disability have brain metastases, and a number of non-metastatic effects of cancer on the nervous system can mimic brain metastasis and lead the unsophisticated observer astray. Posner points out that in many of the earlier treatment studies, the diagnosis of brain metastasis was incorrect in as many as 50% of patients so treated. If the clinical symptoms are considered carefully, the patient is examined by a skilled observer, and appropriate laboratory tests are carried out (sometimes including surgical biopsy), errors should not be made in the diagnosis of brain metastases.

The simplest and most time-honored test for the diagnosis of metastases to the brain is radionuclide imaging. Benua (see Chapter 13) considers the role of this test in the diagnosis of brain metastasis and assesses its current value and some future trends with the use of new, more specific radionuclides.

Benua's discussion indicates that although relatively accurate in defining abnormalities of 2 cm in diameter or less, radionuclide scanning suffers from two disadvantages: it does not identify small lesions, particularly those close to the bony structures at the base of the brain, and because it reveals only areas of blood-brain barrier breakdown, it does not locate normal anatomic structures in the brain. For these reasons, radionuclide scanning for the diagnosis of brian metastases has been nearly replaced by the newer technique of computed x-ray tomography (see Chapter 12). Although the published studies Benua quotes show only marginal advantages for computed tomography over radionuclide imaging, rapid development of new generations of computed tomographic scanners has allowed them to far outstrip the resolving power of conventional radionuclide imaging. At the present time, the major role for radionuclide imaging is for dynamic flow studies in which rapid imaging after an intravenous injection of isotope can reveal abnormalities of cerebral vasculature.

Computed tomographic scanning (CT scanning), a relatively new x-ray technique which can image normal brain, including differentiation of grey and white matter, the normal cerebral ventricles, and tumors as small as 0.5 mm in diameter, has almost replaced other diagnostic techniques for determining the presence of brain metastases. In Chapter 12 Deck presents the usefulness of this test in the diagnosis of brain metastases and also indicates its limitations in the differential diagnosis of brain metastases from other space-occupying lesions such as primary tumors and abscesses. He describes the usefulness of CT scanning for preoperative tumor localization and for postoperative evaluation of treatment for established brain metastasis. At Memorial Hospital, the cost of a CT scan is no greater than that of a radionuclide scan.

Other diagnostic tests (including cerebral angiography, pneumoencephalography and brain biopsy) are not considered in this section be-cause the advent of CT scanning has left them to play a much less impor-tant role in the differential diagnosis of lesions in the brain. These examinations are now reserved for very specific and very limited situa-tions.

In Chapter 14 Raichle discusses a new and exciting scientific tech-nique, positron emission transaxial tomography (PET). This technique al-lows one to measure metabolism in selected areas of the brain by the use of short-lived positron-emitting isotopes. PET complements CT scanning: CT gives an excellent picture of the static anatomy of the brain, and PET allows one to study the dynamic physiology of the brain. Because the CT scan is so effective in identifying the presence of brain metastases, PET will probably play no clinical role, but as a scientific tool for studying the metabolism of brain metastasis and the effects of treatment on that metabolism, PET has a bright future.

TREATMENT

There are four treatment modalities which can be directed against brain metastases: radiation therapy, chemotherapy including adrenocor-ticosteroids, immunotherapy, and surgery. Each of these modalities is considered in the section on treatment. The bulk of this section is devoted to analysis of the benefits of radiotherapy because that modality is the most widely used for brain metastases and is presently the most effective treatment. There have been no significant studies on the use of im-munotherapy to treat brain metastases, and at least some investigators believe that when immunotherapy is used to treat systemic disease, the number of brain metastases increases. Therefore, in Chapter 10 Oettgen and others have chosen to discuss the principles of immunology and its relationship to cancer rather than nonexistent treatment protocols. Chap-ters on chemotherapy and combined chemotherapy and irradiation present the fragmentary data available in this field and point to future hopes rather than present realities.

The results of therapy for brain metastases are difficult to assess. At present, there is no universal language to permit comparison of the results of therapeutic trials among different institutions; such terms as benefit, response and improvement are used interchangeably and have different implications for every observer. The success of treatment is frequently re-ported only as the length of survival without reference to the quality of survival. Even when the term *quality of life* is used, the implications vary widely. In addition, little attempt has yet been made in the United States to systematically select patients for one treatment as opposed to another. Finally, there has been little impetus for most radiotherapists to shorten the course of irradiation in order to permit patients to spend the maximum part of their limited remaining lifetimes outside hospitals. It has therefore been a major goal of this monograph to re-evaluate the state of the art in treating metastases to the brain by inviting contributions from representatives of some of the major American institutions and study groups.

The question of which patients with brain metastases should receive radiation therapy is considered implicitly in each of the chapters on radiation therapy and was discussed explicitly during the informal question and answer period. There was disagreement both among the radiation therapists writing the individual chapters and even among the editors. We believe that every patient suffering a brain metastasis is a candidate for radiation therapy if other treatment modalities (*e.g.*, surgical extirpation) do not appear appropriate. Recognizing that some tumors are less radiosensitive than others and that in some patients with disseminated disease radiation of a brain metastasis may not improve the quality of life, there is no predictability concerning how treatment will affect an individual patient. Occasional patients with highly radioresistant tumors (*e.g.*, malignant melanomas) respond to radiation therapy, and these patients obtain a period of useful remission from neurological disease. Infrequently even widespread and painful metastatic disease responds to treatment of the systemic disease along with radiation therapy of the brain metastasis and the quality of survival improves even though that did not appear to be a likely outcome when treatment was first undertaken.

Because radiation therapy to the brain has no significant deleterious effects beyond the time during which patients are removed from their families, a trial of rapid-course therapy appears indicated in the hope that it will increase both the duration and the quality of survival. At Memorial Hospital the majority of patients who receive radiation therapy to the brain do not die of their brain metastases but of their extracranial disease and the majority of radiated patients develop a desirable and even useful remission in their neurological symptoms.

Brain metastases often occur at the end of the metastatic cascade and are associated with widely disseminated cancer. Radiation therapy directed at the brain metastases, even if successful, may only prolong survival by a few short weeks and may do nothing to enhance the quality of the patient's life because extracranial disease continues to cause symptoms. If a patient must be hospitalized during that time and the treatment is unsuccessful, the treatment itself may prevent a patient from spending the few remaining weeks with family members. Furthermore, radiation therapy is an expensive treatment, particularly if a patient must be hospitalized. Some clinicians believe that it is important to apply resources to those who are more likely to benefit.

Because overt brain metastases occur at the very end of the metastatic cascade and are usually associated with widely disseminated cancer, it is important to understand the extent of extraneurologic metastatic disease and its influence on the life of patients with brain metastases. Brain metastasis becomes the limiting factor for survival in most patients with this complication, and survival is overall 2–6 months. Systemic therapy is useful in treating disseminated testicular, mammary and prostatic cancer, lymphoma, leukemia, and choriocarcinoma. It is minimally beneficial in uterine and kidney cancer, melanoma, bronchogenic carcinoma, and most other cancers, including those of the gastrointestinal tract (Chapter 22).

A few specific examples of the extracranial considerations associated with the treatment of brain metastases follow: In patients with simultaneous brain and bone metastases, prolonging life by treating the brain disease while being unable to control painful bony metastases may be unjustifiably detrimental to the patients' quality of life. In patients with lung cancer, bone metastases are rarely amenable to treatment and therefore may discourage treatment of simultaneous brain metastases. Among patients with breast or prostate cancer in whom the bone disease has been responsive to hormones or chemotherapy, brain treatment is usually worthwhile. Among patients for whom limited, localized bone disease can be adequately treated by local radiotherapy, brain metastases are usually treated. Among patients with both extensive liver involvement and brain metastases, in whom rapidly progressive liver enlargement is causing functional impairment unresponsive to chemotherapy, brain treatment may not be justified. A final example is progressive asthenia with rapid deterioration, excessive weight loss, and inanition. If neurologic improvement occurs due to treatment, the resulting quality of life these patients must face remains very questionable.

The goal of radiotherapy is to control metastasis for a time and to relieve neurologic symptoms. Steroids to relieve the reactive edema are equally important, at least initially (Chapter 23). The radiosensitivity of brain metastases will determine whether they shrink in response to radiation. The lymphomas, testicular tumors (seminomas), breast cancers, choriocarcinomas, and embryonal childhood tumors all respond well to radiation. Cancers of the lung, esophagus, gastrointestinal tract, prostate and other so-called epithelial sites are moderately radiosensitive. Melanoma, hypernephroma, and some sarcomas are usually considered to be radioresistant, and radiation does not shrink them in a predictable sustained manner in any primary or metastatic site. Metastases from carcinomas of the breast and lung, lymphomas, and seminomas respond well, providing the patient presents in an acceptable functional status. These remarks are based on collective experience with irradiation given according to a routine fractionated schedule, usually once a day for several weeks; other schedules of irradiation now being studied may give different results.

In Chapter 15 Order discusses his approach to what our goals should be in attempting palliation of brain metastasis and the factors affecting his decision to treat a patient. He also discusses new treatment regimens such as 600 rads given once a week, which he reevaluates on a weekly basis before administering the next treatment. Other new techniques considered by Order include half-body irradiation, whole-body irradiation with autologous bone marrow transplant, and local irradiation with radioactive isotopes tagged to immunoglobulin for metastases.

After a short review of the development of radiotherapy of brain metastases by Chu (Chapter 16), Wara and Hendrickson (Chapter 18) review the results of the Radiation Therapy Oncology Group (RTOG) studies on brain metastases. They demonstrate that the median survival of the 2,000 patients thus far treated was 15 weeks (21 weeks for ambulatory patients versus 12 weeks for nonambulatory patients). They consider 2,000 rads in one week to be equivalent to more prolonged regimens of irradiation. Only 70% of all patients were improved overall, and 50–60% of these remained improved from the neurologic viewpoint until death. Higher doses of radiation to the brain have not helped any group of patients. In this study 50% of the patients died of their brain metastases. Wara and Hendrickson note that a postirradiation brain syndrome can be confused with tumor recurrence but that recurrence in the brain is almost always in the site of the original tumor. In response to criticisms of the reported study, in which subpopulations of patients who may have benefited from different doses of radiation were obscured when all data were pooled, the RTOG group is planning better controlled studies with more detailed examination of subpopulations of patients under treatment.

Brady and Bajpai (Chapter 17) from the Hahneman Medical College, Philadelphia, present their series of 347 patients, in which they did not find any major variances with the other series presented here in spite of predominantly higher radiation doses.

Fitzpatrick and Keen of the Ontario Cancer Foundation review the history of rapid course irradiation as well as a segment of their own experience in Toronto (Chapter 19). Rapid short-course radiation therapy for brain metastases was pioneered by Dr. Florence Chu of Memorial Sloan-Kettering Cancer Center. Fitzpatrick and Keen emphasize the discrimination between the various factors used to determine appropriate treatment. In their experience, patients receiving short courses of radiation do as well by all response parameters as those receiving more prolonged courses. These investigations indicate that radiation is useful, especially when looking at improvement in neurologic function, but that the overall quality of life did not change much and most patients required hospitalization both before and after treatment. This particular study did not reveal shorter hospitalization with rapid-course irradiation because most of the patients needed continuous hospitalization anyway. This experience is not universal! Most of the brain metastases treated by Fitzpatrick and Keen were multiple, and a smaller percentage of their patients have primary cancer of the lung than in other series. Overall, they recommend a 1-week course of irradiation in patients with adequate neurologic function and a solitary treatment (1000 rads in 1 fraction) for most patients with lung cancer or a poor neurologic functional status.

Gilbert and his colleagues (Chapter 20) note that their own results show a median survival of 3–6 months after radiation therapy with or without steroids. Their patients' survival times and quality of life were related more to their function and neurologic status at presentation rather than primary site or recurrence-free interval to first metastasis.

Radiation of tumors in any part of the body must take into account the response of the surrounding normal tissues. It is therefore pertinent to this volume that in Chapter 21 Wollin and his colleagues discuss the factors that determine the tolerance of central nervous tissues to radiation. They consider the spinal cord to be an excellent model for clinical tolerance. They also discuss the rationale for attributing clinical manifestations of neurologic radiation necrosis to the critical function performed by the neurologic tissue irradiated and not to differential radiation sensitivity. Neurologic susceptibility to irradiation is probably equal in most central nervous sites, but the likelihood of clinical manifestation as a result of radiation damage is very dependent on the irradiation site. Wollin and his co-authors list the most tolerable doses, depending on the volume of neurologic tissue treated although these lower limits must be exceeded in order to be effective in many patients.

The generally depressing status of chemotherapy in the treatment of brain metastases together with the problems of evaluation of such therapy is discussed by Shapiro in Chapter 22. With present techniques, chemoprophylaxis is not effective. A contributory factor to this ineffectiveness is that the blood-brain barrier is probably present and intact early on in the development of brain metastases. Shapiro shows that BCNU alone does not affect clinically obvious brain metastasis from lung cancer and is only questionably effective in melanoma. CCNU appears totally ineffective for most brain metastases. All the other drugs studied also appear relatively ineffective; excluding breast cancer, the cancers generating brain metastases are also notoriously unresponsive to chemotherapy in all extraneurologic sites. Shapiro reviews 40 patients with meningeal carcinomatosis who were treated with chemotherapy and local irradiation; 12 improved. Even during the three-month median survival of those 12 patients who showed disease stabilization or resolution, only five had both better clinical and laboratory (CSF) profiles. Only patients with cancer of the breast and lymphoma did well in terms of the poor overall prognosis.

Many of the symptoms associated with brain metastasis are due to the sensitivity of the brain to space-occupying lesions. In Chapter 23 Ehrenkranz and Posner discuss steroid therapy, which effectively reduces the size of lesions and decreases clinical symptoms.

In Chapter 24 Chan and his colleagues discuss the use of combined chemotherapy and radiation therapy. In their study of 22 patients with lung cancer metastatic to brain, 18 completely responded to treatment and most patients had an improved radionuclide brain scan. In contrast to data given elsewhere in this section, the median survival was 8 months and 8 patients were still alive at 8–18 months. During workshop discussions of these results, Posner noted that one must be aware of false-positive radionuclide brain scans. The study by Chan and others has great potential interest, but as pointed out by the authors, it is a preliminary report only and will require many more patients in a randomized study before any definite conclusions can be drawn.

In view of the usual occurrence of brain metastases late in the course of disseminating cancer, the role of surgical excision is limited. In Chapter 25 Ransohoff describes the factors influencing his decision on whether to explore and resect an apparently solitary brain metastasis. At present only patients with minor neurologic symptoms are candidates for surgery, and extracranial metastases tend to be contraindications. Surgical excision is usually limited to single lesions originating from radioresistant primaries. In Chapter 26 Gamache, Galicich and Posner report a 10-year experience at Memorial Sloan-Kettering Cancer Center in extirpating brain metastases from 94 patients. This chapter emphasizes factors in selecting patients likely to have a long survival after extirpation as well as some of the complications of the surgical procedure itself.

During the workshop discussions, one neurosurgeon described an apparently successful removal of two brain metastases in the same patient although the consensus was against surgery for more than one. Some physicians select patients for surgical excision only when the lesion is single and solitary in the brain, has responded previously to irradiation and steroids, and recurs in the brain alone after a long disease-free period.

Any attempt to present an overall view of the treatment of brain metastases is complicated by various diagnostic criteria in different institutions. There are obvious discrepancies between the stated cause of death by therapists at different centers. To promote standardization of description, Chernik and McDowell's *Neuropathology Workbook*, which is in use at the Memorial Sloan-Kettering Cancer Center, is reproduced in the Appendix. Great care must be taken to separate recurrence within the brain from coma due to extraneurologic causes (such as liver failure). The cause of death cannot be determined in many patients, but in the majority of treated patients, death is not due directly to brain metastases.

Table 1 incorporates a review of the literature on longer term survival in a total of 1,014 patients with treated brain metastases. The data given in these papers indicate that prognosis cannot be made on the basis of primary site alone: generally, the workshop participants found functional status on presentation to be a more critical parameter than site of the primary cancer. They also agreed that longer-term survival is favored by presentation with a single overt brain metastasis without metastases elsewhere—a rare situation found particularly when lung or kidney is the site of primary cancer. In addition, the patient should be a good surgical candidate or the tumor itself should be highly radiosensitive. On the basis of these stringent requirements, the actual members of patients surviving for even the modest periods of time shown in table 1 are understandably small.

In table 2, we review some of the literature describing benefits from treatment. Little information was generally given about the quality of life for most of these patients; the interpretation of each contributor's series was quite subjective. Overall, approximately 70% of all treated patients presented at the workshop appeared to be neurologically improved by irradiation. It appears from the majority of reports that approximately half of all patients who initially benefited from treatment continued to maintain neurologic improvement until death and exhibited no clinically significant recurrence in the brain. These results conflict with the observations of Harwood and Gilbert and their colleagues that 70–90% of all patients with brain metastases die of local recurrence after irradiation; their figures exclude patients with breast cancers, for whom the incidence is 40%. Recurrence did not seem to vary with the irradiation dose or protocol. In general, workshop participants consider 2,000 rads in one week to be as effective as more prolonged, conventional irradiation. The shorter course also permits patients to spend more of their limited expected life outside hospitals. If the disease-free interval is long, the functional status

Table 1

BRAIN METASTASES: LONG-TERM SURVIVAL

Series	Treatment	Survivors	Site of Primary in Survivors
Lang and Slater 1964	Surgery	13% at 2 years	Unknown primary, 8 of 35 patients Breast, 5 of 45 patients Kidney, 6 of 17 patients Lymphoma, 5 of 14 patients Lung, 3 of 100 patients
Posner 1977	Surgery	2% at 4 years 3% at 5 years	
Deeley 1974	Surgery	60% at 1 year	Kidney, 6 of 10 patients
Ransohoff 1975	Surgery and Radiation	20% at 2 years	Lung, 3 of 28 Unknown primary, 2 of 22 Melanoma 3 of 14; breast 3 of 15
Constans et al. 1973	Surgery *or* Surgery and Radiation	25% at 1 year	8 breast, 1 melanoma; 8 GI, thyroid and ovary; 22 of 25 had complete removal of brain metastasis
Deutsch et al. 1974	Radiation	10% at 1 year	Lung (all cell types), 6 Breast, 2
Berry et al. 1974	Radiation	16% at 1 year	Breast at 55 mo., 1 Melanoma at 29 mo., 1 } longest term Lung over 2 yr., none
Gilbert et al., in press	Radiation	3% at 16 months	Breast, 3 of 90 patients

Table 2

FUNCTIONAL RESPONSE TO IRRADIATION

Series	Treatment	Benefited from treatment[*]
Young et al. 1974	3,000 rads/2 weeks	60%
Deeley 1974	3,000–4,000 rads	47%
Order et al. 1968	3,000–4,000 rads	60%
Berry et al. 1974	3,000 rads/2 weeks	41%
Horton et al. 1971	3,000 rods + Decadron	63%
Hendrickson 1977	x-ray therapy	80%
Gilbert et al. 1978	x-ray therapy	50%
Brady et al. 1974	x-ray therapy	50%
Harwood and Simpson 1977	x-ray therapy	60%

[*]Percentage of all treated, *not* percentage of the responders.
[†]NA = Not available

good and the brain metastasis solitary, however, many participants would be inclined to give a potentially curative dose of 5,000 rads over a more prolonged time.

The participants at the workshop who are involved with therapy participated in a survey. The results are summarized in table 3.

Most patients presenting with brain metastases are near death. If left untreated, they often progress to an unresponsive state which is as distressing to them as to their families. These patients can often show a worthwhile response to therapy in terms of restoration of personality, intellect and neuromuscular function. We will not debate whether such therapy should be administered because the relevant decisions are best made by the patients and their families. As physicians, we feel that presently available treatment for brain metastases must not be dismissed simply because it is palliative and does not significantly prolong life. The quality of life remaining to a patient is also important and can be improved in many cases.

	Alive and Improved at 3 months*	Alive and Improved at 6 months*	Survival 1 year*	Mean Survival*
	30%	NA	3%	3 months
	30%	NA	14%	6 months
	NA†	20%	16%	6 months
	NA	20%	NA	4 months
	25%	NA	NA	3 months
	NA	NA	15%	3.5 months
	30–40%	NA	NA	5 months
	NA	NA	NA	3.5 months
	NA	NA	NA	4 months

Table 3

CONFERENCE SURVEY ON IRRADIATION OF BRAIN METASTASES

	Yes	No
Is ambulation the minimal goal of treatment?	3	3
Is one week of irradiation as good as more?	4	2
Is melanoma sufficiently radioresponsive (in other than an anecdotal way) to be usefully palliated by irradiation?	2	4
Is hypernephroma radioresponsive enough to benefit from palliative irradiation (other than anecdotally)?	4	2
Is soft-tissue sarcoma in the adult sufficiently radioresponsive to be usefully palliated by irradiation?	2	4
Do steroid-unresponsive patients respond often enough to irradiation to be usefully palliated by irradiation?	3	3
Are colon cancer metastases to brain sufficiently radioresponsive to be usefully palliated by irradiation?	3	3
Other than for diagnostic purposes, are there any apparently solitary brain metastases that would benefit from primary surgery: Which primary site? Kidney Most Prostate 1 Melanoma Most Thyroid 1 Breast 1 Colon 1 Lung 1		
Are you impressed with the chemoresponsiveness of brain metastases?	0	6
Do you use prophylactic irradiation in any circumstances? Leukemia Oat Cell Cancer of the Lung	6 3	0 3
Do you use steroids alone for treatment in any situation? (usually severe generalized disease)	5	1
Does extraneurologic disease ever alter your therapy?	5	1

REFERENCES

Berry, H. C.; Parker, R. G. and Gerdes, A. J. Irradiation of brain metastases. *Acta Radiol. (Ther.) (Stockh.)* 13:535–544, 1974.

Brady, L. et al. Radiation therapy for intracranial metastatic neoplasia. *Radiol. Clin. Biol.* 43:40–47, 1974.

Constans et al. *Bull. Cancer* 3:301, 1973.

Deeley. *CNS tumors*. London: Butterworth & Co., 1974.

Deutsch et al. *Cancer* 34:1607, 1974.

Gilbert et al. 1978.

Harwood, A. R., and Simpson, W. J. Radiation therapy of cerebral metastases: a randomized prospective clinical trial. *Int. J. Radiat. Oncol. Biol. Phys.* 2:1091–1094, 1977.

Hendrickoom, F. R. Optimum schedule for palliative radiation therapy for metastatic brain cancer. *Int. J. Radiat. Oncol. Biol. Phys.* 2:165–168, 1977.

Horton, J.; Baxter, D.H.; and Olson, K. B. The management of metastases to the brain by irradiation and corticosteroids. *Am. J. Roentgenol.* 111:334–336, 1971.

Lang, E. J., and Slater, J. Metastatic brain tumors: results of surgical and nonsurgical treatment. *Surg. Clin. North Am.* 44:865–872, 1964.

Order, S. E. et al. Improvement in quality of survival following whole brain irradiation for brain metastasis. *Radiology* 91:149–153, 1968.

Posner, J. B. Management of central nervous system metastases. *Semin. Oncol.* 4:81–91, 1977.

Rannohoff, J. Surgical management of metastatic tumors. *Semin. Oncol.* 2:21–7, 1975.

Young, D. F. et al. Rapid course radiation therapy of cerebral metastases: results and complications. *Cancer* 34:1069–1076, 1974.

Part 1

Basic Aspects
of Brain
Metastasis

Brain Metastases:
A Clinician's View

Jerome B. Posner

Cancer is the nation's second leading cause of death. In 1977 there were 690,000 new cases of cancer in the United States and 385,000 deaths, over 1,000 deaths a day (Silverberg 1977). In one autopsy series from a general hospital, almost one-half of the deaths were due to cancer (Rosenblatt et al. 1971). Of those patients who die of cancer and its complications, the majority have suffered metastatic spread (Willis 1973; Hakulinen and Teppo 1977; Viadana et al. 1973, 1978). Willis (1975) found metastatic disease in over 75% of 500 consecutive complete autopsies on patients with malignant disease. Over 10% of patients with cancer die as a direct result of that metastatic spread (Inagaki et al. 1974; Ambrus et al. 1975). In one series, disseminated metastases were the direct cause of death in 20% of patients with cancer, second only to infection (Klastersky et al. 1972).

It is therefore entirely appropriate that metastatic disease be the focus of much clinical and investigative effort. But why devote a monograph to brain metastasis? The brain is a small organ, representing 2% of the body by weight, although in the resting state the brain receives about 15% of the blood flow and consumes about 20% of the body's oxygen uptake and most of the liver's glucose production (Lassen 1959). Several reasons why the brain should be the focus of major efforts by both clinicians and investigators are enumerated in table 1.1. Documentation for the four main statements made in table 1.1 is the purpose of this chapter. Before considering the evidence for these statements, however, the following text defines and classifies brain metastasis as a focus for the remainder of the discussion.

DEFINITIONS

In *Stedman's Medical Dictionary* under the definition of *metastasis*, the following entry appears: "In cancer, the appearance of neoplasms in parts of the body remote from the seat of the primary tumor." One of the sites of metastases is the intracranial contents. For the purposes of this discussion, *intracranial metastasis* is defined as metastatic tumor invading the contents of the intracranial cavity including the dura mater, the leptomeninges, the cranial nerves and the brain itself (table 1.2). Metastases to the skull are

Table 1.1

SOME REASONS FOR SPECIAL ATTENTION TO BRAIN METASTASES

I. Brain metastases are common
  A. Most brain tumors are metastatic
  B. 20% of patients who die of cancer have brain metastasis

II. Brain metastases may be increasing
  A. Recent series have higher frequency than older reports
  B. Steady increase at Memorial Sloan-Kettering Cancer Center
  C. Clinical impression of several investigators

III. Brain metastases are unique
  A. Small lesions produce major symptoms—edema
  B. Symptoms vary with site
  C. Small lesion may be lethal
  D. Blood-brain barrier provides sanctuary

IV. Brain metastases are important
  A. May be initial symptom of cancer
  B. Cause disabling symptoms
  C. CNS destruction is irreversible
  D. A person is his/her brain

Table 1.2

ANATOMIC CLASSIFICATIONS OF INTRACRANIAL METASTASES

I. Skull (if large enough to intrude into intracranial space)
  A. Calvarium
  B. Base of skull

II. Dura Mater
  A. Epidural space (usually extension from skull)
  B. Subdural space
    1. By extension from skull
    2. Direct hematogenous metastases

III. Leptomeninges (arachnoid and pia mater)
  A. Focal (usually by extension from dura of brain)
  B. Diffuse (usually direct metastasis)

IV. Brain

considered intracranial if the tumor is large enough to invade or compress the intracranial contents. Brain metastasis is a form of intracranial metastasis and can be defined as metastatic tumor(s) involving the brain parenchyma either directly (usually by hematogenous spread) or by direct extension from intracranial metastasis in the dura or leptomeninges.

Brain metastases can also be classified by the structure and location of the lesions (see the Appendix). Pathologically, there are several varieties of brain metastases. A brain metastasis can be single (fig. 1.1) with its symptoms being the first suggestion that the patient is suffering from cancer (Rubin and Green 1968) and without any other metastatic manifestation of that cancer. Alternatively, brain metastases may be multiple (fig. 1.2), often occurring as terminal manifestations of widely disseminated systemic disease. Brain metastases are usually found at the junction between gray and white matter (Russell and Rubinstein 1977) and in the fixed specimen have a granular, fleshy appearance with a soft feel (fig. 1.2). They are usually well demarcated, both grossly and microscopically, from the surrounding brain. Despite this apparent demarcation, the surgeon is often unable to remove all of the tumor. Typically, brain metastases are solid but are occasionally hemorrhagic (fig. 1.3) or cystic (fig. 1.4). Very large metastases sometimes undergo central necrosis (fig. 1.5).

Figure 1.

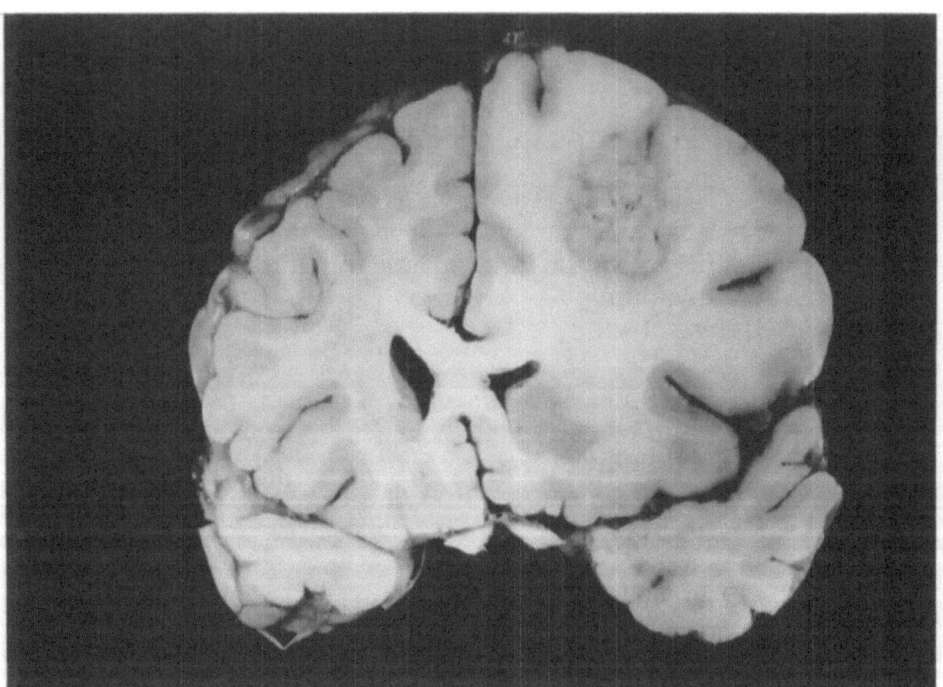

A

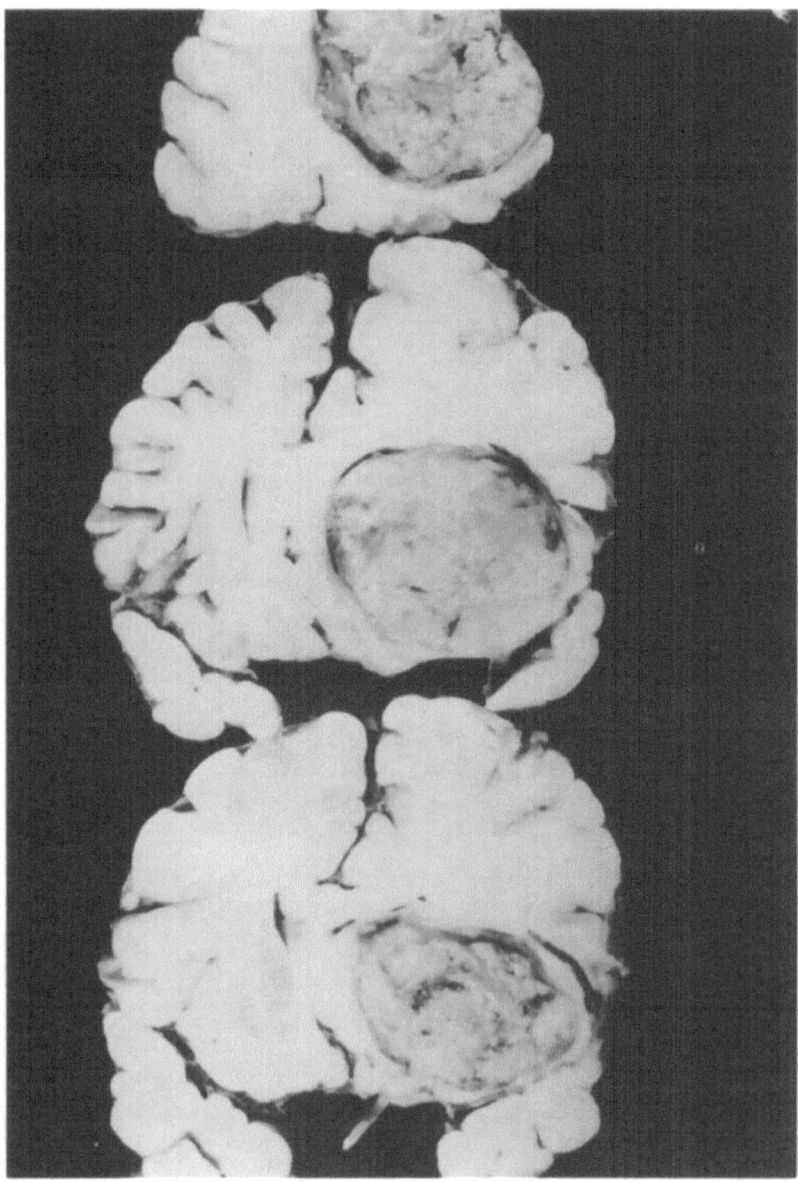

B

Single brain metastasis. A, A small metastasis from carcinoma of the lung. Note the location of the fleshy-appearing tumor at the junction of the gray and white matter, its clear demarcation from the surrounding brain, massive edema of the white matter of the entire hemisphere, and the poor demarcation between gray and white matter in the involved hemisphere. B, A metastasis from carcinoma of the thyroid. Note that despite the much larger tumor than in A, there is little swelling in the hemisphere. The shift is a direct mass effect of the tumor.

Figure 1.2.

Multiple metastases. A, Malignant melanoma with multiple lesions in both cerebral hemispheres and in the cerebellum. Most of the tumors are in the white matter, but as with many patients with melanoma, there are gray matter lesions as well.

B, Malignant melanoma with an uncountable number of gray matter metastases. In this patient, the white matter is largely spared. There is diffuse spread of tumor through the gray matter of the cerebral cortex and the basal ganglia. The pineal gland is also involved with tumor (arrow).

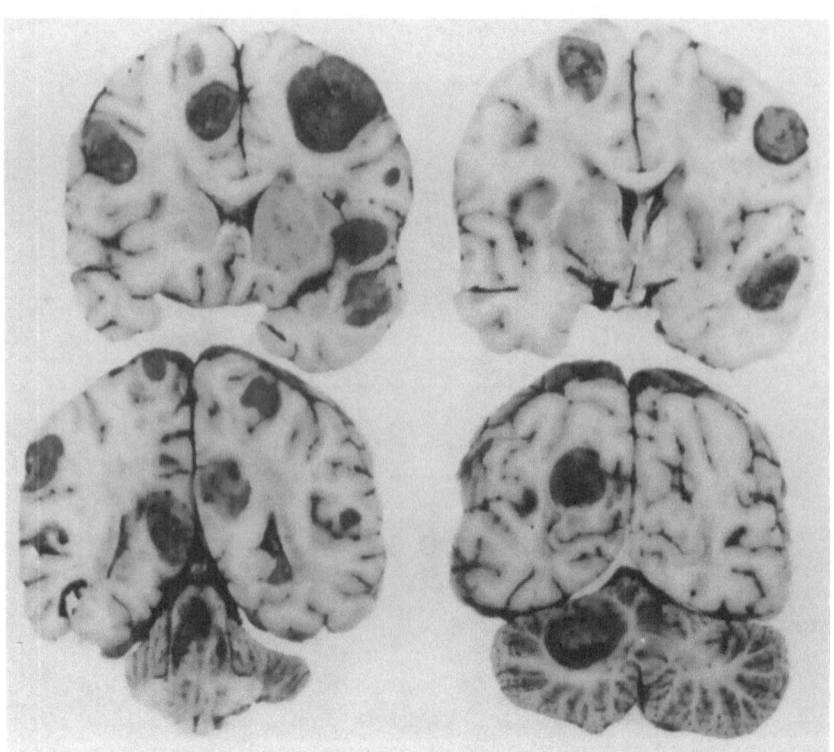

B, Malignant melanoma with an uncountable number of gray matter metastases. In this patient, the white matter is largely spared. There is diffuse spread of tumor through the gray matter of the cerebral cortex and the basal ganglia. The pineal gland is also involved with tumor (arrow).

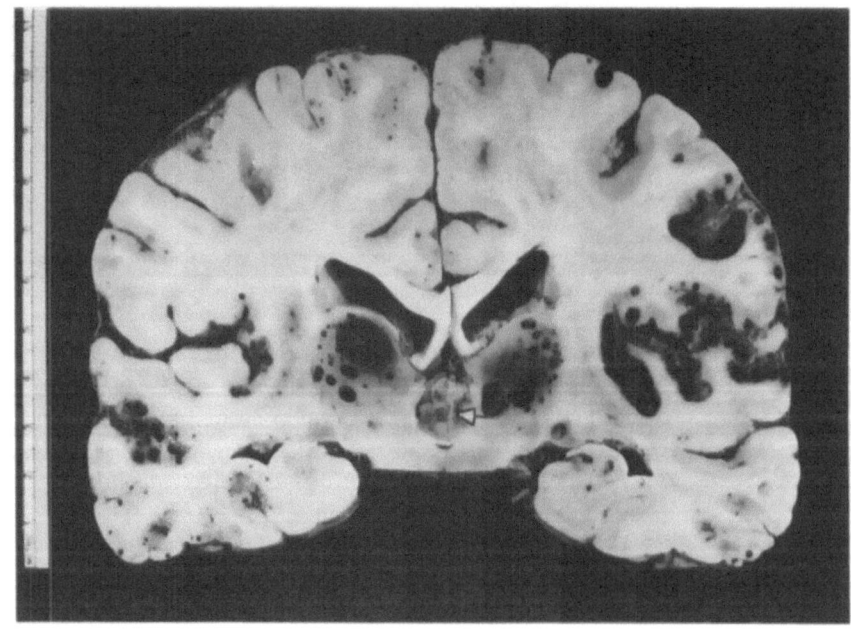

Figure 1.3.

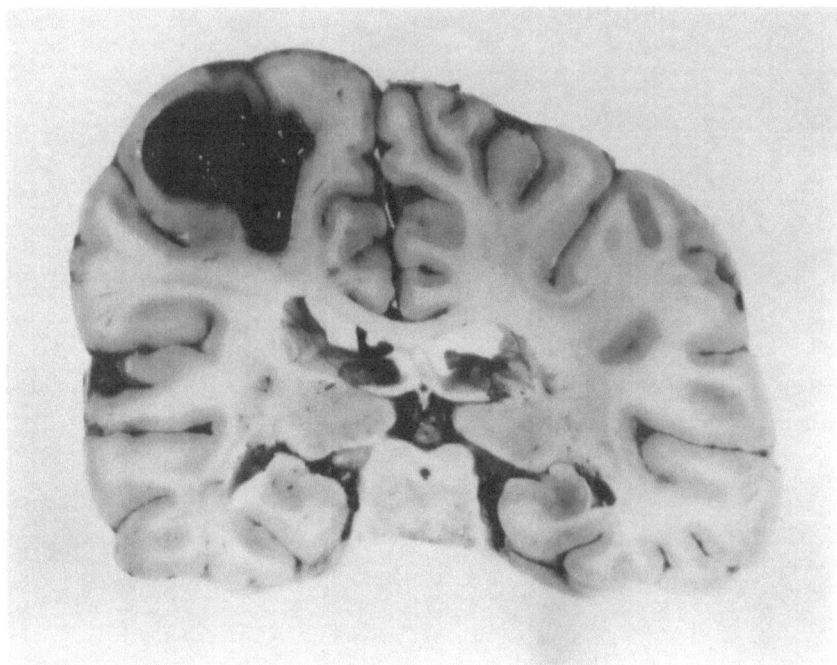

Hemorrhagic metastasis. This patient with malignant melanoma presented with sudden onset of hemiplegia. Location of the lesion at the gray matter /white matter junction suggests hemorrhage into a metastasis. Although no tumor is visibly grossly, a microscopic tumor was present within the hemorrhage.

Figure 1.4.

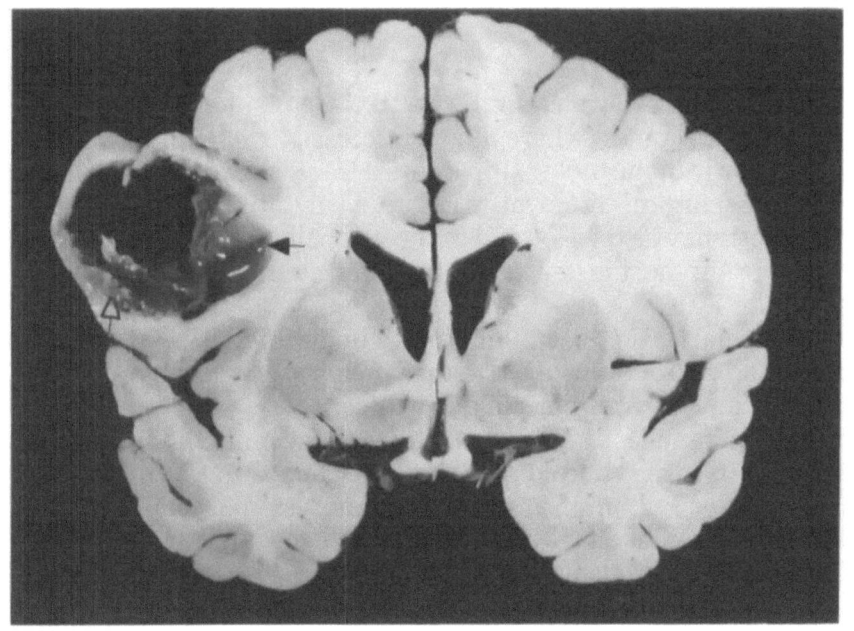

Cystic metastasis. This patient had carcinoma of the breast. Metastatic tumor is visible grossly on the underside of the cyst (open arrow). Most of the fluid from the cyst has been lost. A small area of loculated fluid is visible at the right of the lesion (closed arrow). The tumor itself was small and would probably not have caused symptoms.

Figure 1.5.

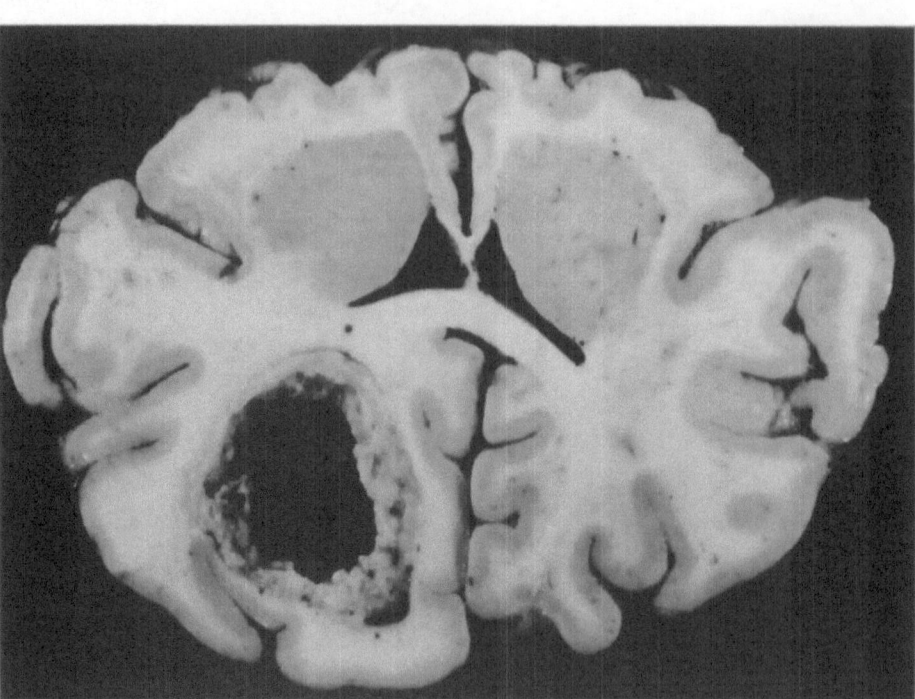

Central necrosis in a metastasis. In this patient with carcinoma of the breast, a large metastasis became centrally necrotic. The tumor is visible surrounding the entire necrotic core. There was no evidence of cyst formation.

Single metastases are usually located in the cerebral hemispheres, at times in the frontal or occipital poles (where they are accessible to surgical removal) but more frequently in the motor strip or most frequently of all in the parietal lobe where surgical removal is more likely to produce neurologic deficit. Tumors may also be located in the cerebellum (fig. 1.6), a surgically accessible area in most instances, or the brain stem where removal is not possible (fig. 1.7).

A typical cerebral metastasis is surrounded by edema (fig. 1.1). At times, the edematous fluid surrounding even a small metastasis is so massive that lethal complications result from the edema itself.

Less common than brain metastases are metastases to the pineal body (fig. 1.8) (Ortega et al. 1951), to the choroid plexus of the lateral and fourth ventricle, and to other tumors within the central nervous system. Metastases from systemic primary cancers have been reported to intracranial meningiomas (Doring 1975), to acoustic neuromas (Le Blanc 1974), and to malignant astrocytomas and ependymomas (Long 1970). Even rarer is a metastasis from one primary tumor to a brain metastasis from another primary tumor.

Figure 1.6.

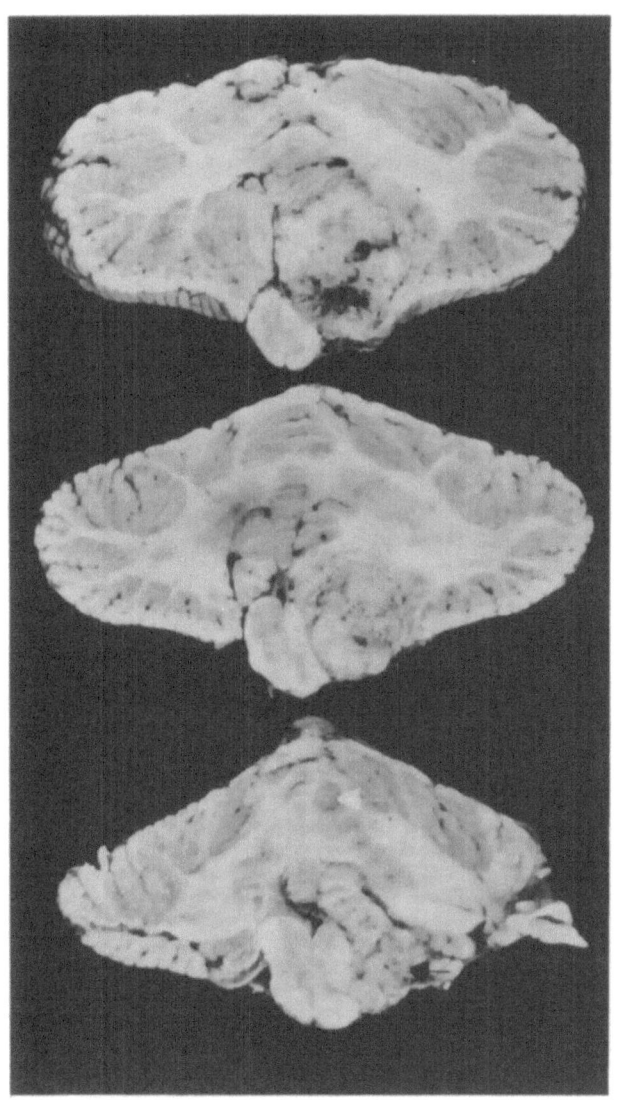

A

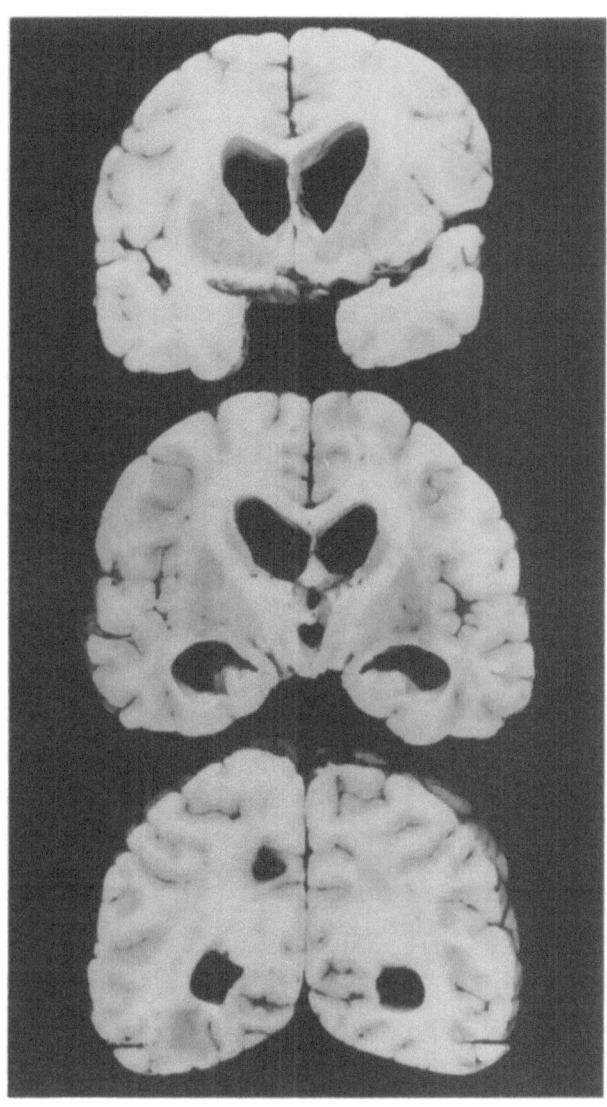

B

Cerebellar metastasis. A. This patient had carcinoma of the breast. A large metastasis is visible in the cerebellar tonsil (black arrow). A smaller one is present superiorly (white arrow). The metastasis is occluding the outflow foramina of the fourth ventricle thus obstructing CSF flow. B. The cerebral hemispheres from the same patient show marked hydrocephalus. Both lateral ventricles including the temporal horns and the third ventricle are enlarged. A small metastatic lesion is visible in one occipital lobe.

Figure 1.7.

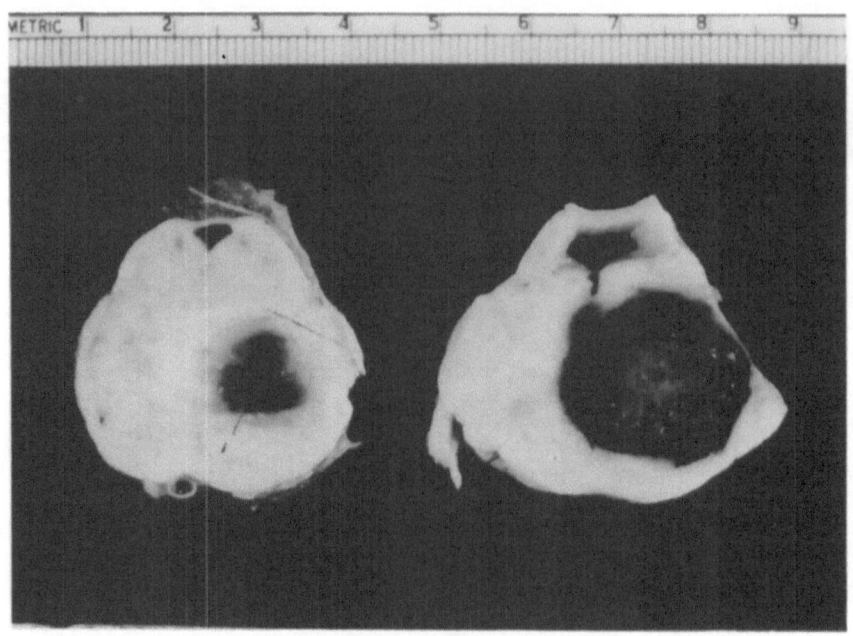

Figure 1.8.

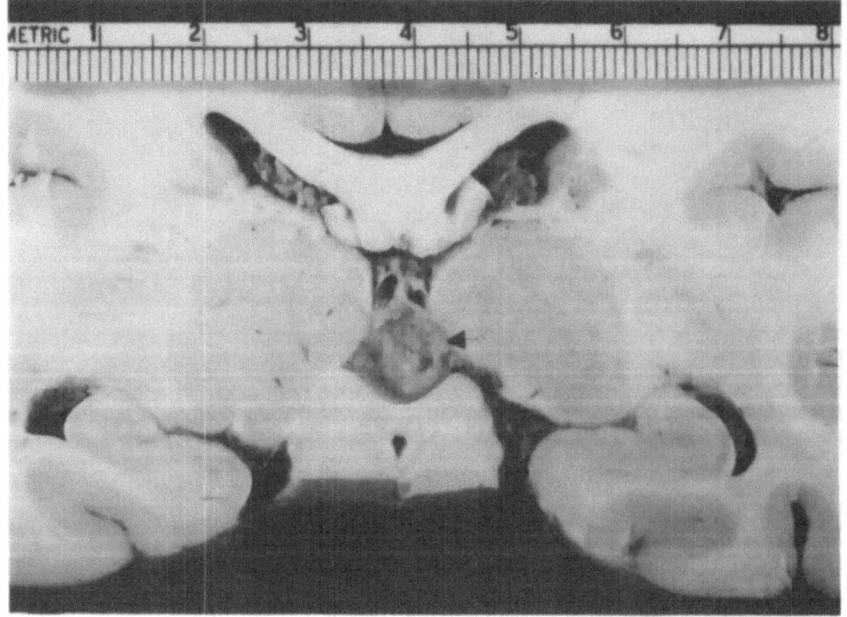

The microscopic appearance of a brain metastasis is generally quite similar to that of the primary tumor from which it arose. The metastasis grows in the brain in two general forms: as a discrete lesion, fairly well demarcated from the surrounding brain and replacing all normal brain tissue in its wake; or as an infiltrating tumor generally invading by growing along the perivascular (Virchow-Robin) spaces and infiltrating brain tissue rather than replacing it. In the second form there may be extensive microscopic metastasis throughout the brain without evidence of gross tumor. Metastatic brain tumors are usually highly vascular despite the fact that most appear to be avascular on arteriographic study. The blood vessels within brain tumors (primary, metastatic, or experimental) differ from those of the normal brain in two ways: the tight junctions which characterize normal brain substance are often absent (Long 1970; Vick and Bigner 1972) and fenestrated vessels are often present (Hirano and Matsui 1975; Hirano and Zimmerman 1972).

CLASSIFICATION OF BRAIN METASTASIS

Using these definitions, brain metastases can be classified in several ways, each of which gives a different perspective on the biology or clinical aspects of the illness (table 1.3). Brain metastases can be classified by mode of spread. In the majority of instances, tumor reaches the brain by hematogenous (arterial) spread; the tumor embolus lodges and later grows at the junction between gray and white matter, the site of most cerebral emboli (Russell and Rubinstein 1977). The distribution of brain metastases is roughly proportional to the blood supply to a given area of the brain. In our study of 106 single brain metastases, 81% were in the cerebrum which receives approximately 85% of the brain blood flow; 16% were in the cerebellum which receives about 10% of the brain blood flow; and 3% were in the brainstem which receives about 2% of the brain blood flow (Posner and Chernik 1978). Hematogenous spread of metastasis to the brain through the vertebral venous system has been proposed by Batson (1940) and supported by others (Onuigbo 1975; Vider et al. 1977), but its numerical importance is controversial, and the weight of evidence appears to be against it (Onuigbo 1975) (see Chapter 4). We have encountered occasional patients with head and neck cancers in whom there appears to be spread of tumor to the brain via the jugular vein and sagittal sinus. In a smaller number of patients, tumor extends into the brain from adjacent structures such as the skull or the dura mater.

Brain metastases can be classified clinically by the nature and extent of the patient's disease (table 1.3). The nature of the primary tumor has important diagnostic and prognostic implications in patients with brain metastases; for example, melanomas and choriocarcinomas, and renal cell carcinomas have a propensity for causing hemorrhage in the brain. The rate of growth of the tumor may determine its symptoms. The sensitivity of the primary tumor to various treatment modalities also has a major role in determining the clinical approach to the brain metastasis. Classification of brain metastases by the systemic condition of the patient has important therapeutic implications: that is, is the patient otherwise free of systemic disease?

All of these forms of classification must be considered for an individual patient because they have significant clinical, therapeutic, and physiologic implications.

Table 1.3

CLASSIFICATION OF BRAIN METASTASES

I. By Mode of Spread to Brain
   A. Hematogenous
      1. Arterial
      2. Venous
         a. Vertebral veins (Batson's plexus)
         b. Jugular veins

   B. Direct Extension
      1. Skull
      2. Dura
      3. Leptomeninges

II. By Structure and Location of Lesion(s)
   A. Gross pathology
      1. Number of lesion(s)
         a. Single
         b. Multiple

      2. Site of Lesion(s)
         a. Cerebrum
            Left
            Right
         b. Cerebellum
         c. Brainstem

      3. Appearance of Lesion(s)
         a. Solid
         b. Necrotic
         c. Cystic
         d. Hemorrhagic

   B. Microscopic Pathology
      1. Discrete
      2. Infiltrating—perivascular

Table 1.3

(*Continued*)

III. Clinical Classification
   A. Nature of Primary Tumor
      1. Histologic type
      2. Rate of growth
      3. Treatability
         Surgery
         Radiation therapy
         Chemotherapy
         Immunotherapy

   B. Time of Occurrence of Metastases
      1. After diagnosis and treatment of primary (metachronous)
      2. Simultaneous with appearance of primary (synchronous)
      3. Before primary is identified (precocious)

   C. Extent of Systemic Disease
      1. Free of systemic disease
      2. Not free of systemic disease
         a. Primary tumor unknown
         b. Systemic disease present but controlled
         c. Systemic disease uncontrolled

WHY A MONOGRAPH ON BRAIN METASTASIS?

Brain Metastases Are Common

Frequency of Brain Metastasis   The exact frequency of brain metastases in the cancer population is unknown. There are three general approaches to estimating their frequency: epidemiologic studies, clinical studies, and autopsy studies. Only a few epidemiologic studies have addressed the frequency of metastatic brain tumors. Guomundsson (1970) surveyed central nervous system tumors in Iceland between 1954 and 1963. The average annual incidence of metastatic brain tumors was 2.8/100,000 population; the prevalence was 1.6/100,000 population. He indicated that these data probably underestimated the true incidence and prevalence because of failure to identify all patients with metastatic brain tumors. Percy and colleagues (1972) surveyed central nervous system neoplasms in Olmstead County, Minnesota. They reported an annual incidence of 11.1/100,000 population—nearly equal to the incidence of primary central nervous system tumors (12.5/100,000 population). They also suggested that the rate of metastatic tumors was underestimated because of inadequate reporting. After a survey of neurologic disease in an English city, Brewis and colleagues (1966) reported an average annual incidence of metastatic brain tumors of 5.4/100,000 population. In all of these epidemiologic studies, both the true annual incidence and prevalence and the frequency of disability caused by intracranial metastases are underestimated because death certificates, although indicating the primary cancer, do not usually specify the site of even symptomatic metastases. Consequently, most cancer patients suffering from brain metastases are not identified. Without adjusting for the underestimation of these incidence figures, the study of Percy and colleagues indicates that brain metastases are at least as common as primary brain tumors.

Several reports of the clinical frequency of brain metastases come from neurologic and neurosurgical centers where the patients present with signs and symptoms of brain tumor. In these reports, the number of brain metastases is expressed as a fraction of the total number of brain tumors of all types encountered. There has been an increase in the representation of metastatic brain tumors in these series in recent years (table 1.4). Thus Cushing reported that metastases comprised 4.2% of brain tumors in 1932. Stortebecker reported 3.5% in 1954; Simionescu, 6.7% in 1960; Richards and McKissock, 10% in 1963; and Arseni and Constantinescu, 13% in 1965. In a series of reports from the neurosurgical center of St. Anne's Hospital in Paris, the relative frequency of brain metastases among central nervous system tumors was 4.8% in 1943, 14.8% in 1953, and 21% in 1963 (Paillas and Pellet (1976). Paillas and Pellet estimate that of 100 patients presently hospitalized for brain tumor, 20 will be suffering from a metastasis, and of these 20, half will be judged operable. In these series the true incidence of brain metastases is likewise underestimated because only symptomatic patients who are potential surgical candidates are included.

A third method of estimating the frequency of brain metastases is by autopsy study. Such studies can accurately define the frequency, site and multiplicity of metastatic brain tumors from each of the individual primary tumors. Several autopsy studies are listed in table 1.5. A series reported by Posner and Chernik (1978) is representative. Of 2,375 patients who died of cancer between 1969 and 1976 at Memorial Sloan-Kettering Cancer Center and whose autopsy included examination of the central nervous system, 361 (15%) suffered from brain metastases. Of these, 225 or 9% of the total patients at autopsy had brain metastases without other intracranial lesions. The other 136 suffered from a combination of brain metastasis and other intracranial metastasis, such as metastases to the dura or leptomeninges. The distribution of other intracranial metastases in this series is indicated in table 1.6. The accuracy of such incidence figures is limited only by the skill and persistence of the neuropathologist and the frequency with which the central nervous system is examined at autopsy.

Autopsy studies suffer because they are done on selected patients—those who die in particular hospitals (often attracted to that hospital for

Table 1.4

FREQUENCY OF BRAIN METASTASES ON NEUROLOGIC SERVICES

Source	Number of Brain Tumors	Percentage Metastatic
Meagher and Eisenhardt 1931	1,850	3.0
Cushing 1932	2,023	4.7
Elkington 1935	805	9.0
Livingston et al. 1948	1,256	4.1
Christensen 1949	2,023	3.9
Zulch 1949	3,000	4.0
Stortebecker 1954	4,444	3.5
Papo and Tritapepe 1957	—	6.3
Simionescu 1960	195	6.7
Richards and McKissock 1963	3,890	10.0
Petit-Dutaillis et al. 1956	594	25.0 (of malignant brain tumors)
van Eck et al. 1965	904	13
Arseni and Constantinescu 1965	15,821	13
Paillas and Pellet 1976	Not stated	12

treatment of a brain metastasis) rather than those who die at home. Furthermore, some of the lesions detected at autopsy were asymptomatic during life and thus had little clinical significance. Hildebrand (1978) estimates that 25% of brain metastases are not suspected before autopsy, a figure similar to our own 25–33% asymptomatic brain metastasis. Another drawback of autopsy studies is that many of them do not differentiate the various types of intracranial metastases. Some studies include dural lesions, others exclude them. Some include leptomeningeal lesions and others exclude them. Thus comparisons among the studies are not entirely valid. Despite these drawbacks, autopsy series probably offer the most accurate estimates of the true incidence of brain metastases. A reasonable figure taking all of the studies listed in table 1.4 into consideration would be that 24% of patients dying of cancer have intracranial metastases (including dural metastases). Approximately 20% of cancer patients have metastatic disease involving either the leptomeninges or brain itself, and as many as 10% of patients who die of cancer have brain metastases without involvement of either dura or leptomeninges.

Although selection factors in these autopsy data probably overestimate the incidence of brain metastases to the extent they can be applied to the general population, they indicate that of the 385,000 patients dying yearly of cancer, 92,400 (385,000 × 24%) suffer from intracranial metastases, 77,000 (385,000 × 20%) suffer from brain and leptomeningeal involvement, and 38,500 (385,000 × 10%) suffer from brain metastases in the absence of other intracranial involvement.

Site of Primary Cancer As important as the frequency of brain metastases is the site of origin of the tumor. This problem can be addressed in two ways: by determining the most frequent tumors metastatic to the brain and by determining the frequency with which a given cancer metastasizes to the brain. The primary origin of metastatic brain tumors is indi-

Table 1.5

CNS METASTASIS IN PATIENTS WITH CANCER (SOME AUTOPSY STUDIES)

Series	Number of Cases	Intracranial Metastases Number	Intracranial Metastases Percentage	Comment
Willis 1973	461	23	5	
Lesse and Netsky 1954	595	207	35	Includes dura; terminal care hospital
Earle 1954	710	79	10	No dural metastases
Earle 1955	1,399	167	12	No dural metastases
Chason et al. 1963	1,096	200	18	Includes spinal and pituitary metastases; no epidural
Aronson et al. 1964	2,406	397	16.5	No dura
Posner and Chernik 1978	2,375	572 / 467	24 / 20	Includes dura / No dural metastases

cated in table 1.7. In most series carcinoma of the lung is the most common primary site and the breast is the next most common. At Memorial Sloan-Kettering melanomas, leukemias, and lymphomas are also common offenders, but this finding differs from other series. The difference is partially due to the relatively low incidence of melanoma. It appears that patients with such tumors are attracted to major cancer centers. In addition, leukemias and lymphomas, although commonly metastatic to the nervous system, are usually not treated at neurosurgical centers where most of these series originate. In every series reported from clinical units, brain metastases of unknown origin are important (see Chapter 25).

Certain primary tumors commonly metastasize to the brain and others do not (table 1.7). Spread to the brain is the rule in patients who die

Table 1.6

INTRACRANIAL METASTASES IN 2,375 PATIENTS WITH CANCER:
MEMORIAL SLOAN-KETTERING CANCER CENTER 1970–1976

Type of Tumor	Number of Patients	Percentage of Total Patient Population
Total intracranial metastases	572	24
Intradural metastases*	467	20
Brain metastases	361	15
Brain metastases only	225	9
single	106	47 (of intracerebral metastases)
cerebrum	86	81
cerebellum	17	16
brainstem	3	3
multiple	119	53
Leptomeningeal metastases	184	8
Leptomeningeal metastases only	68	3
Dural metastases	202	9
Dural metastases only	105	4

*Brain + leptomeninges.

of melanoma, common but less frequently so in patients who die of carcinoma of the lung or breast, and relatively rare among patients who die of prostatic cancer (Catane et al. 1976), ovarian carcinomas, or certain sarcomas. The implication of these findings is not clear. Willis (1973) reviews the evidence for the so-called fertile soil theory or the propensity of certain tumors to grow in the brain once malignant cells have reached the brain via the bloodstream. A contrary view is that the varying incidence of brain metastasis is a result of the propensity of the lungs and then the systemic circulation as opposed to spreading by lymphatics or venous circulation (see Chapter 4). These considerations are discussed in more detail elsewhere in this monograph.

The site of metastasis in the intracranial cavity once tumor cells reach the central nervous system is also interesting. Certain primary cancers such as prostate carcinoma and neuroblastoma invade intracranial structures such as the dura mater commonly (usually by spread from skull lesions) but are rare in the brain. Other primary tumors such as pulmonary carcinomas and melanoma more commonly metastasize to the brain than to other intracranial structures. For example, in one group of 49 patients who died of prostatic carcinoma, 13 (27%) had intracranial metastases which were restricted to the dura mater and no patients had intracranial metastases restricted to the brain (Catane et al. 1976). On the other hand, of 125 patients with malignant melanoma, only 5 (4%) had intracranial metastases restricted to the dura mater whereas 50 (40%) had metastases restricted to the brain (Posner and Chernik 1978). The high incidence of brain metastases in malignant melanoma has been emphasized in other series as well (Chason et al. 1963; Aronson et al. 1964; Meyer and Reah 1953).

Number of Brain Metastases Most metastatic brain tumors are multiple. In several autopsy studies single metastases accounted for only 14–35% of cases (Chason et al. 1963; Espana et al. 1978; Posner and Chernik 1978). In our own studies (table 1.8), 52% of patients dying with brain metastases but without other intracranial metastases had more than one lesion in the brain and only 48% had a single brain metastasis. The likelihood of multiple metastases varied with the nature of the primary tumor. Single metastases were more common in patients suffering from breast and renal primaries; multiple metastases were more common in patients suffering from carcinoma of the lung or malignant melanoma.

The site of a single brain metastasis has important therapeutic implications and has been studied several times (Paillas and Pellet 1976; Lesse and Netsky 1954; Chason et al. 1963; Aronson et al. 1964; Meyer and Reah 1953). The brain can be divided into three large segments: cerebrum, cerebellum and brainstem. The site of a single metastasis appears to relate to the blood flow to that particular portion of the brain. Two other important factors are the anatomy of the blood vessels (metastatic brain tumors like cerebral emboli are slightly more common to the left hemisphere than to the right hemisphere) and the terminal distribution of the blood vessels. Thus, Pail-

Table 1.7

SITE OF PRIMARY TUMOR FOR 572 PATIENTS WITH
INTRACRANIAL METASTASIS

Tumor	Intracranial Metastasis		Brain and Leptomeningeal Metastasis		Brain Metastasis Only	
	Number of Patients	Percentage of Total	Number of Patients	Percentage of Total	Number of Patients	Percentage of Total
Lung	101	18	95	20	61	26
Breast	98	17	75	16	33	14
Melanoma	90	16	85	18	50	21
Leukemia	66	12	58	12	10	4
Lymphoma	55	10	38	8	4	2
Testes	21	4	20	4	17	9
Neuroblastoma	20	3	8	2	2	1
Renal	14	2	13	3	11	5
Other	107	18	75	17	47	20
TOTALS:	572	100%	467	100%	235	100%

las and Pellet (1976) document that there are more metastatic brain tumors in the postcentral gyrus representing the end distribution of the middle cerebral artery than in the central or precentral areas of the brain.

All of the foregoing data indicate that brain metastases commonly occur in about 25% of patients who die of cancer and are worthy of careful study on the basis of their frequency alone.

Brain Metastases May Be Increasing in Frequency

Many oncologists believe that they are seeing more patients with brain metastases now than in prior years. Documentation for this anecdotal belief is not fully available, but there are supporting hints in the literature. Gercovich, Luna and Gottlieb (1975) have reported an increasing incidence of brain metastases in patients with sarcoma, which they attribute to more effective chemotherapy for the systemic tumor. Espana, Chang and Wiernik (1978) have reported a similar increasing incidence among their patients with nonhematologic sarcomas. Mayer, Berkowitz

Table 1.8

FREQUENCY OF METASTASES TO BRAIN FROM SELECTED
PRIMARY TUMORS

Primary Tumor	Total Patients	Brain Metastases*	
		Patients	Percentage
Breast	324	33	10
Lung	297	61	21
Melanoma	125	50	40
Kidney	52	11	21
Ovary	60	3	5
Colon	130	6	5
Osteogenic sarcoma	39	4	10
Others	1,061	57	
TOTALS	2,088	225	11

*None of these 225 patients had leptomeningeal or dural metastases.

and Griffiths (1978) have suggested an increasing incidence of brain metastases in patients with ovarian carcinoma that occurs because of longer survival of patients with metastatic disease.

Our own data (fig. 1.9) suggest that at Memorial Sloan-Kettering Cancer Center the incidence of all kinds of intracranial metastases has increased within the years 1970 through 1977. We believe our data are accurate because during this time the entire central nervous system was examined in all patients for whom such examination was not proscribed. Examination of the central nervous system was standardized throughout this period under the supervision of the same neuropathologist. (See the Appendix for *Neuropathology Workbook*.) Interpretation of the data from this series is difficult, however. Selection factors may have played an important role because many patients are referred to this center because of intracranial metastasis and the number of such referrals has probably increased over the years.

When one compares the overall incidence of intracranial metastases between 1970 and 1977 in this series with those found in the older litera-

	Location			
	Cerebrum Only	Cerebellum Only	Brainstem Only	Multiple Sites
	18	1	0	14
	20	4	1	36
	16	3	0	31
	7	3	0	1
	3	0	0	0
	1	1	0	4
	2	1	0	1
	19	4	2	32
	86	17	3	119

ture, the more recent series appear to have no more brain metastases than the older ones. If one restricts the comparison to the years 1976 and 1977, our own series appears to have a greater incidence than any older series except that of Lesse and Netsky (1954). Thus, some evidence suggests that brain metastases are increasing in incidence, but it is not firm and further studies are clearly indicated.

If brain metastases are increasing in incidence, what is the reason? Some possibilities which must be considered include: (1) A greater clinical recognition of brain metastasis may lead to more accurate diagnosis during life and more careful examination of the brain after death. (2) Longer survival in some patients may lead to a greater period of time for metastatic disease to disseminate and in turn to produce more widespread metastases throughout the body including the brain. If most metastases reach the brain by a cascade effect (Viadana et al. 1978) (see Chapter 4), then the

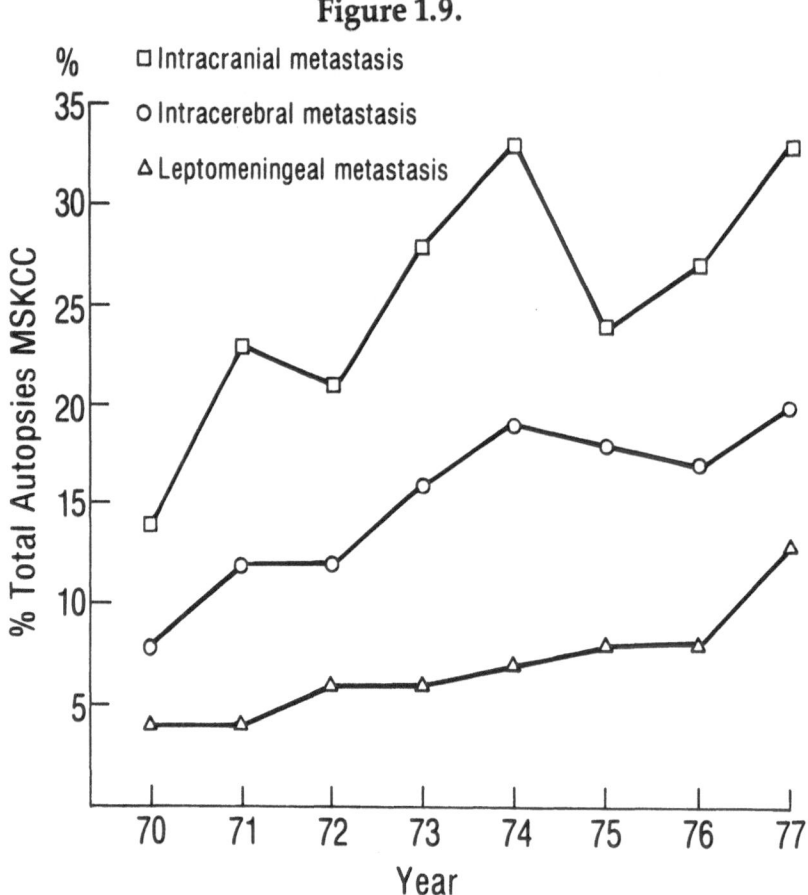

Figure 1.9.

Frequency of intracranial (brain) and leptomeningeal metastases encountered at autopsy at Memorial Sloan-Kettering Cancer Center between 1970 and 1977. There has been a steady increase in the frequency of all varieties of intracranial metastases during this time.

longer the patients live after pulmonary metastases develop the more likely those pulmonary metastases are to disseminate via the arterial systems to several organs including the brain. (3) The brain may provide a sanctuary for neoplastic cells controlled elsewhere by systematic therapy.

According to this view, an increase in brain metastasis recapitulates the experience with leptomeningeal metastasis from acute lymphoblastic leukemia. A similar situation appears to be developing in leukemias other than childhood acute lymphoblastic leukemia as systemic chemotherapy becomes more effective and patients are living longer (Wolk et al. 1974). Malignant cells are presumably given sanctuary in the central nervous system when the blood-brain barrier prevents many water-soluble chemotherapeutic agents from entering the central nervous system. Central nervous system metastases, including brain metastases and leptomeningeal tumors, produce neovascularization, however, and the newly formed blood vessels do not have the tight junction which is responsible for the blood-brain barrier. Thus, there is no blood-brain barrier in a brain metastasis, a phenomenon which makes radionuclide scans reliable in identifying these metastases. There is evidence that in small brain metastases, the barrier to the entrance of chemotherapeutic agents still exists, allowing the tumors to reach sizable proportions before systemic chemotherapeutic agents can reach them (Blasberg et al. 1979). The blood-brain barrier is discussed extensively in Chapter 6.

Brain Metastases Are Unique

The biology of metastases in the brain differentiates them from metastasis of the same tumor to other organs of the body. Most of these unique aspects of brain metastases relate to the anatomy of the central nervous system (table 1.9). The brain and its surrounding membranes are encased in a rigid box, the skull, which effectively prevents expansion of the intracranial contents. Within the skull are the brain, its blood supply, and the cerebrospinal fluid (CSF). The CSF fills the ventricles in the center of the brain and the subarachnoid space over the surface of the brain. An increase in the size of one compartment of the brain can only occur if there is a decrease in the size of one of the other compartments. When new tissue such as a brain metastasis is introduced into the intracranial cavity, the other tissues must accommodate by decreasing their quantity or elevated pressure will shift intracranial structures and compromise the blood supply to the brain.

The brain is also unique in that it has no lymphatics. As a result, unwanted materials which cross into the extracellular cerebral spaces are more difficult to remove than in other organs. They must be reabsorbed by bulk flow of the extracellular fluid into the CSF and thence into the venous drainage of the brain. Finally, the endothelial cells of arterioles and capillaries of the brain are connected by tight junctions that effectively exclude from the brain most molecules of protein size and many smaller polar molecules. These tight junctions are the mechanism for the so-called blood-brain barrier, which excludes from the brain many agents which might be deleterious to brain function. Because a metastasis in the brain disrupts the blood-brain barrier, edema develops around the tumor. Because there are no lymphatics in the brain, drainage is poor and the edematous fluid tends to accumulate. Cerebral edema by itself and by the production of shifts or herniations of cerebral substances can produce severe brain dysfunction. Thus, in many instances small brain tumors which might otherwise be asymptomatic produce severe cerebral symptoms because marked edema surrounds the tumor. This unique aspect of the brain has a potentially happy obverse side: to the degree that edema can be displaced (see Chapter 23), symptoms can be relieved even though the metastasis itself is not directly treated.

Another unique aspect of the brain is the formation and absorption of CSF. CSF is largely formed in the lateral ventricles and, in order to be reabsorbed, must pass through the third ventricle, the narrow aqueduct of Sylvius and the fourth ventricle and into the subarachnoid space. The fluid then returns to the general circulation by reabsorption through arachnoid villi over the surface of the hemisphere. A strategically located brain metastasis, even a very small one, can interfere with the absorption of CSF and cause an increase in CSF volume (hydrocephalus). Hydrocephalus can cause increased intracranial pressure and severe neurologic symptoms. The brain metastases which usually cause hydrocephalus are located in the cerebellum and brainstem. Even without treatment of tumor, drainage of the ventricle by a shunt often eliminates all of the neurological symptoms.

Table 1.9

SOME UNIQUE ASPECTS OF BRAIN METASTASIS

    I. Closed Skull
        A. Increased intracranial pressure
        B. Cerebral herniations

    II. Blood-Brain Barrier
        A. Cerebral edema
        B. Exclusion of chemotherapeutic agents
        C. Exclusion of toxic substances

    III. No Lymphatics
        A. Poor drainage of edema
        B. ? poor drainage of toxic substances

    IV. No Regeneration
        signs may not reverse

A final unique characteristic of the brain is the fact that neurons do not reproduce. This fact has several implications. If neurons are damaged or destroyed, either by the metastasis itself or by treatment, function of that neuron is lost forever and regeneration cannot take place. On the obverse side, because neurons do not reproduce, they are considerably less sensitive to some of the agents used to treat tumors—agents whose effectiveness depends on destroying cells in the reproductive phase.

Brain Metastases Are Clinically Important

The main justification for a monograph devoted to brain metastases is not their frequency (whether increasing or remaining the same) but the severity and intractability of the symptoms they produce. A small metastasis in most organs of the body is asymptomatic. Metastases to organs other than the central nervous system rarely cause symptoms unless they destroy or replace a considerable portion of the organ to which they have metastasized. The situation is different in the brain. If strategically placed, a metastasis no more than 1 or 2 cm in diameter may destroy the ability to speak or to comprehend speech and effectively disable the patient. Even smaller metastases in the cerebral cortex may cause disabling focal or generalized seizures. Symptoms of brain metastases are discussed in more detail elsewhere in this monograph. Suffice it to say that the major symptoms which include paralysis, disorders of language, abnormalities of intellectual function and seizures, are among the most frightening and disabling from which a patient can suffer. Thus brain metastases like primary brain tumors are feared by both patients and physicians alike.

Most central nervous system tissue regenerates poorly, and neurons once dead cannot be replaced. Thus, once an area of brain is destroyed by metastatic tumor, even effective treatment of the tumor is not likely to restore the patient's functions. Patients whose optic nerves are invaded by carcinoma of the breast benefit little from destruction of the tumor by radiation therapy. If a patient is already blind when radiation is begun, that patient will remain blind. As an example from elsewhere in the nervous system, when the spinal cord is compressed even by a radiosensitive metastatic tumor, the response to therapy depends on the patient's clinical state at the time therapy is begun (Gilbert et al. 1978). Thus, radiation therapy can maintain ambulation in patients who are walking at the time treatment is undertaken but restores ambulation in fewer than 10% of patients who are paralyzed before treatment.

In the final analysis, brain metastasis is so important because a person is his/her brain. Many patients, even with widespread metastatic disease, can live useful and rewarding lives. With chemotherapeutic agents, radiation therapy, analgesic drugs and a variety of other supportive measures, the period of useful living after systemic metastasis has developed appears to be lengthening. Once the brain is invaded by tumor, however, the situation changes dramatically. Patients who previously were functional now become paralyzed, demented or threatened by recurrent seizures. Patients who otherwise might have remained at home or even at work often become bedridden or require a hospital or terminal care home. For many patients brain metastases represent the end of the line. To the degree that the clinician is able to reverse the course by early diagnosis and vigorous therapy, a great service is offered even to those patients with widespread and incurable disease. In a sense this is the rationale for this monograph since by learning from each other where we stand and where we are going in our understanding of the basic science and clinical manifestations of brain metastases, we may make our patients' lives more useful and bearable.

REFERENCES

Ambrus, J. L. et al. Causes of death in cancer patients. *J. Med.* (Basel) 6:61–64, 1975.

Aronson, S. M.; Garcia J. H.; and Aronson, B. E. Metastatic neoplasms of the brain: their frequency in relation to age. *Cancer* 17:558–563, 1964.

Arseni, C., and Constantinescu, A. I. Considerations on the metastatic tumours of the brain with reference to a statistics of 1217 cases. *Schweizer Arch. Neurol.* 17:179–195, 1965.

Batson, O. V. Function of vertebral veins and their role in spread of metastasis. *Ann. Surg.* 112:138–149, 1940.

Blasberg, R. G. et al. Metastatic brain tumors: local blood flow and capillary permeability. Neurology, in press.

Brewis, M. et al. Neurological disease in an English city. *Acta Neurol. Scand.* 42 (Suppl 24):1–89, 1966.

Catane, R. et al. Brain metastasis from prostatic carcinoma. *Cancer* 38:2583–2587, 1976.

Chason, J. L.; Walker, R. B.; and Landers, J. W. Metastatic carcinoma in the central nervous system and dorsal root ganglia. *Cancer* 16:781–787, 1963.

Christensen, E. Intracranial carcinomatous metastases in a neurosurgical clinic. *Acta Psychiatr. Scand.* 24:353–361, 1949.

Cushing, H. *Intracranial tumors. Notes upon a series of two thousand verified cases with surgical mortality. Percentages pertaining thereto.* Springfield, Ill.: Charles C Thomas, 1932.

Doring, L. Metastasis of carcinoma of prostate to meningioma. Virchows Arch. [*Pathol. Anat.*] 87:366–369, 1975.

Earle, K. M. Metastatic and primary intracranial tumors of the adult male. *J. Neuropathol. Exp. Neurol.* 13:448–454, 1954.

Earle, K. M. Metastatic brain tumors. *Dis. Nerv. Syst.* 16:86–92, 1955.

Elkington, J. S. C. Metastatic tumors of the brain. *Proc. R. Soc. Med.* 28:1080–1096, 1935.

Espana, P.; Chang P.; and Wiernik, P. H. Increasing incidence of brain metastases in sarcoma patients. *Proc. ASCO* 19:370, 1978.

Gercovich, R. G.; Luna, M. A.; and Gottlieb, J. A. Increased incidence of cerebral metastases in sarcoma patients with prolonged survival from chemotherapy. Report of cases of leiomyosarcoma and chondrosarcoma. *Cancer* 36:1843–1851, 1975.

Gilbert, R. W.; Kim, J. H.; and Posner, J. B. Epidural spinal cord compression from metastatic tumor: diagnosis and treatment. *Ann. Neurol.* 3:40–51, 1978.

Guomundsson, K. R. A survey of tumours of the central nervous system in Iceland during the 10-year period 1954–1963. *Acta Neurol. Scand.* 46:538–552, 1970.

Hakulinen, T. and Teppo, L. Causes of death among female patients with cancer of the breast and intestines. *Ann. Clin. Res.* 9:15–24, 1977.

Hildebrand, J. *Lesions of the nervous system in cancer patients.* New York: Raven Press, 1978.

Hirano, A., and Zimmerman, H. M.: Fenestrated blood vessels in a metastatic renal carcinoma in the brain. *Lab. Invest.* 26:465–468, 1972.

Hirano, A., and Matsui, T. Vascular structures in brain tumors. *Hum. Pathol.* 6:611–621, 1975.

Inagaki, J.; Rodriguez, V.; and Bodey, G. Causes of death in cancer patients. *Cancer* 33:568–573, 1974.

Klastersky, J.; Daneau, D.; and Verhest, A. Causes of death in patients with cancer. *Eur. J. Cancer* 8:149–154, 1972.

Lassen, N. A. Cerebral blood flow and oxygen consumption in man. *Physiol Rev.* 39:183–238, 1959.

Le Blanc, R. A. Metastasis of bronchogenic carcinoma to acoustic neurinoma. *J. Neurosurg.* 41:614–617, 1974.

Lesse, S., and Netsky, M. G. Metastasis of neoplasms to the central system and meninges. *Arch. Neurol. Psychiatr.* 72:133–153, 1954.

Livingston, K. E.; Horrax, G.; and Sachs, E. Metastatic brain tumors. *Surg. Clin. North Am.* 28:805–810, 1948.

Long, D. M. Capillary ultrastructure and the blood-brain barrier in human malignant brain tumors. *J. Neurosurg.* 32:127–144, 1970.

Mayer, R. J.; Berkowitz, R. S.; and Griffiths, C. T. Central nervous system involvement by ovarian carcinoma. *Cancer* 41:776–783, 1978.

Meagher, R., and Eisenhardt, L. Intracranial carcinomatous metastases. *Ann. Surg.* 93:132–140, 1931.

Meyer, P. C., and Reah, T. G. Secondary neoplasms of the central nervous system and meninges. *Br. J. Cancer* 7:438–447, 1953.

Onuigbo, W. I. B. Batson's theory of vertebral venous metastasis. *Oncology* 32:145–150, 1975.

Ortega, P.; Malamud, N.; and Shimkin, M. B. Metastasis to pineal body. *Arch. Pathol.* 52:518–528, 1951.

Paillas, J. E., and Pellet, W. Brain metastases. In *Handbook of Clinical Neurology*, ed. P. J. Vinken and G. W. Bryn. New York: American Elsevier Publishing Co., 1976.

Papo, I., and Tritapepe, R. Considerazioni su 162 casi di metastasi endocraniche verificate. *Minerva Chir.* 12:269–285, 1957.

Percy, A. K. et al. Neoplasms of the central nervous system. *Neurology* 22:40–48, 1972.

Petit-Dutaillis, D.; Messimy, R.; and Berdet, H. Considerations sur les metastases intracraniennes, d'apres 107 cas histologiquement verifies. *Rev. Neurol.* (Paris) 95:89–115, 1956.

Posner, J. B., and Chernik, N. L. Intracranial metastases from systemic cancer. *Adv. Neurol.* 19:575–587, 1978.

Posnikoff, J., and Stratford, J. Carcinoma metastasis to malignant glioma. *Arch. Neurol.* 3:559–563, 1960.

Richards, P., and McKissock, W. Intracranial metastases. *Br. Med. J.* 1:15–18, 1963.

Roger, H.; Cornil, L.; and Paillas, J. Étude anatomique et pathogenique des tumeurs cerebrales metastatiques. *Rev. Neurol.* (Paris) 72:137–148, 1939.

Rosenblatt, M. B. et al. Causes of death in 1,000 consecutive autopsies. *N. Y. State J. Med.* 71:2189–2193, 1971.

Rubin, P., and Green, J. *Solitary metastases*. Springfield: Charles C Thomas, 1968.

Russell, D. S., and Rubinstein, L. J. *Pathology of tumours of the nervous system*. 4th ed. Baltimore: Williams and Wilkins Co., 1977.

Silverberg, E. *Cancer statistics 1977*. Cancer 27:26–41, 1977.

Simionescu, M. E. Metastatic tumors of the brain. A follow-up study of 195 patients with neurosurgical considerations. *J. Neurosurg.* 17:31–373, 1960.

Stedman's medical dictionary. 23rd ed. Baltimore: Williams and Wilkins Co., 1976.

Stortebecker, T. P. Metastatic tumours of the brain from a neurosurgical point of view (a follow-up study of 158 cases). *J. Neurosurg.* 11:84–111, 1954.

Van Eck, J. H. M.; Go, K. G.; and Ebels, E. J. Metastatic tumours of the brain. *Psychiatr. Neurol. Neurochir.* 68:443–462, 1965.

Viadana, E. et al. An autopsy study of metastatic sites of breast cancer. *Cancer Res.* 33:179–181, 1973.

Viadana, E.; Bross, I. D. J.; and Pickren, J. W. The metastatic spread of cancers of the digestive system in man. *Oncology* 35:114–126, 1978.

Vick, N. A., and Bigner, D. D. Microvascular abnormalities in virally-induced canine brain tumors. *J. Neurol. Sci.* 17:29–39, 1972.

Vider, M.; Maruyama, Y.; and Narvaez, R. Significance of the vertebral venous (Batson's) plexus in metastatic spread in colorectal carcinoma. *Cancer* 40:67–71, 1977.

Willis, R. A. *The spread of tumours in the human body*. 3d ed. London: Butterworths and Co., 1973.

Wolk, R. W. et al. and Co. The incidence of central nervous system leukemia in adults with acute leukemia. *Cancer* 33:863–869, 1974.

Zulch, K. J. *Brain tumors; their biology and pathology*. 2d ed. New York: Springer Publishing Co., Inc., 1949.

2

The Cell Periphery and Metastasis

Leonard Weiss

The phenomenon of cancer involves the internal contents of malignant cells and their environment as well as interactions between the two. One such interaction is metastasis, and the site of primary interaction is the cell periphery. It is reasonable, therefore, to seek correlation between the nature of the cancer cell periphery and metastasis.

Periodically, reports appear claiming clearcut differences between the peripheries of cancer cells and their so-called normal counterparts. On examination, the data for these often sweeping generalizations usually identify differences between a very few cells of dubious normalcy (such as 3T3) and a virus transformant (such as SV40-3T3). In these studies, the characterization of malignancy by transplantation into animals is usually more impressive than the criteria used to establish normalcy. Repeatedly the generalizations on purported differences between the two classes of cells have to be retracted when more extensive surveys reveal a considerable overlap between so-called normal and malignant physicochemical and functional characteristics (Weiss and Poste 1976). At present, I am unaware of any absolute qualitative or quantitative differences between the peripheries of all normal and all malignant cells. Upon reflection, this is hardly surprising because there are more than 270 histologically identifiable cancers in humans. The possession of these distinct histologic features implies distinct biologic behavioral patterns, some of which are probably related to the physicochemical nature of the cancer-cell periphery. To group together all cancer cells regardless of their individual expressions of malignancy, ranging from nonmetastatic basal-cell carcinomas to highly metastatic melanomas, implies a curious combination of optimism and ignorance. It would be much more to the point to compare the peripheral structure of the basal carcinoma cells with the malignant melanoma cells in order to seek correlations with nonmetastasis and metastasis respectively.

In this chapter some salient features of metastasis are examined in relation to some properties of malignant-cell peripheries. The list is not

30

exhaustive and is not primarily concerned with whether these properties are unique to cancer cells. An attempt is made to identify peripheral properties which favor metastasis and those which do not.

THE PRIMARY CANCER

The cellular heterogeneity of solid tumors is well recognized among pathologists, who discriminate between cancer cells and noncancerous constituents, including stromal elements and parts of the defense system (including lymphocytes, polymorphonuclear leukocytes and macrophages). A more subtle question is whether the cancer cells within a primary tumor fall into subpopulations with respect to metastasis—in terms of the whole metastatic process or individual components of it (Weiss 1967).

This idea is not new (Green 1965; Leighton 1965; Zeidman 1965). Foulds (1969) has used the label *tumor progression* to indicate a continuous development in cancer-cell populations toward increased malignancy (metastasis), and studies by Robotti (1959) and Yamada and others (1966) have revealed karyotypic differences between certain primary cancers and their metastases. Interpretations of such comparisons are difficult: even when specimens of primary and metastatic lesions are obtained at the same time, the time of metastatic seeding in relationship to the development of primary lesions is unknown. This may have considerable importance in view of studies of the karyotypes of cells obtained in effusions from a single patient with pseudomycoma peritonei over a period of one month (Sandberg and Yamada, 1966). During this time, the karyotype of cells released directly into the peritoneal cavity from a primary ovarian carcinoma varied from two distinct marker chromosomes in 40% of examined cells to over 90%. These changes represent shifts in karyotype of the primary cancer and exceed differences often noted between primary and metastatic lesions.

Another complicating factor in interpreting differences in site-associated characteristics of cancer cells lies in determining whether pre-existing differences were responsible for the development of tumors in specific sites, or whether site-induced, epigenetic changes were responsible for the differences. For example, Cook and others (1963) have shown significant differences in the mean net surface negativities of murine sarcoma 37 cells from the same primary source grown either in an (abdominal) ascites form or as a subcutaneous tumor. Treatment of cells with neuraminidase showed a highly significant reduction in electrophoretic mobility for the ascites type but no detectable change occurred in cells from the subcutaneous tumors even though sialic acids were released from both forms by the enzyme. The differences were reversible and were judged to be due to a site-induced change in the populations rather than a selective process: no evidence of a bimodal distribution of electrophoretic mobilities was found in the original inocula.

More recently, Fidler (1976) and Nicolson and colleagues (1976) have shown differences in arrest patterns of injected cell lines developed in vitro and those grown in tumors of different organs in mice, and Fidler (1978) has developed high and low metastatic clones of the B16 mouse melanoma from the same initial tumor-cell population. In an interesting variation of these selection experiments, Tao and Burger (1977) selected nonmetastasizing variants from metastasizing B16 melanoma cells by repeated in vitro exposure to wheat germ agglutinin, which binds specifically to cell-surface carbohydrates. In the clones developed from surviving lectin-treated cell cultures, the metastasizing capacity of the cells injected into animals decreased as lectin binding and agglutination decreased. Because the ability of all clones to form tumors diminished little, there was discrimination between metastatic potential and tumorgenicity, and a relationship was established between a specific property of the cell periphery (that is, high lectin binding) and high metastatic capacity.

Continuing observations of the in vivo and in vitro properties of these clones of B16 cells are obviously required in order to determine the permanency of the subpopulations. Possibly comparisons of the surface properties of high and low metastatic clones of these and other types of tumor cells may help elucidate those surface properties relevant to metastasis, and such studies have indeed been started. Tao and Burger's observations illustrate some of the interpretative and correlative problems in this field. In their population of B16 melanoma cells in the mouse, lectin agglutin ability correlated with a higher degree of malignancy or metastatic capacity. Lectin agglutinability does not invariably correlate with malignancy, however, and nonagglutinability does not invariably correlate with normalcy. Nonetheless, Tao and Burger's observation appears reasonable in terms of the common malignant background of the B16 cells. It is also known that wheat germ agglutinin demonstrates sugar specificity for N-acetyl-D-glucosamine. On the given data, however, it cannot be inferred that the low metastatic line of B16 cells has fewer N-acetyl-D-glucosamine surface groups than the high metastatic line because there is no simple or constant relationship between the numbers of lectin molecules bound to a cell and its relative lectin agglutinability (Nicolson 1974).

Quite apart from this interpretative problem, the fundamental problem lies in ascribing functional and mechanistic properties to the lectin binding sites. Does metastatic potential really directly correlate with these sites, or is the correlation indirect? Are lectin agglutination and metastatic potential related through some other, yet unspecified cell-periphery property such as membrane fluidity? The real issue is that although such observations as those of Tao and Burger may well provide a useful approach to the problem of correlating peripheral properties of cancer cells with metastasis, they do not at present indicate whether the properties described are directly involved in the metastatic process. If they are, is this cause or effect, and what are their specific functional roles?

Another approach to this problem is a study by Pimm and Baldwin (1977) of antigenetic differences between primary methylcholanthrene-induced rat sarcomas and their recurrences after surgical resection of the primary lesions. These investigators concluded that secondary tumors arose by clonal amplification of separate subpopulations of highly polymorphic primary lesions in which there are demonstrably different tumor-rejection antigens at the cancer-cell peripheries. Whether or not tumor rejection antigens play a part in the natural history of metastasizing cancers in humans is open to question (Rapp 1977). The observation does suggest that surface differences among subpopulations of cancer cells expressed in terms of varying antigenicity could stimulate some kind of endogenous control of the metastatic process at those developmental stages during which weak immunologic stimuli are effective. Although many cell peripheral components are usefully categorized by their ability to act as antigens, this does not mean that their primary function is immunologic.

If cancer cells in metastases are in some way different from those of their parent primary cancers, then the important therapeutic consequences of these differences demand examination of a number of nonexclusive mechanisms for these differences (fig. 2.1). In the natural development of cancer, metastases may arise by means of a random survival of cells going through all of the various steps of the metastatic cascade. Such chance survival, which is common to many biologic events, is most usefully described in statistical terms, and the concept of subpopulations is inappropriate in this context. This type of selection may be interposed in all of the models shown in figure 2.1A, between the primary lesions and the metastases.

A second mechanism (fig. 2.1B), is the development of metastases from a small metastatic subpopulation. It is difficult to reconcile organ-specific subpopulations (Nicolson et al. 1976) with the clinical data summarized by Bross in Chapter 4 in the cascade theory, in which brain metastases occur largely from other organs.

A third mechanism (fig. 2.1C) involves the different peripheral properties of cancer cells observed in various metabolic states and in relationship to proliferative and degenerative events elsewhere in the tumor and host. These changes move the cells into so-called transient metastatic compartments at different times. In other words, the cancer cells participating in some or all of the steps in the metastatic cascade are temporarily different from at least some of the cells remaining in the primary tumor. The term *subpopulation* is inappropriate for this type of phenotypic variability. This mechanism would account for a dynamic heterogeneity in the cancer cells of both primary and secondary tumors.

A fourth mechanism (fig. 2.1D) departs from the concepts of both metastatic subpopulations and transient metastatic compartments. It depends on site-induced modulation and in essence claims that local interactions of cancer cells with the organ to which they have metastasized result in differences between them and the cells in the parent cancer. Thus, the cancer cells in a metastasis are different from those in the primary lesion because of interactions with the metastatic site; these cells do not form metastases because of pre-existing differences.

A fifth comprehensive mechanism (fig. 2.1E) combines features of the previous mechanisms in that cells move into a transient metastatic compartment, survive trauma as described in statistical terms, and establish themselves in a target organ, in which they respond to local environmental interactions.

From the clinical data presented elsewhere in this book, it is not all clear that there are true differential responses to therapy among primary cancers of the lung and breast and melanomas, and their brain metastases. Awareness of the possibility, however, may stimulate fresh clinical observations and experiments.

Figure 2.1.

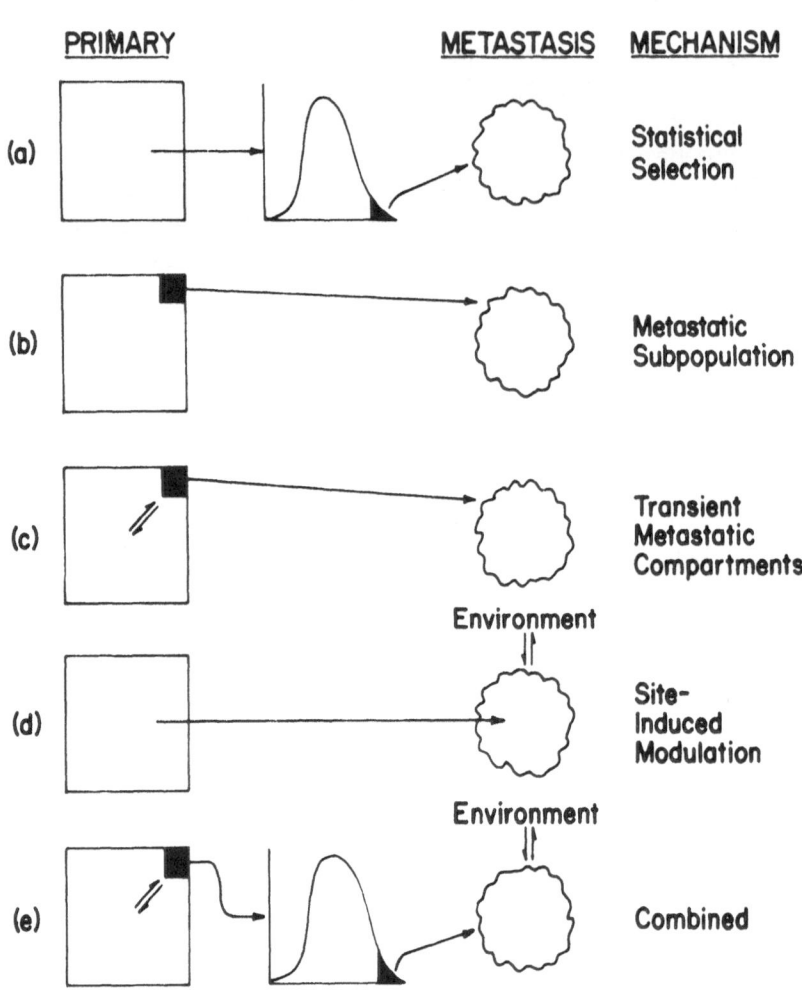

Mechanisms to account for possible differences between cells in primary cancers and their metastases.

CELL DETACHMENT

One of the initial steps in the metastatic process is the detachment of single cancer cells or clusters of cancer cells from the parent cancer. This step may occur before or after penetration of blood channels by the tumor. Thus the blood channels may consist of clefts within the tumor, lined by cancer cells which exfoliate into it. Alternatively, the tumor may grow into a vein which may be part of the neovasculature, and detachment of tumor emboli may occur under the influence of hemodynamic forces. Detached cells may also migrate through tissue spaces and gain access to lymphatic channels or nearby veins. This phase of metastasis emphasizes cell detachment and cell movement.

Cell detachment is one of the best misunderstood facets of metastasis! It is usually confused with cell adhesion, which is an interfacial phenomenon occurring between cell surfaces and their substrata. The plane of cell detachment is unlikely to correspond to the plane of cell adhesion and involves cohesive failure in parts of the cell periphery or its substratum (Weiss 1976a). Cancer cells in general are not less adhesive to each other as originally postulated by Coman (1953), and as shown later in this chapter, the detachment of cancer cells from each other is a dynamic event associated with other internal and environmental changes. In our efforts to define the chemical properties of the cell periphery, its mechanical properties should not be overlooked nor should the interrelationship between these two.

A common feature of tumors reaching the size at which metastasis becomes increasingly frequent is that in some regions active growth is predominant, while in other regions of the same tumor degenerative processes are occurring. In vitro studies have shown that increasing growth rate facilitated cell detachment from solid surfaces (Weiss 1964), and in vitro cells commonly detach during the rounding-up process associated with metaphase. Other factors often associated with growth also facilitate cell detachment including activation of lysosomes (Weiss 1965a), increased endocytosis (Weiss 1964), and changes in membrane permeability (Weiss and Huber 1974). In an attempt to determine the overall effect of increased growth rate on cell-from-cell separation, Weiss (1977a) studied the mechanically induced in vitro separation of parenchymal cells from cylinders punched out of regenerating mouse livers during the six days following partial (53%) hepatectomy. Regeneration was assessed by liver wet weight, protein content and mitotic indices. Under the conditions of these experiments, the maximal regenerative response occurred during the second to fourth postoperative days. Associated with these changes, significantly more cells were detached from the partially hepatectomized groups on the second and third postoperative days than from the sham-operated groups. These experiments show that accelerated growth in a noncancerous tissue is in fact associated with facilitated release of its constituent cells. Regardless of the actual mechanisms involved, these results suggest that one factor contributing to the release of malignant cells from solid cancers may be their abnormally high growth rate independent of their cancer-specific properties.

Additional factors facilitating the release of cancer cells include enzyme activity (Weiss 1963). After the in vitro demonstration that factors activating lysosomes (such as antisera) facilitated cell detachment and that factors stabilizing lysosomes (such as hydrocortisone) inhibited this facilitation (Weiss 1965a) it was suggested that lysosomal enzymes released from malignant cells themselves or surrounding nonmalignant cells may have considerable importance in releasing cells from solid tumors. Support for this suggestion comes from the observation that high levels of vitamin A, which activates lysosomes, cause the release of lysosomal enzymes which act on the pericellular regions and thus facilitate cell detachment from solid substrata in vitro (Weiss 1967). In addition, studies of hypervitaminotic A animals with mammary adenocarcinomas revealed an association between the increased numbers of cells shaken free from excised tumors and a higher incidence of pulmonary metastasis, compared with appropriate controls (Weiss and Holyoke 1969). Any process releasing lysosomal enzymes, including therapeutic measures, may thus promote the release of cells from tumors.

Degeneration is a universal feature of parts of solid tumors over a few millimeters in diameter. Recently the effects of necrotic material on cell-from-cell detachment in both tumors and normal surrounding tissues have been investigated by a standardized in vitro shaking procedure (Weiss 1977b). In cystic tumors of the liver, greater volumes of viable cells are detached from the innermost regions of the walls adjacent to regions of central necrosis than from the outermost parts of the tumor. More liver parenchymal cells are shaken free of liver adjacent to a tumor interface than from regions 0.5 and 1.0 cm from it. Detachment of tumor and liver cells is also enhanced by prior incubation of tissue samples with necrotic extracts. It appears that necrotic regions of tumors or the diffusion of products derived from them facilitate cell detachment.

The effects of these various growth and degenerative processes on the detachment of malignant cells from their parent tumors are good illustrations of the dependence and dynamic nature of underlying cellular peripheral mechanical properties on both internal and external events and suggest how these events when reflected at the cell periphery, can promote the detachment phase of metastasis. Because facilitation of cell separation involves a mechanical weakening of the cell periphery and intercellular material, separation of liver cells by a tumor which they surround indicates a reduction in the strength of the intercellular planes which might also facilitate their invasion by the tumor.

CELL MOVEMENT

When fibroblasts crawling over coverslips bump into each other in vitro, movement in the direction of contact ceases, a phenomenon termed *contact inhibition of movement* by Abercrombie (1975). If sarcoma cells are confronted by fibroblasts, however, movement of the sarcoma cells is not paralyzed by contact but movement of the fibroblasts is. This loss of contact inhibition of movement by malignant cells was suggested as one basis for their invasiveness. Another basis was the vis a tergo generated by tumor growth. At present, Abercrombie (1975) is not prepared to generalize on correlations between malignancy, loss of contact inhibition of movement, and invasion. Regardless of its specificity, however, in vitro malignant cells are known to migrate actively from tumor explants, and single tumor cells are capable of active movement. Wolff (1967) has shown that if tumor fragments are cultured on top of embryonic organs, where tumor pressure is directed upward along the path of least resistance to invasion by the main tumor mass, single cancer cells migrate through the organ. It has therefore been suggested that one mechanism whereby cancer invades normal tissues is by active movement of single cancer cells. Even in invasion of tissues by tumor projections or the whole tumor front, this could conceivably be mediated by active movements of cells at the advancing edge of a cancer.

In essence then, many observations show that cancer cells are capable of active translocatory movements and that it is feasible that such movements can play a role in invasion in vivo; however, the direct evidence for this is sparse. Apparently single malignant cells are commonly observed some distance from multicellular cancer foci and appear to be actively migrating through the normal tissues. Streaming of cells from malignant melanoma through the dermis and the presence of single carcinoma cells in the stomach wall in linitis plastica are familiar examples. Before such cases can be accepted as evidence for the involvement of active cell movement in invasion of this type, serial sections must be examined to verify that the apparently single cells are not part of a multicellular assembly. In addition, special staining techniques should be used to verify that the malignant cells apparently observed in tissue spaces are not in fact being carried passively inside small blood or lymphatic vessels which are not discerible in standard sections (Friedell and Parsons 1962). When these two selective criteria are applied, the histologic evidence for active movements of single cancer cells in invasion is not impressive. In order to move actively over or through tissues, or any other substratum, a mammalian cell must

(1) make contact with and adhere to the substratum, to obtain a hold against which it can push or pull,
(2) generate the necessary locomotive energy, and
(3) break contact in regions of adhesion with its substratum.

The peripheries of malignant cells in general were once believed to have an inherent defect which prevented their adhesion. This is incorrect and should not be confused with the common observation that with respect to applied forces cells detach easily from regions of some but certainly not all solid tumors. This so-called nonadherence of cancer cells was partially attributed to failure to form adhesive "calcium bridges" with other cells; more recent work provides no support for the generality that cancer cells have low binding capacities for calcium or that intercellular calcium bridges bind cells together.

Another explanation postulated for the nonadherence of cancer cells was that their abnormally high net surface charge prevented them from making contact with other cell surfaces by mutual electrostatic repulsion. In general, cancer cells exhibit no higher average net surface negativity than normal cells, and like other parameters the negativity of cancer cells varies with mitotic and metabolic events. Although charge patterns on individual cell surfaces may determine where cells will not adhere, there appears to be space between charge clusters for adhesion to occur (Weiss et al. 1975). This surface heterogeneity may be responsible for the lack of correlation between adhesiveness or nonadhesiveness and the average surface charge (Weiss 1968). Examination of many metastasizing tumors confirms that the cells of solid cancers adhere to each other and to non-malignant cells. Thus, the first criterion for active movement is met. It is true that the physicochemical nature of the cell periphery determines its mode of adhesion, but there appear to be no clearcut differences between normal and malignant cells in this regard.

The role of locomotive energy in cell movement is undisputed and is provided by contractile, intracellular filaments which are attached to the inner aspect of the cell membrane. No qualitative or quantitative differences have been reported between normal and malignant cells in this respect, however (Sträuli and Weiss, 1977), and attempts to measure locomotive energies in mammalian cells (macrophages) have revealed a demand and supply system whereby within defined limits cells generate enough locomotive energy to maintain a constant velocity in environments of different viscosities (Folger et al. 1978).

The role of localized cell detachment in movement has been demonstrated with macrophages in vitro by showing a correlation between the effects of migration-inhibiting factors and decreased macrophage detachment (Weiss and Glaves 1975).

In summary, malignant cells are capable of active crawling movements although the role of these movements in tissue invasion needs careful assessment. There appears to be nothing unique in the mechanisms of movement of malignant cells, and at present the invasiveness of malignant cells cannot be associated with cancer-specific cell-surface properties. The other side of the coin is not the moving cell, however, but the tissues through which it moves. My own studies on the liver surrounding Walker 256 tumors in rats suggest that intercellular infiltration would be easier in this location (Weiss 1977b).

CIRCULATING CANCER CELLS

Circulating cancer cells are subjected to mechanical and biochemical trauma. The mechanical trauma consists of repetitive squeezing through small blood vessels. The painstaking experiments of Sato and Suzuki (1976) in a series of rat tumors have shown that the higher the cellular resistance to deformation, the higher the percentage of cells killed by one pulmonary passage. Generalizations on cell deformability and cell survival in the circulation are difficult. Erythrocytes, which are the least deformable of mammalian cells (Weiss 1976b), have an average lifetime of 120 days. Monocytes, which are the most deformable of cells (Weiss et al. 1966), have a lifetime of 12–102 hours (Volkman 1976); mature granulocytes, which are less easily deformable than macrophages, have an average lifetime of a few hours; lymphocytes survive for days; and memory cells survive for years. All of these survival times coexist with circulation times of 10–20 seconds, which implies approximately 200 transpulmonary passages/hour. The malignant cells are less well-suited than normal cells to withstand hemodynamic trauma, but within comparable populations of tumor cells, the most easily deformable cells have the greatest chance of survival.

Direct comparisons between the lifetimes of circulating cells could be misleading. For example, the granulocyte population consists of two approximately equal parts, the circulating and so-called marginal pools. The latter adhere to the vascular endothelium where there is reduced blood flow, such as the postcapillary venules, and the two pools are in equilibrium (Athens 1961). In contrast, the majority of mononuclear cells reside in the tissues, and at any one time only a small proportion of them are found in the circulation. The periods spent in circulation may thus be traumatic, and those spent out of circulation may be regarded as a rest and recovery period.

Stoker (1968) has suggested from in vitro studies that one surface-dependent difference between normal and malignant cells is that the former require attachment to a solid substrate in order to survive and thrive (anchorage dependence) whereas cancer cells do not. Anchorage independence cannot be accepted as an absolute criterion of malignancy even in vitro, and the failure of circulating cancer cells to survive for long in vivo suggests that it is a minor consideration in metastasis. Possibly some explanation of differential survival can be offered in terms of marginal pools of cells. Interestingly Donald and others (1977) found attached cancer cells on a sclerosed mitral valve in a patient with no other signs of cancer, either at the time or 15 months later. These cancer cells survived at rest even though they were exposed to a high bloodflow presumably while other circulating cells from a clinically covert lesion did not.

Cytotoxic factors in the serum have been recognized for many years, but in a recent review of the literature (Weiss 1978), it was impossible to discriminate between often ill-defined humoral immunologic phemonena and nonimmunologic cytotoxic agents. Thus, circulation is a traumatic experience for metastasizing cells from which the major escape route is arrest.

Before examining the anatomy of the arrest process, some short-term dynamic aspects of the detachment-arrest cycle merit consideration. A feeling for the early phases of the detachment-arrest cycle comes from studies on cells labeled with [125]IUdR injected into mice. After tail-vein injections, a high proportion (depending on host, cell type and number) of the initially injected cells is usually arrested in the lungs. Over the course of hours or even minutes, however, the number of retained cells falls sharply (Weiss and Glaves 1978); it is not known whether retention is a selective process. Of those arrested cells released, a considerable number are destroyed by transpulmonary passage, which in humans can occur approximately every 15 seconds. It is not known whether the same proportion of cancer cells is killed by each passage through the lungs, leading to exponential decay in circulating cells, or whether most cells are killed within a given number of passages. Extrapulmonary metastases may arise only from a pre-existing fraction of the total circulating cancer-cell population with a high resistance to transpulmonary passage or they may arise from a statistical selection.

Due to technical difficulties, there is sparse information on the deformability of malignant cells, but the short series of Sato and Suzuki (1976) does suggest a meaningful relationship between deformability and capacity for metastasis. The deformability of individual cells probably varies during different phases of their lifetime; for example, Lichtman and Weed (1976) have suggested that increased cell deformability as maturation progresses in granulopoiesis plays a vote in the egress of these cells from the bone marrow. In some malignant cells, there is increased surface density of sialic acid at the G2 phase of the mitotic cycle (Mayhew 1966), and in some cells there is a short-term sialic acid-dependent increase in surface negativity associated with increased metabolic rate (Weiss 1966). Since incubation with neuraminidase has been shown to reduce cell-surface negativity and increase cell deformability in some cancer cells (Weiss 1965b), actively metabolizing or G2-phase cells, by virtue of being less deformable, may be more susceptible to mechanical trauma during the circulatory phase of metastasis. Because metastasis is most marked during the active growth phases of some tumors, decreased cancer-cell deformability may have a controlling influence and act to reduce the number of metastases.

Interestingly, when exponentially growing fibrosarcoma 1233 cells, synchronized by fractionation according to cell size, were injected intravenously into mice, lung colony-forming efficiency correlated with the cycle stage of the injected cells: efficiency was highest at S phase, declined at G2, and was lowest at G1 (Suzuki et al. 1977). Due to the complexity of the metastatic cascade, this observation does not permit unequivocal correlation of cycle phase with survival in the circulation or arrest. Nonetheless, the results do indicate the potential temporal variability of cells released from the same primary cancer to form metastases.

A recent summary of studies on alteration of cancer-cell deformability noted that some enzymes acting on the cell periphery can increase deformability (Weiss 1976b). The large range of lysosomal enzymes in many cancers make them prime candidates for this function, and these hydrolases may originate in the cancer cells themselves or any of the other cellular components of the tumor. It thus appears reasonable that enzymes promoting cell detachment will also facilitate cell deformation. The hematogenous phase of metastasis appears to involve at least those peripheral properties of cancer cells determining their deformability and their resistance to rather ill-defined cytotoxic factors.

ARREST OF CIRCULATING CANCER CELLS

Arrest is a necessary and obvious step in the formation of metastases and appears to be a necessary prerequisite for survival of circulating cancer cells.

All mammalian cells carry a net negative surface charge, and the resulting electrostatic repulsion between cancer cells and the vascular endothelium tends to prevent their adhesion. From this consideration alone, the incorrect generalization that cancer cells carry a higher net negative surface charge than their normal counterparts would argue against arrest and metastasis rather than for it. Details of the physical bases of contact between cells in general (Weiss 1971; Weiss and Harlos 1971) deal with the problems of relating cell contact and adhesion to the average physical parameters of cell periphery. In addition to electrostatic repulsion, boundary layers generated by blood flow make direct collisions and adhesion between a circulating tumor cell and the vascular endothelium of the microcirculation unlikely. Electron microscopy of cationic particles adsorbed to a number of normal and malignant cells suggests, however, that the charges are arranged in surface clusters and that contact takes place at surface regions where the density of charges is low (Weiss and Subjeck 1974). Contact is made by cellular exudates (Maslow and Weiss 1972) or macromolecular hairs (Weiss et al. 1975). In the special case of circulating malignant cells, blood coagulation components may substitute for the exudates seen in vitro.

THROMBOSIS AND CELL ARREST

Some tumor cells, particularly from adenocarcinomas, tend to become associated with platelets and varying degrees of thrombus formation either just before or just after arrest (Warren 1970; Chew et al. 1976). Because disseminated intravascular coagulation (DIC) often occurs in patients with carcinoma, correlations have been made between the arrest of circulating cancer cells and hypercoagulability and thromboplastin release from tumor cells or platelets with which they interact. This provides the basis for the use of anticoagulants as prophyllactic therapy in metastasis, a practice for which there is little evidence of success.

The conversion of tumor emboli to thrombi raises the question of whether cancer cells have coagulation activity associated with their peripheries either as exudates or structural components. Thromboplastic activity has been associated with tumors, leading O'Meara (1958) to postulate the existence of a cancer coagulative factor, and Frank and Holyoke (1968) showed that more thromboplastin activity was associated with fluid obtained from the peripheries of Lewis sarcoma than from the normal tissues. More detailed in vitro studies at a cellular level provided no evidence for a unique cancer coagulative factor but suggested rather that thromboplastin activity arose from degenerative processes in both normal and malignant tissues consequent to tumor growth (Holyoke et al. 1972). Attempts by my colleagues and myself to provoke in vitro fibrinogenic interactions between intact tumor cells and plasma or intact platelets have been largely unsuccessful. Although fibrinogenic reactions appear to be associated in some way with the adhesion of some tumor emboli to vascular endothelium, such interactions have not been demonstrated to be directly associated with the nature of the intact cancer-cell surface.

In attempts to provide a meaningful model for the early arrest patterns of circulating cancer cells, my colleagues and I have studied radiolabeled cells injected into the systemic circulation of normal, tumor-bearing and tumor-sensitized syngeneic mice (Weiss et al. 1974; Glaves and Weiss 1976; Weiss and Glaves 1976). The results were revealing: each of three injected tumors studied showed a different initial retention pattern of intravenously injected cancer cells in the lungs in response to sensitization. The numbers of cells retained in the lungs at a given time after administration in part represented the summation of the efficiency of the trapping system and the loss due to cell detachment. The changes in observed retention patterns were immunospecific (Weiss and Glaves 1976) and were in addition to any nonspecific, general effects of tumor bearing.

Dynamic studies with injected labeled cells have shown that after initial organ arrest most tumor cells are released. Some of these are dead, others are later destroyed in the circulation, and others are distributed to other organ sites. Short-term arrest-release reactions of this type are expected to reduce the overall efficiency of the metastatic process in terms of cancer cells. Detachment of arrested cells involves the general mechanisms described previously. In addition, in those cases in which tumor emboli are arrested by mechanisms involving fibrogenesis, it is worthy of note that fibrinolytic activity has long been associated with tumors on the evidence that cancer fragments cultured in plasma clots frequently digest the fibrin and the fragment then detaches from the surface on which it was cultured. Although it now appears that plasminogen activation is not a unique property of malignant cells, the relevant point is that by release of plasminogen activators, malignant cells do have the potential to facilitate their release when fibrin plays a major role in their arrest. Other enzymes facilitating the release of arrested cancer cells may be released by platelets, leukocytes, macrophages and vascular endothelial cells as well as the tumor cells themselves.

With regard to the effects of immune status on tumor-cell arrest, it should also be remembered that antibodies may stimulate the release of lysosomal enzymes from cells, promoting their nonlateral detachment (Weiss 1965), and that antibody-antigen complexes may also result in similar release of enzymes from malignant cells or be associated with them.

DEVELOPMENT OF METASTASES

In my opinion, we currently know least about that critical phase of metastasis, the development of small foci of arrested cancer cells into "clinical" metastases. It is generally accepted that cell growth and metabolism are in part regulated by the cell periphery. Compared with their so-called normal counterparts, a relatively small number of different types of cancer cells have peripheral properties favorable to growth. These properties, which are not cancer-specific, include increased capacities for sugar and amino-acid transport, increased Na^+K^+ ATPase activity, and reduced adenylate cyclase activity (Poste and Weiss 1976). In addition, in contrast to their usual counterparts, very few tumor cells injected into suitable animals grow rapidly into overt cancers.

Along with others, I have frequently observed that mice and rats, bearing a large variety of transplanted subcutaneous, intramuscular, or intraperitoneal (ascites) tumors, succumb to the cancers or their sequelae without developing pulmonary metastases visible either to the naked eye or in stained serial sections. When pieces of these lungs are transplanted into the peritoneal cavities of fresh animals, however, the lung tissues are rapidly replaced by the same tumors which involve the peritoneal cavities. Thus, within the lifetime of their hosts, operationally dormant micrometastases, which have survived trauma, do not develop into overt or "clinical" metastases. Parenthetically, operational definitions of dormancy do not discriminate between a true dormant state, in which cancer cells are not dividing, and a pseudodormant state, in which an increase in cell numbers is matched by cell loss. The phenomena of minimal metastasis in patients with some cancers and the sudden development of many pulmonary metastases in patients long after removal of their primary lesions or in the terminal stages of disease are probably manifestations of the development of, or emergence from, dormancy. In addition to considering the role of the cancer-cell periphery in the growth of arrested cells, its role should also be examined in the maintenance and departure from dormancy.

The dormant tumor state with respect to metastasis has been discussed by Alexander (1976) and by Wheelock and others (1977). A number of host defense mechanisms clearly are involved in dormancy, but it remains to be determined whether factors retarding development of a tumor transplant at the primary innoculation site also maintain a distant metastasis in the dormant state.

A considerable body of evidence from experimental animals supports the view that dormant metastases become manifest on immunosuppression (Barnes et al. 1957; Fisher et al. 1969; Eccles and Alexander 1974) and that this effect is due to a T-lymphocyte deficiency. Extrapolating immunologic data from experimental animals to humans is uncertain. Nonetheless, the emergence and rapid growth of dormant metastases in patients on the point of dying with cancer could be reasonably ascribed to a terminal immune deficiency. In nonterminal patients, current technology does not permit general statements about immune status although "in a variety of assessments patients with solid tumors show, on average, a significantly greater immunological reactivity to their tumors than do normal controls. The specificity seems usually to be for tumor type rather than on the individual tumor." (Stevenson and Laurence 1975). This fickleness is compatible with the observations of Wheelock and others (1977) on rodent tumors: dormancy is an unstable state and in individual animals it was impossible to predict whether a transplanted tumor would become dormant or not.

Many tumors shed so-called cell-surface antigens (Price and Baldwin 1977). The fact that these antigens are present in the cell periphery and are secreted or shed by their cells of origin as a nonlethal event in no way detracts from their designation as legitimate components of the cancer-cell periphery. A major conceptual error was to claim cancer specificity for many of these oncofetal antigens such as carcinoembryonic antigen (CEA) and α-feto proteins; more recent studies (Holyoke 1976) have shown them to be present in people without cancer, albeit on occasion in smaller amounts. The important biologic point is that cancer cells liberate this material regardless of its specificity and that it may generate the production of antibodies with which it combines to form immune complexes, which then adsorb to macrophages, which on contact either kill cancer cells or convert them to a dormant state. Thus operational dormancy results from cytolysis or cytostasis. Macrophage activation may also follow exposure to lymphokines produced by interaction of lymphocytes with oncofetal antigens.

In addition to these essentially antimetastatic activities, antigen-antibody complexes also serve as blocking factors which adsorb to cancer cells and protect them from attack by cell-mediated immune mechanisms. It is conceivable, therefore, that shed material from a primary cancer could protect a small metastasis. Upon removal of the primary lesion, the metastasis would be left relatively unprotected. Thus, in an indirect manner, constituents of cancer-cell surfaces may maintain a delicate balance in the status of metastases by initiating dormancy by cytolysis or cystostasis on the one hand or by protecting metastases from cell-mediated attack on the other. Like other constituents of the cell periphery, the oncofetal antigens by virtue of their physicochemical properties will partially determine whether or not contact takes place between the malignant and other cells and, if contact takes place, which regions of the individual cells are involved in the process.

CONCLUSIONS

The metastatic process is obviously complex, and in terms of cancer cells it is inefficient and costly. Fewer than 0.1% of malignant cells released from a solid tumor appear to survive the trauma of metastatic cascade and actually form metastases. If the survivors are highly selected subpopulations of cancer cells, studies of the peripheries of cells from primary tumors are much more likely to explain why metastasis does not occur than why it does. If metastasis in fact occurs by selective modifications of the peripheries of cells from which they derive, studies of cell clones derived from metastases are likely to hold the clue to successful metastasis. Thus, by comparisons between cells of primary tumors and their metastases using the high- and low-metastatic clones developed by Fidler (1977), Nicolson and others (1976) and Tao and Burger (1977), new comparisons should be more meaningful than the traditional comparisons between so-called normal cells and their malignant counterparts.

When comparing or describing the peripheries of any cells, their malignant or genetic status, their metabolic and mitotic status, and the consequences of their direct and indirect interactions with their cellular and noncellular environments must be taken into account. All of these factors considerably broaden the repertoire of the cell periphery with respect to its physicochemical structure and function. With a few notable exceptions, most studies to date of so-called cancer-specific properties of the cell periphery have not assessed these variables and it is hardly surprising that they have provided few explanations of the metastatic process.

Metastases are assumed to occur because of some as yet undefined peripheral properties of cancer cells. Considerations of the economics of metastasis lead to the diametrically opposite view, however: metastasis occurs in spite of these properties, which tend to make metastasis a rare event in comparison with the numerous cancer cells released from primary tumors (Liotta et al. 1974; Butler and Gullino 1975).

REFERENCES

Abercombie, M. The contact behavior of invading cells. In *Cellular membranes and tumor cell behavior*. Baltimore: Williams and Wilkins Co., 1975.

Alexander, P. Dormant metastases which manifest on immunosuppression and the role of macrophages in tumours. In *Fundamental aspects of metastasis*, ed. L. Weiss. Amsterdam: North-Holland Publishing Co., 1976.

Athens, J. W. Leukokinetic studies. III. The distribution of granulocytes in the blood of normal subjects. *J. Clin. Invest.* 40:159–164, 1968.

Barnes, D. W. H. et al. Tissue transplantation in the radiation chimera. *J. Cell Comp. Physiol.* 50(Suppl. 1):123–138, 1957.

Butler, T. P., and Gullino, P. M. Quantitation of cell shedding into efferent blood of mammary adenocarcinoma. *Cancer Res.* 35:512–516, 1975.

Chew, E. C.; Josephson, R. L.; and Wallace, A. C. Morphologic aspects of the arrest of circulating cancer cells. In *Fundamental aspects of metastasis*, ed. L. Weiss. Amsterdam: North-Holland Publishing Co., 1976.

Coman, D. R. Mechanisms responsible for the origin and distribution of blood-borne tumor metastases: a review. *Cancer Res.* 13:397–404, 1953.

Cook, G. M. W.; Seaman, G. V. F.; and Weiss, L. Physicochemical differences between ascitic and solid forms of sarcoma 37 cells. *Cancer Res.* 23:1813–1818, 1963.

Donald, K. J.; Chalk, S.; and Sullivan, J. J. Fibrin-bound tumour cells on a sclerosed mitral valve. *Pathology* 9:195–198, 1977.

Eccles, S. A., and Alexander, P. Macrophage content of tumours in relation to metastatic spread and host immune reaction. *Nature* 250:667–669, 1974.

Fidler, I. J. Patterns of tumor cell arrest and development. In *Fundamental aspects of metastasis*, ed. L. Weiss. Amsterdam: North-Holland Publishing Co., 1976.

Fidler, I. J. The heterogeneity of metastatic neoplasms. In *Pulmonary metastasis*, eds. L. Weiss and H. A. Gilbert. Metastases Monograph Series, Vol. 1. Boston: G.K. Hall and Co., 1978.

Fisher, B.; Soliman, O.; and Fisher, E. R. Effect of antilymphocyte serum on parameters of tumor growth in a syngeneic tumor host system. *Proc. Soc. Exp. Biol. Med.* 131:16–18, 1969.

Folger, R. et al. Translational movements of macrophages through media of different viscosities. *J. Cell Sci.* 31:245–257, 1978.

Foulds, L. Neoplastic Development. London: Academic Press, 1969.

Frank, A. L., and Holyoke, E. D. Tumor fluid thromboplastin activity. *Int. J. Cancer* 3:677–682, 1968.

Friedell, G. H., and Parsons, L. Blood vessel invasion in cancer of the cervix. *Cancer* 15:1269–1274, 1962.

Glaves, D., and Weiss, L. Initial arrest patterns of circulating cancer cells: effects of host sensitization and anticoagulation. In *Fundamental aspects of metastasis*, ed. L. Weiss. Amsterdam: North-Holland Publishing Co., 1976.

Greene, H. S. N. Discussion of paper by Zeidman. *Acta Cytol.* 9:138, 1965.

Holyoke, E. D. Oncofetal antigens and metastasis monitoring. In *Fundamental aspects of metastasis*, ed. L. Weiss. Amsterdam: North-Holland Publishing Co., 1976.

Holyoke, E. D.; Frank, A. L.; and Weiss, L. Tumor thromboplastin activity in vitro. *Int. J. Cancer* 9:258–263, 1972.

Keller, R. Mechanisms by which activated normal macrophages destroy syngeneic rat tumour cells in vitro. *Immunology* 27:285–298, 1974.

Krahenbuhl, J. L., and Remington, J. S. Inhibition of target cell mitosis as a measure of the cytostatic effects of activated macrophages on tumor target cells. *Cancer Res.* 37:3912–3916, 1977.

Leighton, J. Inherent malignancy of cancer cells possibly limited by genetically differing cells in the same tumor. *Acta Cytol.* 9:139–140, 1965.

Lichtman, M. A., and Weed, R. J. Cellular deformability of normal and leukemic hematopoietic cells: a determinant of marrow and vascular egress. In *Fundamental aspects of metastasis*, ed. L. Weiss. Amsterdam: North-Holland Publishing Co., 1976.

Liotta, L. A.; Kleinerman, J.; and Saidel, G. M. Quantitative relationships of intravascular tumor cells, tumor vessels, and pulmonary metastases following tumor implantation. *Cancer Res.* 34:997–1004, 1974.

Maslow, D. E., and Weiss, L. Cell exudation and cell adhesion. *Exp. Cell Res.* 71:204–208, 1972.

Mayhew, E. Cellular electrophoretic mobility and the mitotic cycle. *J. Gen. Physiol.* 49:717–725, 1966.

Nicolson, G. L. The interactions of lectins with animal cell surfaces. *Int. Rev. Cytol.* 39:89–190, 1974.

Nicolson, G. L.; Winkelhake, J. L.; and Nussey, A. C. An approach to studying the cellular properties associated with metastasis: some in vitro properties of tumor variants selected in vivo for enhanced metastasis. In *Fundamental aspects of metastasis*, ed. L. Weiss. Amsterdam: North-Holland Publishing Co., 1976.

O'Meara, R. A. Q. Coagulative properties of cancer. *Irish J. Med. Sci.* 394:474–479, 1958.

Pimm, M. V., and Baldwin, R. W. Antigenic differences between primary methylcholanthrene-induced rat sarcomas and post surgical recurrences. *Int. J. Cancer* 20:37–43, 1977.

Poste, G., and Weiss, L. Some considerations on cell surface alterations in malignancy. In *Fundamental aspects of metastasis*, ed. L. Weiss. Amsterdam: North-Holland Publishing Co., 1976.

Price, M. R., and Baldwin, R. W. Shedding of tumor cell surface antigens. *Cell Surface Rev.* 2:423–472, 1977.

Rabotti, G. Ploidy of primary and metastatic human tumors. *Nature* 183:1276–1277, 1959.

Rapp, H. J. Of cavies and men: the propriety and rationality of "cancer immunotherapy." *J. Nat. Cancer Inst.* 59:1577–1579, 1977.

Sandberg, A. A., and Yamada, K. Chromosomes and causation of human cancer and leukemia. I. Karyotypic diversity in a single cancer. *Cancer* 19:1869–1878, 1966.

Sato, H., and Suzuki, M. Deformability and viability of tumor cells by transcapillary passage, with reference to organ affinity of metastasis in cancer. In *Fundamental aspects of metastasis*, ed. L. Weiss. Amsterdam: North-Holland Publishing Co., 1976.

Stevenson, G. T., and Lawrence, D. J. R. Report of a workshop on the immune response to solid tumours in man. *Int. J. Cancer* 16:887–896, 1975.

Stoker, M. G. P. Anchorage dependence. *Nature* 218:234–236, 1968.

Sträuli, P., and Weiss, L. Cell locomotion and tumor penetration. *Europ. J. Cancer* 13:1–12, 1977.

Suzuki, N. et al. Cell cycle dependency of metastatic lung colony formation. *Cancer Res.* 37:3690–3693, 1977.

Sylven, B. Biochemical factors accompanying growth and invasion. In *Endogenous factors influencing host-tumor balance*, eds. R. W. Wissler, T. L. Dao and S. Wood. Chicago: University of Chicago Press, 1967.

Tao, T. W., and Burger, M. M. Non-metastasizing variants selected from metastasizing melanoma cells. *Nature* 270:437–438, 1977.

Volkman, A. Monocyte kinetics and their changes in infection. In *Immunobiology of the macrophage*, ed. S. D. Nelson. New York: Academic Press, 1976.

Warren, B. A. The ultrastructure of platelet pseudopodia and the adhesion of homologous platelets to tumour cells. *Br. J. Exp. Pathol.* 51:570–580, 1970.

Weiss, L. Studies on cellular adhesion in tissue-culture. V. Some effects of enzymes on cell-detachment. *Exp. Cell Res.* 30:509–520, 1963.

Weiss, L. Studies on cellular adhesion in tissue culture. VII. Surface activity and cell detachment. *Exp. Cell Res.* 33:277–288, 1964.

Weiss, L. Studies on cell adhesion in tissue-culture. VIII. Some effects of antisera on cell detachment. *Exp. Cell Res.* 37:540–551, 1965a.

Weiss, L. Studies on cell deformability. I. Effects of surface charge. *J. Cell Biol.* 26:735–739, 1965b.

Weiss, L. Effect of temperature on cellular electrophoretic mobility phenomena. *J. Nat. Cancer Inst.* 36:837–847, 1966.

Weiss, L. *The cell periphery, metastasis and other contact phenomena.* Amsterdam: North-Holland Publishing Co., 1967.

Weiss, L. Studies on cellular adhesion in tissue culture. X. An experimental and theoretical approach to interaction forces between cells and glass. *Exp. Cell Res.* 53:603–614, 1968.

Weiss, L. Biophysical aspects of initial cell interactions with solid surfaces. *Fed. Proc.* 30:1649–1657, 1971.

Weiss, L. Biophysical aspects of the metastatic cascade. In *Fundamental aspects of metastasis*, ed. L. Weiss. Amsterdam: North-Holland Publishing Co., 1976a.

Weiss, L. Cell deformability: some general considerations. In *Fundamental aspects of metastasis*, ed. L. Weiss. Amsterdam: North-Holland Publishing Co., 1976b.

Weiss, L. Cell detachment and metastasis. *Cancer Res.* 20:25–35, 1977a.

Weiss, L. Tumor necrosis and cell detachment. *Int. J. Cancer* 20:87–92, 1977b.

Weiss, L. Factors leading to the arrest of cancer cells in the lungs. In *Pulmonary metastasis*, eds. L. Weiss and H. A. Gilbert. Boston: G. K. Hall & Co., 1978.

Weiss, L.; Mayhew, E.; and Ulrich, K. The effect of neuraminidase on the phagocytic process in human monocytes. *Lab. Invest.* 15:1304–1309, 1966.

Weiss, L., and Holyoke, E. D. Some effects of hypervitaminosis A on metastasis of spontaneous breast cancer in mice. *J. Nat. Cancer Inst.* 43:1045–1054, 1969.

Weiss, L., and Harlos, J. P. Short-term interactions between cell surfaces. *Progr. Surface Sci.* 1:355–405, 1971.

Weiss, L.; Glaves, D.; and Waite, D. A. The influence of host immunity on the arrest of circulating cancer cells and its modification by neuraminidase. *Int. J. Cancer* 13:850–862, 1974.

Weiss, L., and Huber, D. Some effects of antimetabolites on cell detachment. *J. Cell Sci.* 15:217–220, 1974.

Weiss, L., and Subjeck, J. R. Interactions between the peripheries of Ehrlich ascites tumor cells as indicated by the binding of colloidal iron hydroxide particles. *Int. J. Cancer* 13:143–150, 1974.

Weiss, L., and Glaves, D. Effects of migration inhibiting factor(s) on the in vitro detachment of macrophages. *J. Immunol.* 115:1362–1365, 1975.

Weiss, L. et al. Long-distance interactions between Ehrlich ascites tumour cells. *J. Theor. Biol.* 51:439–454, 1975.

Weiss, L., and Glaves, D. The immunospecificity of altered initial arrest patterns of circulating cancer cells in tumor-bearing mice. *Int. J. Cancer* 18:774–777, 1976.

Weiss, L., and Poste, G. The tumour cell periphery. In *Scientific foundations of oncology*, eds. T. Symington and R. L. Carter. London: Heinemann, 1976.

Weiss, L., and Glaves, D. Alterations in the arrest patterns of circulating lymphosarcoma cells in tumor-bearing mice produced by previously injected cell suspensions. *Br. J. Cancer* 37:363–368, 1978.

Wheelock, E. F. et al. The tumor dormant state. *Progr. Cancer Res. Ther.* 5:105–116, 1977.

Wolff, E. Le mechanisme de l'invasion du cancer en culture organotypique. In *Mechanisms of invasion in cancer*, ed. P. Denoix. New York: Springer-Verlag, 1967.

Yamada, K.; Takagi, N.; and Sandberg, A. A. The chromosomes and causation of human cancer and leukemia. II. Karyotypes of human solid tumors. *Cancer* 19:1879–1890, 1966.

Zeidman, I. The fate of circulating tumor cells. *Acta Cytol.* 9:136–138, 1965.

3

Experimental Brain Metastasis

Kenneth W. Brunson
Garth L. Nicolson

Tumor metastasis is a complex, multistep process that appears to be dependent upon a number of host and tumor properties (Fidler 1975a; Weiss 1977a; Fidler and Nicolson 1979; Nicolson 1978a). First, emergent malignant tumor cells must be able to survive and grow in a potentially hostile environment and proliferate to form a primary tumor. Once a primary tumor is established, invasion of surrounding normal tissues may take place by mechanical infiltration (Eaves 1973), enzymatic digestion (Dresden et al. 1972), or both. If a primary tumor is able to penetrate blood vessels, malignant cells can be transported to distant sites. Several factors probably influence tumor-cell detachment (Weiss 1977b) and survival in the circulation. While in the blood, tumor cells (or cell emboli) can interact with a variety of humoral or cellular components (such as lymphocytes, platelets, endothelial cells). The hostile environment of the circulatory system probably causes the death of most blood-borne malignant cells originating from solid tumors; only a small percentage of tumor cells actually survive to form secondary tumors (Fidler 1970, 1976). Survival at a distant site appears to involve successful implantation in the microcirculation, extravasation and establishment of a proper environment for subsequent vascularization and growth.

PATTERNS OF EXPERIMENTAL METASTASIS

The distributions of viable malignant cells in the blood and formation of secondary metastases are not necessarily based on circulatory pathways or the first vascular capillary bed encountered by the blood-borne tumor cells. Circulating malignant cells or emboli can be temporarily arrested in the first capillary bed contacted, but at this point the cells may die, survive to form a secondary tumor at this site, invade and survive at extravascular sites, or deform and recirculate to be arrested at other sites. This last phenomenon has been experimentally demonstrated in a variety of animal tumor systems. Transpulmonary capillary passage of both V2 and Brown-Pearce carcinoma cells was documented by Zeidman (1957, 1961) and Zeidman and Buss (1952), who suggested that the higher incidence of passage through the lungs by viable Brown-Pearce carcinoma cells might correlate with the greater tendency of these cells to metastasize to extrapulmonary organs. In contrast to Brown-Pearce carcinoma cells, V2 carcinoma colonization generally was restricted to lungs.

A number of animal metastatic systems have yielded nonrandom distributions of experimental metastases forming from blood-borne malignant tumor cells. Sugarbaker (1952) reported different patterns of organ selectivity for tumor colonization after arterial inoculation of rats with suspensions of carcinoma or sarcoma cells. The distributions of tumor metastases in the various organs appeared to be unique to the type of tumor cell used for injection. Dunn (1954) observed that a variety of neoplasms involving lymphatic or hemopoietic tissue possessed somewhat distinct patterns of organ distribution in the mouse. Using the plasmacytoma X5563, Potter and others (1957) observed that while the regional lymph nodes were infiltrated and colonized, the spleen was rarely involved and the liver and kidneys never contained metastases. A reticulum-cell sarcoma (type B) injected intravenously was found to specifically colonize the spleen and lymph nodes without involving other organs (Parks 1974). This reticulum-cell sarcoma displayed a similar pattern of metastasis from subcutaneous sites, forming tumors only in the draining regional lymph nodes and spleen (Pilgrim 1969).

One of the more remarkable demonstrations of organ specificity by tumor metastasis was reported by Kinsey (1960), who noted that the Cloudman S91 melanoma specifically formed spontaneous metastases in lungs or trocar transplants of lung tissue. Fragments of lung tissue from newborn DBA / 2 mice were placed into one thigh of adult DBA / 2 animals. As controls, the other thigh received tissue fragments from other organs such as kidney, spleen, brain or heart or was traumatized by mock surgery. Ten days after tissue-fragment transplantation, the animals received S91 melanoma cells intravascularly. Subsequent tumor formation after 3–4 weeks occurred only in the lungs or transplanted lung fragments; no melanoma colonies were found in other organs or transplanted tissue fragments.

DEVELOPMENT OF EXPERIMENTAL MODELS FOR MALIGNANT MELANOMA

A murine melanoma which commonly forms lung metastases is the B16 malignant melanoma which arose spontaneously in C57BL / 6 mice. This tumor-cell line was used by Fidler (1973) to develop an animal tumor system for studying melanoma lines of low or high metastatic potential. In order to obtain melanoma lines of high metastatic potential, parental B16 melanoma cells were suspended and injected intravenously into groups of syngeneic mice to select for lung implantation, survival and growth. Pigmented melanoma pulmonary colonies that formed during the first lung selection were adapted to tissue culture and designated line B16-F1 (Fidler

1973). Single-cell suspensions of line B16-F1 were reinjected into mice, and three weeks later melanomatous pulmonary nodules were removed, cultured in vitro, and designated line B16-F2. B16-F2 was further sequentially selected in vivo for lung colonization, and after ten such selections tumor-cell line B16-F10 was obtained. Melanoma line B16-F10 yielded significantly more gross experimental metastases in the lungs than B16-F1 (Fidler 1973, 1975b; Fidler and Nicolson 1976, 1977).

Lung specificity of line B16-F10 was assessed by following the kinetic distributions of ^{125}IUdR-labeled melanoma cells after intravenous (tail vein) or left ventricle intracardiac injection (Fidler and Nicolson 1976). By the latter route, extrapulmonary arrest, detachment and recirculation are necessary in order to reach the lung microcirculation. Organs and blood from the animals were analyzed for viable ^{125}I-labeled B16 cells. Although the kinetic distributions of blood-borne melanoma cells were different in blood and all organs within 2 minutes after injection by these two routes, by one day the same numbers of viable B16-F10 cells were found in the lungs independent of the route of entry into the circulation. When animals were sacrificed after two weeks and the numbers of gross melanoma nodules counted in the lungs and at other sites, similar numbers of pulmonary metastases were found in mice receiving melanoma cells via the tail vein (9 ± 3 and 79 ± 16 nodules for B16-F1 and B16-F10, respectively, per 25,000 input cells) or left ventricle (10 ± 2 and 83 ± 10 for B16-F1 and B16-F10, respectively, per 25,000 input cells) (Fidler and Nicolson 1976).

B16-F10 extrapulmonary metastases were not found, indicating that initial blood-borne tumor-cell distribution and arrest may have little bearing on subsequent metastatic colonization. In these experiments significantly more cells from the highly metastatic B16-F10 line implanted, survived and grew to detectable lung metastases compared to line B16-F1, and B16-F1 but not B16-F10 cells formed a variety of extrapulmonary metastases (Fidler and Nicolson 1976, 1977; Nicolson and Brunson 1977). Although the initial tumor-cell distributions, rates of vascular entry and first organ capillary beds encountered were different, the ultimate outcome of metastatic colonization was unchanged. Tumor cells entering into the circulation via the left ventricle and temporarily arresting in the extrapulmonary microcirculation were able to detach, recirculate and ultimately reach the lungs to implant and survive forming the same number of tumor colonies as melanoma cells entering the lung microcirculation first after tail vein injection. These data indicate that implantation and survival of bloodborne malignant cells are not random and that recirculation of once-arrested tumor cells can lead to efficient metastatic colonization (Fidler and Nicolson 1976, 1977; Nicolson and Brunson 1977).

SELECTION AND PROPERTIES OF BRAIN-COLONIZING MELANOMA VARIANTS

One of the most clinically troublesome sites of metastasis is the brain (Posner 1977). About 18% of patients with systemic cancer have intracranial metastases observable at autopsy (Posner and Shapiro 1975), and in one retrospecive study of autopsy-proven melanoma, 44% of the patients had central nervous system lesions (Beresford 1969). Thus, it would be useful to develop an animal model for studying brain metastasis, particularly from malignant melanoma, in an effort to understand the predilection of certain tumors to spread to the central nervous system.

Animal models for brain metastases were not available until the recent development of B16 melanoma lines that preferentially colonize brain (fig. 3.1) (Nicolson and Brunson, 1977; Brunson et al. 1978; Nicolson et al. 1978). Brain-colonizing B16 melanoma lines were selected in a sequential fashion

Figure 3.1.

IN VIVO SELECTION FOR METASTATIC
B16-B MELANOMA LINES

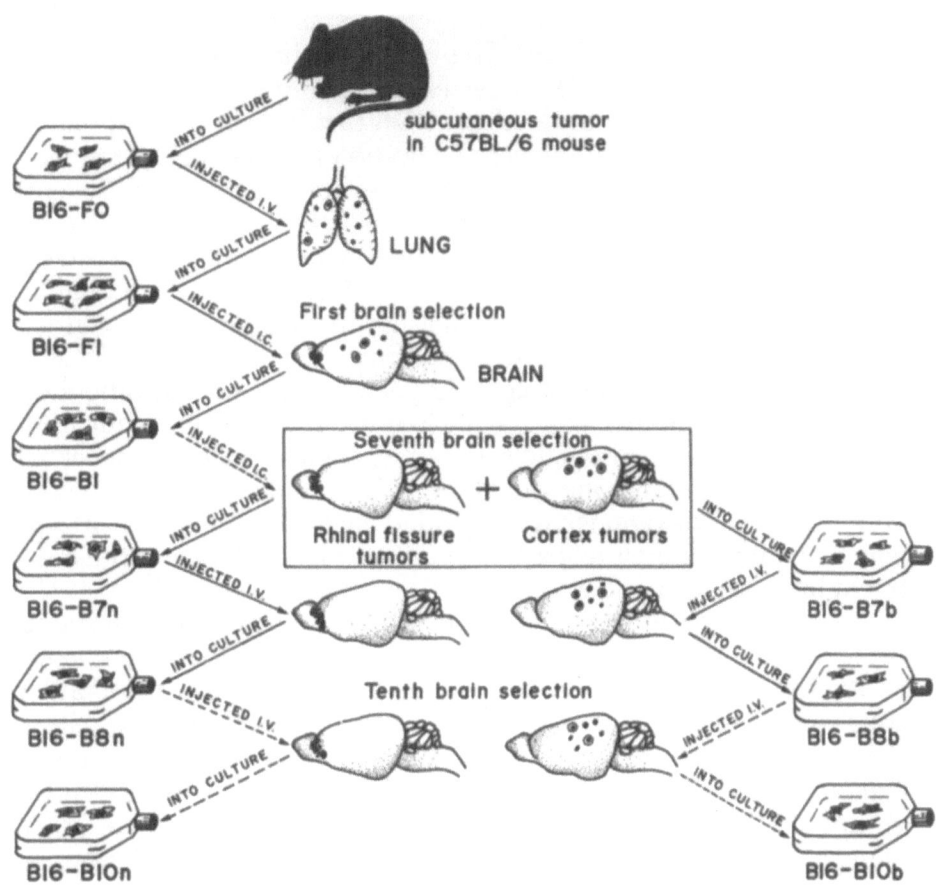

In vivo selection for brain-colonizing metastatic B16-B melanoma lines. Scheme for selecting brain-colonizing B16 melanoma lines. One type of selection yielded line B16-B10N, which colonizes the rhinal and longitudinal fissure region; another yielded B16-B10B, which colonizes the meninges of the dorsal cerebral cortex.

using the melanoma line B16-F1, which was originally selected for lung implantation, survival and growth. For initial in vivo selections, it was necessary to employ large tumor-cell inocula (200,000–400,000 viable B16-F1 melanoma cells per mouse), which were administered into the left cardiac ventricle of syngeneic C57Bl / 6 female recipients in order to obtain enough viable B16 cells from brain to culture in vitro. Brain tumors were located as pigmented (melanotic) nodules, and the first successful line cultured from a brain lesion was designated B16-B1 (fig. 3.1). Cells from line B16-B1 were then reinjected intracardially into syngeneic hosts to yield line B16-B2. After four in vivo selections via the intracardiac route for successful cerebral metastasis, subsequent brain colonization selections were performed employing intravenous injections with gradually decreasing numbers of tumor-cell inocula until only 20,000–40,000 cells were used for brain selections B16-B8 through B16-B10.

We found that with successive in vivo selections, tumor-cell lines were obtained which were more efficient in brain colonization with fewer intravenous injected B16-B cells. This could only have occurred if the B16-B cells traversed the lung capillary system more efficiently because this is the first capillary bed encountered and because fewer B16-B pulmonary nodules were found with increased selection for brain colonization.

Two regions of brain colonization were apparent after the seventh in vivo selection (fig. 3.2) (Nicolson and Brunson 1977; Nicolson 1978a; Brunson et al. 1978; Nicolson et al. 1978). One B16 melanoma variant line, B16-B7N, formed melanoma nodules almost exclusively in the forebrain in an area primarily restricted to the rhinal fissure with an occasional tumor nodule within the olfactory bulb. Another B16 variant line, designated B16-B7B, formed pigmented tumors in the meninges surrounding the dorsal cerebrum. Mice inoculated with line B16-B7N but not with B16-B7B exhibited apparent neurologic symptoms, such as staggering gait, tilted head and poor balance and orientation. Three subsequent in vivo selections via the intravenous route yielded lines B16-B10N and B16-B10B, which maintained their respective specificities for colonizing the two different brain regions.

Biologic assays were performed after intravenous injections of single-cell suspensions of brain-selected B16 melanoma lines, and we found that sequential in vivo selection of brain-preferring melanoma variants yielded increasingly brain-specific cell lines as the in vivo selections progressed (table 3.1). For these assays 2–5×10^4 cells of each variant B16 melanoma line were injected intravenously into age- and weight-matched groups of 10 animals each at essentially the same time so that a direct comparison of organ colonization was possible. These parallel assays were necessary because some variability in the numbers of tumors formed was noted in different groups of animals. In these assays animals were sacrificed after 3–4 weeks instead of 2 weeks in order to insure that all micrometastases could grow to visually detectable size. Lines B16-F1 and B16-B1 yielded large numbers of pulmonary tumors and few brain tumors, whereas lines B16-B5 and B16-B10N formed four and nine times, respectively, the number of brain lesions compared to B16-F1 while forming

Figure 3.2.

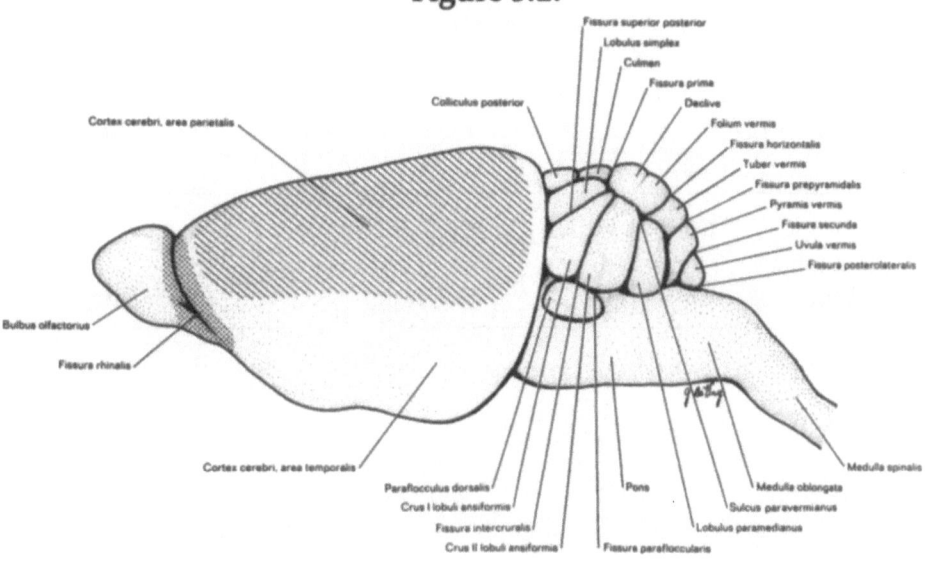

Lateral View   A

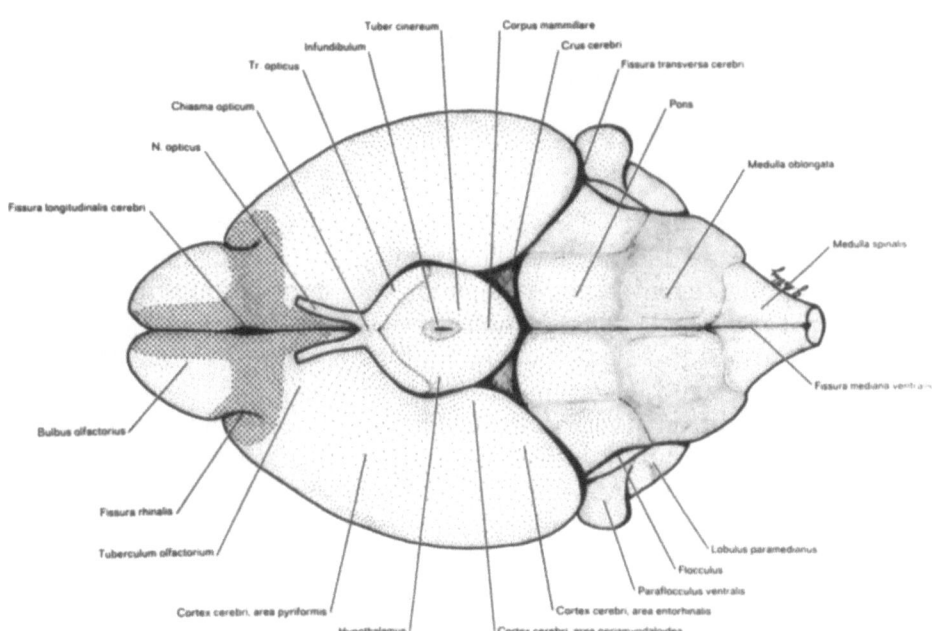

Ventral View   B

Lateral (A) and ventral (B) views of a mouse brain showing regional areas of experimental metastatic involvement of B16-B10N (heavily dotted section) and B16-B10B (slanted line section) melanoma variant lines.

Table 3.1

EXPERIMENTAL METASTASES FOUND AFTER
INTRAVENOUS INJECTION OF B16 MELANOMA VARIANT LINES
SELECTED BY THE VASCULAR ROUTE

Melanoma Line	Median Brain Tumors/Mouse (range)	Median Lung Tumors/Mouse (range)	Other Sites
B16-F1	1 (0–3)	74 (31–97)	6/10 thoracic cavity 2/10 ovary 1/10 adrenal
B16-B1	1 (0–2)	85 (32–95)	6/9 thoracic cavity 3/9 ovary 1/9 lumbar spine
B16-B5	4 (0–11)	1 (0–9)	5/10 thoracic cavity
B16-B10N	9 (3–28)	0 (0–1)	1/10 ovary

Single-cell suspensions ($2-5 \times 10^4$ cells) of viable B16 melanoma cells were injected into tail veins of syngeneic C57B1/6 mice (9–10 animals/melanoma line), and pigmented melanoma colonies were counted after 3–4 weeks.

fewer extracranial tumors. Line B16-B10N formed almost exclusively brain tumors, even though B16-B10N cells were injected into the tail veins of test animals and initially arrested in the lungs before recirculation to the brain (Brunson et al. 1978). When melanoma lesions from brains of mice bearing B16-B10N tumors and displaying neurologic symptoms were examined histologically, the tumors appeared to reside almost exclusively in the rhinal and longitudinal fissures of the forebrain with fingers occasionally extending into the cortex along vascular routes (fig. 3.3).

Because the brain-preferring B16 melanoma lines were selected by intravenous injections of tumor-cell suspensions, a process that circumvents growth, invasion and detachment at the primary site, the following experiment was designed to test whether the B16-B lines were metastatic from primary sites. Groups of mice were injected subcutaneously in the midpart of the ear with an inoculum of 50,000–100,000 viable tumor cells. A few weeks later the ears bearing tumors were amputated, and the incidence of spontaneous metastasis to lymph nodes and organs was subsequently scored (Fidler 1978). Although line B16-F1 is quite heterogeneous and spontaneously metastasizes at a low rate, it formed metastases in

Figure 3.3.

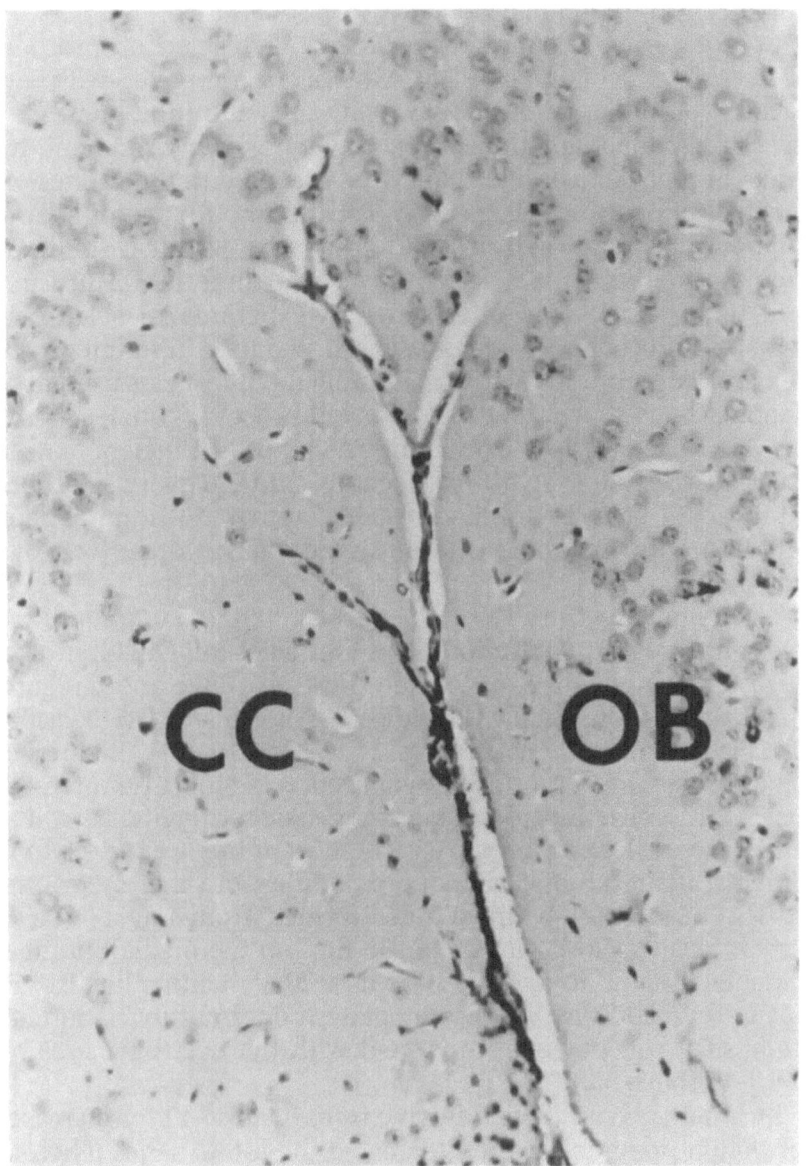

Histologic section of mouse brain demonstrating the rhinal fissure region with a B16-B10N tumor. The section is a sagittal cut through the forebrain exposing the cerebral cortex (CC) and the olfactory bulb (OB) in the region of the median sagittal rhinal fissure. The melanoma cells appear to extend along a vascular pathway into the cerebrum. (Haematoxylin-eosin stain, X600.)

the lung and at several other organ sites (Fidler 1978). In similar experiments line B16-B10N overwhelmingly formed brain metastases, a few thoracic metastases, and some lymph node tumors (K. W. Brunson and G. L. Nicolson, preliminary data).

In order to determine whether the in vivo selection procedures described above actually selected variant tumor cells with enhanced capacities for implantation, survival and growth in the brain, or alternatively selected for adaptation in a particular organ environment, two other types of in vivo control selections were carried out. One series of experimental selections was designed to test the importance of adaptation of melanoma cells for growth in brain tissue (the so-called soil hypothesis) and employed sequential selections by direct intracerebral implantation of B16-F1 tumor cells. The other series of experimental selections tested whether B16-F1 could be sequentially selected for a different organ preference of colonization. In this latter control line B16-F1 was used to select for melanoma lines that preferentially colonized ovary instead of brain or lung. Approximately the same numbers of B16-F1 melanoma cells were used as described for the B16-B selections, and the ovary selections paralleled those for brain in duration, route of tumor-cell administration, and length of in vitro cultivation except that the target organ was ovary, not brain.

Melanoma line B16-F1 was selected for brain adaptation by repeated direct intracerebral inoculation. The first selection for brain adaptation yielded a melanoma line designated B16-ICer1. Five and ten subsequent sequential selections resulted in lines B16-ICer5 and B16-ICer10, respectively. Lines B16-ICer1, B16-ICer5 and B16-ICer10 were compared to B16-F1 in biologic assays after intravenous injection of single tumor-cell suspensions (2×10^4 cells / inoculum) into syngeneic recipients. Few, if any, differences were noted in the capacity of lines in the ICer series to form experimental brain tumors, pulmonary nodules, or other metastases (table 3.2). The number of brain nodules formed from any of the B16-ICer selected lines was low, similar to B16-F1, and the median number of experimental lung tumor colonies was near 20 with either line B16-F1 or line B16-ICer10. In addition, no distinct pattern of tumor formation in various visceral sites was obvious, consistent with the heterogeneous nature of line B16-F1 (table 3.2).

Melanoma lines selected in vivo from line B16-F1 for increased ovary colonization preference were designated the B16-O series (Nicolson et al. 1978; Brunson and Nicolson 1980). In the initial ovary selections large numbers of animals were utilized in order to recover some ovarian tumor nodules. The ovary-colonizing B16 cells were then grown in tissue culture to form line B16-O1, and this process was repeated five and ten times to obtain ovary colonizing lines B16-O5 and B16-O10, respectively. Because these latter B16-O lines produced less melanin with sequential in vivo selections (Brunson and Nicolson 1980), it was difficult to accurately assess experimental brain metastasis with line B16-O10; however, no visible tumors or neurologic symptoms were noted in recipient mice bearing any of the B16-O tumors. We did find a considerable enhancement in the ability of the B16-O lines to implant, survive and grow in the ovaries with sequential selection for ovary colonization (table 3.3). Although no experimental ovarian metastases were found in animals injected with B16-F1 tumor cells in this series of assays, a few tumors were noted in the ovaries of mice receiving B16-O1 cells, and approximately 70% and 80% of the animals injected with B16-O5 or B16-O10 melanoma cells, respectively, exhibited ovarian tumors. With increasing sequential selection of melanoma lines for ovarian preference, pulmonary tumor formation decreased although the differences were not as striking as seen with the B16-B series. The B16-O10 melanoma line has maintained its ability to form tumors at nonovarian sites beside the lungs, in contrast to the fairly strict brain colonization preference of line B16-B10N (Brunson and Nicolson 1980).

These experiments suggest that the B16-B melanoma lines selected for blood-borne implantation, survival and growth in the brains of syngeneic recipients may be unique in their capacities to form experimental brain metastases after intravenous inoculation of single-cell suspensions. In comparison, the B16-ICer melanoma series selected by direct intracerebral

Table 3.2

EXPERIMENTAL METASTASES FOUND AFTER
INTRAVENOUS INJECTION OF B16 MELANOMA VARIANT LINES
SELECTED BY DIRECT BRAIN IMPLANTATION

Melanoma Line	Median Brain Tumors/Mouse (range)	Median Lung Tumors/Mouse (range)	Other Sites
B16-F1	2 (0–3)	24 (0–76)	1/12 thoracic cavity 1/12 ovary 2/12 pancreas 2/12 mesentery
B16-ICer1	2 (0–5)	40 (3–49)	1/11 thoracic cavity
B16-ICer5	2 (0–5)	22 (0–63)	1/11 pancreas 3/11 thoracic cavity
B16-ICer10	3 (0–6)	19 (0–46)	1/11 thoracic cavity

Single-cell suspensions (2×10^4 cells) of viable B16 melanoma cells were injected into tail veins of syngeneic C57Bl/6 mice (11–12 animals/melanoma line), and pigmented colonies were counted after 3–4 weeks.

Table 3.3

EXPERIMENTAL METASTASES FOUND AFTER
INTRAVENOUS INJECTION OF B16 MELANOMA VARIANT LINES
SELECTED BY THE VASCULAR ROUTE

Melanoma Line	Positive Ovary Tumors*	Median Lung Tumors/Animal (range)	Other Sites*
B16-F1	0/10 0/10	61 (31–91)	10/10 thoracic cavity 3/10 thoracic cavity
B16-01	0/10 3/10	53 (1–256)	6/10 thoracic cavity 3/10 thoracic cavity
B16-05	8/10 6/10	32 (4–155)	0/10 thoracic cavity 2/10 thoracic cavity
B16-010	7/9 8/10	7 (1–17)	No other metastases 1/10 adrenal, 3/10 liver

*Two experiments.
NOTE: Single-cell suspension (2–5 × 10⁴ cells) of viable B16 melanoma cells were injected into tail veins of syngeneic C57B1/6 mice. Pigmented and nonpigmented melanoma colonies were located and counted after 3–4 weeks.

inoculations does not share this property. Thus, we conclude that the procedures employed do not simply result in selection for tumor-cell variants with enhanced adaptation for brain survival and growth.

CELL-SURFACE PROTEINS OR SPECIFIC ORGAN-PREFERRING MELANOMA VARIANTS

The surfaces of cells from the B16-B, B16-O and B16-F series of melanoma lines have been examined for differences in exposed cell-surface proteins by the lactoperoxidase-catalyzed ¹²⁵I-iodination procedures of Marchalonis and others (1971). Cell suspensions obtained from subconfluent cultures of brain-, ovary- or lung-selected melanoma lines were used for surface labeling. Radiolabeled cells were then treated with detergent (0.5% Nonidet P-40) to disrupt plasma membranes, and the solubilized radiolabeled membrane preparations were electrophoresed on 7.5–10% linear gradient polyacrylamide slab gels (Nicolson et al. 1977; Robbins et al. 1977; Brunson et al. 1978). Autoradiograms prepared from the dried gels were then scanned with a densitometer to reveal possible differences in the exposure of surface proteins between the various B16 melanoma-cell lines.

When analyzed by this technique, cell-surface differences were noted among the B16-B and B16-O series when compared to line B16-F1 (Nicolson 1978b; Brunson et al. 1978). In the brain-selected lines the major differences observed were increased exposure of two surface-labeled components having molecular weights of approximately 95,000 (95K) and 100,000 (100K) daltons. Sequential in vivo selection for enhanced experimental brain metastasis resulted in increased labeling of both the 95K and 100K exposed surface proteins when compared to line B16-F1. The 95K and 100K components incorporated slightly more ^{125}I in B16-B1 than B16-F1, higher levels in B16-B5, and the highest amount of exposure in the B16-B10N melanoma line. Moreover, the ratio of radiolabeling between the 95K and 100K surface-exposed proteins changed with sequential in vivo selection for brain colonization. The 95K component was more highly labeled compared to the 100K component in lines B16-B1 and B16-F1; both components were labeled about equally well in line B16-B5, and the 100K component incorporated more ^{125}I compared to the 95K protein in line B16-B10N, the most brain-specific line.

The cell-surface-exposed proteins of melanoma lines selected for other organ sites were unique. B16 melanoma variant cells of the ovary-selected lines (B16-O series) did not display increased exposure of 95K and 100K surface proteins compared to the parental B16-F1 line, but modifications were noted in two other cell-surface components with approximate molecular weights of 140,000 (140K) and 150,000 (150K) daltons. The amount of ^{125}I label incorporated during lactoperoxidase-catalyzed iodination of 140K and 150K surface proteins on the in vivo ovary-selected melanoma lines correlated with enhanced experimental ovarian metastasis. The degree of exposure of the 140K and 150K components increased slightly in the line B16-O1 when compared to B16-F1, was higher in line B16-O5, and was highest in line B16-O10, the melanoma line most successful in ovarian colonization. These differences were not found in brain- or lung-selected B16 lines (Nicolson et al. 1977; Nicolson 1978b). These results suggest that variant cell lines possessing unique cell-surface properties are obtained by the sequential selection procedures for organ preference and colonization.

IN VITRO DRUG SENSITIVITIES OF SPECIFIC ORGAN-PREFERRING MELANOMA VARIANTS

Another test for the unique character of the selective melanoma variant lines is whether these tumor-cell lines are affected differently by chemotherapeutic drugs. In addition to tests demonstrating the heterogeneous response of tumor-cell populations to drugs, Fidler (1978) has also suggested that efforts to design effective therapeutic agents and protocols would be aided by studying the few but often fatal metastatic subpopulations that exist within a tumor.

Several investigators have utilized analogs of vitamin A (retinoids) for prevention and therapy of benign and malignant tumors (Sporn 1977), and we have found that retinoids such as retinoic acid are effective chemotherapeutic agents against murine malignant melanomas such as B16 (Lotan and Nicolson 1977; Lotan et al. 1978). Therefore, we examined the ability of retinoids to inhibit in vitro proliferation of the B16 parental cell line and the in vivo selective variants with differing metastatic potential, particularly the brain- and ovary-selective series of variant lines.

Most B16 melanoma lines proliferate rapidly in culture with a doubling time of 14–16 hours. Exceptions are line B16-B10N (17–18 hours) and B16-O10 (18–19 hours). Subculturing B16 cell lines in the presence of retinoic acid did not decrease their plating efficiency but did decrease their growth rates in a dose-dependent manner compared to controls (Lotan and Nicolson, unpublished results, 1978). After a 5-day exposure to 10^{-5}M retinoic acid, growth of the parental B16 line (B16-F0), line B16-F1, and several clones obtained from the parental line was inhibited 80–90%. In contrast, similar experiments utilizing lines B16-F10, B16-O10 and B16-B10N retinoic acid-inhibited growth by $42\pm4\%$, $48\pm2\%$ and $75\pm3\%$, respectively. Comparison of the concentrations of retinoic acid required for a 50% inhibition of growth in the B16 lines yielded even greater differences. Growth of parental B16-FO and line B16-F1 was inhibited 50% at concentrations in excess of 10^{-8}M, whereas lines B16-F10, B16-O10 and B16-B10N were inhibited 50% at about 10^{-5}M, 10^{-6}M and 10^{-7}M retinoic acid (Lotan and Nicolson 1979). This indicates that there is almost a thousand-fold difference in the sensitivity to retinoic acid between parental B16 melanoma and some but not all of the in vivo selected lines. Irrespective of the exact mechanism which accounts for the heterogeneous response of the B16 cell lines to retinoic acid, these studies suggest that malignant cells growing at secondary sites may possess different sensitivities to chemotherapeutic drugs, probably because these cells represent tumor-cell subpopulations with various properties differing from the primary tumor.

Conclusion

A series of complex interactions between tumor cells and cells of the host are involved in metastatic tumor spread. The unique properties of malignant tumor cells determine, in part, whether they can successfully metastasize to form secondary tumors as shown by our studies with melanoma. Variant melanoma cell lines were selected in vivo for their abilities to implant, survive and grow in specific host organs. Using the procedures described in this chapter, we have been able to select brain-preferring B16 melanoma lines that possess unique cell-surface properties, drug sensitivities and potentials to form experimental brain metastasis.

These brain-colonizing tumor lines should prove valuable in studying tumor-cell and host properties important in metastases and in designing new therapeutic procedures to treat brain metastases.

REFERENCES

Beresford, H. R. Melanoma of the nervous system. *Neurology* 19:59–65, 1969.

Brunson, K. W.; Beattie, G.; and Nicolson, G. L. *In vivo* selection of malignant melanoma for organ preference of experimental metastasis. *J. Cell Biol.* 75:209a, 1977.

Brunson, K. W.; Beattie, G.; and Nicolson, G. L. Selection and altered properties of brain-colonising metastatic melanoma. *Nature* 272:543–545, 1978.

Brunson, K. W., and Nicolson, G. L. Selection of malignant melanoma variant cell line for ovary colonization. *J. Supramol. Struct.*, 1980.

Dresden, M. H.; Heilman, S. A.; and Schmidt, J. D. Collagenolytic enzymes in human neoplasms. *Cancer Res.* 32:993–996, 1972.

Dunn, T. B.; Normal and pathologic anatomy of the reticular tissue in laboratory mice, with a classification and discussion of neoplasms. *J. Natl. Cancer Inst.* 14:1281–1433, 1954.

Eaves, G. The invasive growth of malignant tumors as a purely mechanical process. *J. Pathol.* 109:233–237, 1973.

Fidler, I. J. Metastasis: quantitative analysis of distribution and fate of tumor emboli labeled with ^{125}I-5-iodo-2'-deoxyuridine. *J. Natl. Cancer Inst.* 45:775–782, 1970.

Fidler, I. J. Selection of successive tumor lines for metastasis. *Nature* [*New Biol.*] 242:148–149, 1973.

Fidler, I. J. Mechanisms of cancer invasion and metastasis. In *Cancer: a comprehensive treatise*. Biology of Tumors: Surfaces, Immunology, and Comparative Pathology, ed. F. F. Becker, Vol. 4. New York: Plenum Press, 1975a.

Fidler, I. J. Biological behavior of malignant melanoma cells correlated to their survival *in vivo*. *Cancer Res.* 35:218–224, 1975b.

Fidler, I. J. Patterns of tumor cell arrest and development. In *Fundamental aspects of metastasis*, ed. L. Weiss. Amsterdam: North-Holland Publishing Co., 1976.

Fidler, I. J. Tumor heterogeneity and the biology of cancer and metastasis. *Cancer Res.* 38:2651–2660, 1978.

Fidler, I. J., and Nicolson, G. L. Organ selectivity for implantation, survival and growth of B16 melanoma variant tumor lines. *J. Natl. Cancer Inst.* 57:1199–1202, 1976.

Fidler, I. J., and Nicolson, G. L. Fate of recirculating B16 melanoma metastatic variant cells in parabiotic syngeneic recipients. *J. Natl. Cancer Inst.* 58:1867–1872, 1977.

Fidler, I. J., and Nicolson, G. L. The immunobiology of experimental metastatic melanoma. *Cancer Biol. Rev.*, 1980.

Kinsey, D. L. An experimental study of preferential metastasis. *Cancer* 13:674–676, 1960.

Lotan, R. et al. Characterization of the inhibitory effects of retinoids on the *in vitro* growth of two malignant murine melanomas. *J. Natl. Cancer Inst.* 60:1035–1041, 1978.

Lotan, R., and Nicolson, G. L. Inhibitory effects of retinoic acid or retinyl acetate on the growth of untransformed, transformed and tumor cells *in vitro*. *J. Natl. Cancer Inst.* 59:1717–1722, 1977.

Lotan, R., and Nicolson, G. L. Heterogeneity in growth inhibition by retinoic acid or metastatic B16 melanoma clones and *in vivo* selected cell variant lines. *Cancer Res.* 39:4767–4771, 1980.

Marchalonis, J. J.; Cone, R. E.; and Santer, V. Enzymatic iodination: a probe for accessible surface proteins of normal and neoplastic lymphocytes. *Biochem. J.* 124:912–927, 1971.

Nicolson, G. L. Experimental tumor metastasis: characteristics and organ specificity. *BioScience* 28:441–447, 1978a.

Nicolson, G. L. Cell surface proteins and glycoproteins of metastatic murine melanomas and sarcomas. In *Biological markers in neoplasia: basic and applied aspects*, ed. R. W. Ruddon. New York: North-Holland Publishing Co., 1978b.

Nicolson, G. L. et al: Cell interactions in the metastatic process: some cell surface properties associated with successful blood-borne tumor spread. In *Cell and tissue interactions*, ed. J. Lash and M. M. Burger. New York: Raven Press, 1977.

Nicolson, G. L., and Brunson, K. W. Organ specificity of malignant B16 melanomas: *in vivo* selection for organ preference of blood-borne metastasis. *Gann. Monogr. Cancer Res.* 20:15–24, 1977.

Nicolson, G. L.; Brunson, K. W.; and Fidler, I. J. Specificity of arrest, survival and growth of selected metastatic variant cell lines. *Cancer Res.*, 38:4105–4111, 1978.

Parks, R. C. Organ-specific metastasis of a transplantable reticulum cell sarcoma. *J. Natl. Cancer Inst.* 52:971–973, 1974.

Pilgrim, H. I. The kinetics of the organ-specific metastasis of a transplantable reticuloendothelial tumor. *Cancer Res.* 29:1200–1205, 1969.

Posner, J. B. Management of central nervous system metastases. *Semin. Oncol.* 4:81–91, 1977.

Posner, J. B., and Shapiro, W. R. Brain tumor. Current status of treatment and its complications. *Arch. Neurol.* 32:781–784, 1975.

Potter, M.; Fahey, J. L.; and Pilgrim, H. I. Abnormal serum protein and bone destruction in transmissible mouse plasma cell endoplasm. *Proc. Soc. Exp. Biol. Med.* 94:327–333, 1957.

Robbins, J. C. et al. Cell-surface changes in a *Ricinus communis* toxin-resistant variant of a murine lymphoma. *J. Natl. Cancer Inst.* 58:1027–1033, 1977.

Smith, R. T., and Landy, M. *Immune Surveillance*. New York: Academic Press, 1971.

Sporn, M. B. Retinoids and carcinogenesis. *Nutr. Rev.* 35:65–69, 1977.

Sugarbaker, E. D. The organ selectivity of experimentally induced metastasis in rats. *Cancer* 5:606–612, 1952.

Weiss, L. A pathobiologic overview of metastasis. *Semin. Oncol.* 4:5–19, 1977a.

Weiss, L. Cell detachment and metastasis. *Gann. Monogr. Cancer Res.* 20:25–35, 1977b.

Zeidman, I. Metastasis: a review of recent advances. *Cancer Res.* 17:157–162, 1957.

Zeidman, I. The fate of circulating tumor cells. I. Passage of cells through capillaries. *Cancer Res.* 21:38–39, 1961.

Zeidman, I., and Buss, J. M. Transpulmonary passage of tumor cell emboli. *Cancer Res.* 12:731–733, 1952.

4

The Role of
Brain Metastases
in Cascade Processes:
Implications for Research
and Clinical Management

Irwin D. J. Bross

During the past decade, hundreds of millions of dollars have been spent each year on research and clinical technology with the purpose (or more accurately, the hope) of curing human cancer. In terms of objective criteria such as the long-term survival of patients, there is not very much to show for this expenditure of medical resources. One of the main reasons for this record of few successes and many failures is the strategic mistake that most clinicians make: the problem with cancer is not what the clinician can see but what the clinician cannot see. The problem of cancer is the problem of metastases, particularly remote occult metastases.

If substantial progress is to be made toward curing cancer, we must deal with hard realities, not vague hopes. Once human cancer has become generalized through the body, there is little in the present or forseeable armamentarium of the clinician that offers any appreciable chance of cure. So the crucial question for effective decision-making in patient management is: has the cancer reached the generalized stage? Answering this question is not simply a matter of clinical skill or technology. Equally important is a clear understanding of the steps in generalization of human cancer—in what is here called the *cascade process*. From my studies in the past five years with Dr. Enrico Viadana and Dr. John Pickren (Bross et al. 1975a and b; Viadana et al. 1976a and b, 1978), a clear picture of the cascade process at almost every major site of cancer has emerged. The principal results are not difficult to understand and in retrospect may seem obvious, but they contradict many doctrines and dogmas about cancer that have dominated research and treatment in this century.

A comprehensive report covering all of the principal sites of cancer and the cascade process for each of these sites was included in a previous symposium volume (Viadana et al. 1978). In that report detailed statistical tables give the basic data from the survey of metastatic sites at autopsy that

66

my colleague Dr. Pickren has been carrying out for many years. These data are a unique resource, and although we have already learned a great deal from them, there is much more to be learned. For instance, there is much more that could be learned about the lymphatic routes of dissemination.

The biostatistical technology for the analysis of this data, which can be called *cascade analysis*, is relatively simple. It uses a combination of two well-known statistical techniques, chi-square and sign tests. Implementation of the statistical analyses, however, was a task which took Dr. Viadana about a year, even with our computerized procedures. In the end, the patterns coalesced into the relative simple pictures presented here, but this was a fortunate and somewhat unexpected result. We did not try to force any pattern onto the autopsy data—only to try to read the patterns in the actual data.

In this presentation, no attempt will be made to re-examine in detail the tabular and statistical material in the publications cited above. The present aim is to show the general picture, rather than go into specific details. However, those who wish to use the results to develop rational therapeutic regimens for cancer at specific sites and have the incentive to carry out this demanding task may do so.

When this survey was initiated, there was no focus on the brain metastases although we already were aware that they came toward the end of the cascade process. Between the primary sites and these late sites are the so-called generalizing or key sites. They involve metastasis from a metastasis, an effect which cascade analysis brings out very clearly and which is crucial to a rational policy for the treatment of cancer. Contrary to what is sometimes supposed, cancer rarely generalizes throughout the body directly from the primary site but rather proceeds stepwise through a cascade process.

THE NATURE OF THE CASCADE PROCESS

The picture of the cascade process emerged from detailed analysis of 4,728 consecutive autopsies of single-primary cancer patients reported by the Pathology Department at Roswell Park Memorial Institute (Viadana et al. 1978). In general, the main conclusions are (1) the overwhelming majority of cancers are disseminated by a multistep process; (2) generalized disease (such as brain metastases) does not ordinarily occur directly from the primary; (3) there are one or more key generalizing sites that are specific for a given primary; (4) these sites depend largely on the drainage of the venous blood; (5) the generalized disease is produced by secondary metastases from the key sites; and (6) the similarity of the cascade processes at so many different sites reflects a similar underlying process of generalization through the blood system. To all such general points there are occasional exceptions, but the patterns in the cascade process are comprehensible and consistent and can provide a reliable basis for the development of therapeutic strategies for cancer.

The details of the cascade processes for most of the major primary sites of solid tumors are shown in schematic representations (figs. 4.1, 4.2, and 4.3). The discontinuous lines in all figures show the spread of malignant cells from the primary cancer to the key disseminating organ. The thin continuous lines follow the route of metastases from the first to the second key disseminating site (fig. 4.2). The thick continuous lines show the metastatic spread from the key disseminating organs to anywhere else in the body. The solid black areas, symbolizing organs, indicate the primary cancer sites, hatched areas indicate the key disseminating sites, and the unshaded, white areas represent metastases in the endocrine system and in the central nervous system (when cancer is already generalized).

For simplicity, metastases in the cortex cerebri are used as representatives of malignant cells in the entire central nervous system (which includes the gray and white matter of the cerebrum, cerebellum, pons, medulla, leptomeninges, and spinal cord). The thyroid gland represents the entire endocrine system. All primary cancer sites, as well as metastases in the lungs, are shown as unilateral, and the figures describe only the commonest disseminating routes. They do not show rare occurrences, such as a transorgan passage of the lungs or anomalous routes of dissemination via the lymphatic system.

The head and neck cancers (fig. 4.1) spread metastases from the lungs to the liver, endocrine glands, and central nervous system. Testicular seminomas, skin melanomas, osteochondrosarcomas, renal clear-cell carcinoma, and cancers of the endocrine glands produce pulmonary metastases as the first step in the cascade. Subsequently the cancer disseminates from the lungs to the liver, endocrine glands, and brain. Combining all head and neck cancers shows this metastatic pattern even more clearly on a statistical basis. The lungs disseminate tumor cells to the liver, brain, and endocrine system.

Figure 4.2 depicts the metastatic spread of primary gastrointestinal cancers in the pancreas, stomach, colon, and rectum. Malignant cells move from the primary cancer to the liver, which in turn disseminates metastases throughout the body via the lungs. Rectal adenocarcinomas appear to seed the liver and lungs independently.

In a similar manner, combining all the gastrointestinal cancers brings out even more clearly the pattern by which metastases to the liver generate metastases to the lungs which, in turn, disseminate metastases to both the endocrine system and central nervous system.

Figure 4.3 describes the metastatic spread of esophageal, bladder, and female genital cancers (ovaries, cervix, and corpus uteri). The lung and liver parenchyma are seeded independently of each other in this group of malignant tumors with the exception of ovarian adenocarcinomas in which the liver seeds the lungs. The lungs disseminate metastases to the brain whether or not there are hepatic metastases, but they seed the endocrine system only when there are hepatic metastases. This may mean that the lungs disseminate metastases to the endocrine glands only when the disease is so far advanced that the liver is also seeded.

Figure 4.1.

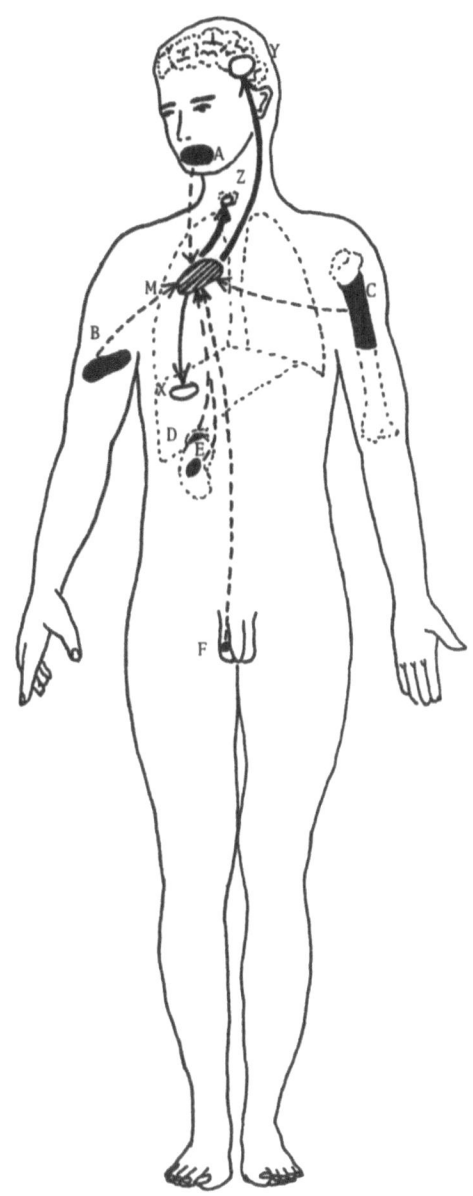

Cancers generalized by lung metastases with dissemination to the liver, endocrine glands, and central nervous system. Dark areas indicate primary tumors. A = primary cancers of head and neck; B = primary skin melanoma; C = primary osteochondrosarcoma; D = primary cancers of the adrenals; E = primary cancers of the kidney; F = testicular seminoma. Cross-hatched area indicates the key disseminating organ. M = lung as key disseminating site. Unshaded areas identify generalized metastases. X = metastases in liver; Y = central nervous system metastases; Z = endocrine system metastases. Lung metastases are presented as unilateral for simplicity in the drawing.

Figure 4.2.

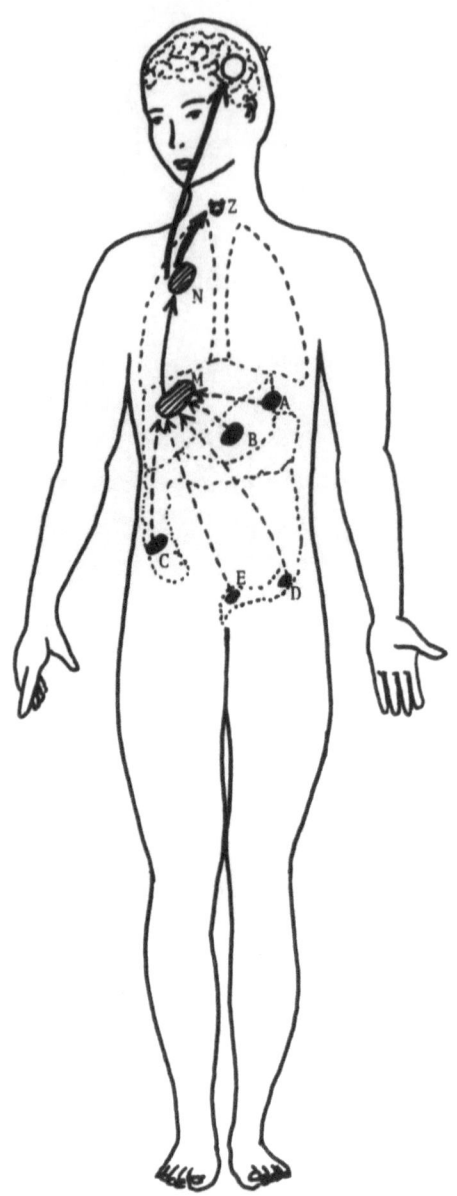

Cancers generalized by liver metastases (through the lungs) with dissemination to the endocrine glands and central nervous system. Dark areas indicate primary tumors. A = primary cancer of pancreas; B = primary cancer of stomach; C = primary cancer of coecum; D = primary cancer of colon; E = primary cancer of rectum. Cross-hatched areas indicate the key disseminating organs. M = liver, as first key disseminating site; N = lung as second key disseminating site. Unshaded areas identify generalized metastases. Y = central nervous system metastases; Z = endocrine system metastases. Lung metastases are presented as unilateral for simplicity in the drawing.

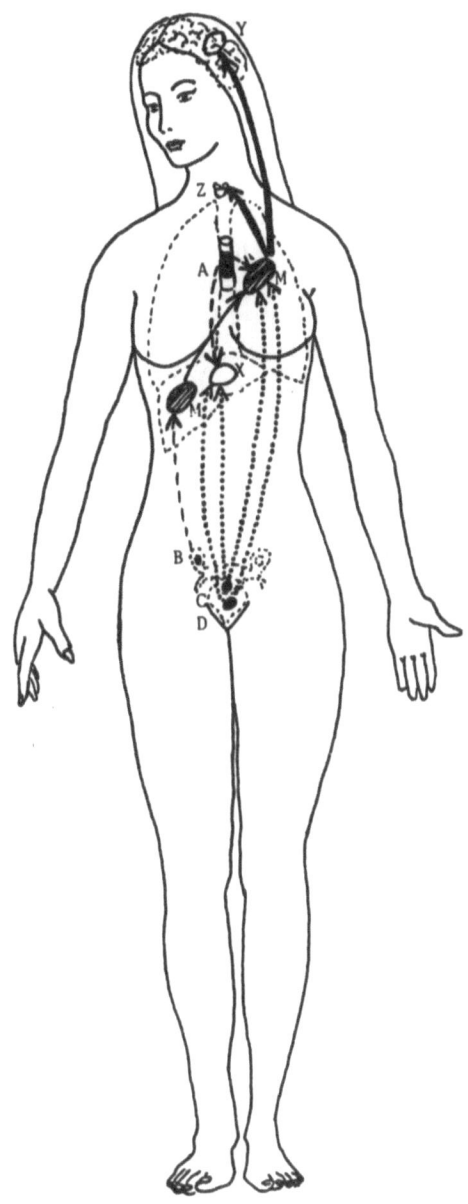

Cancers generalized either by lung metastases only or by the liver via the lungs (ovarian cancer only) with dissemination to the endocrine glands and central nervous system. Dark areas indicate primary cancers. A = primary cancer of esophagus; B = primary cancer of ovaries; C = primary cancer of uterus (cervix or corpus); D = primary cancer of bladder. Cross-hatched areas indicate key disseminating organs. M = liver as first key disseminating site only for ovary adenocarcinomas; M = lung as key disseminating site for esophagus, cervix, corpus uteri and bladder carcinomas, and lung also as second key disseminating site for ovarian tumors. Unshaded areas identify generalized metastases. Y = central nervous system metastases; Z = endocrine system metastases. Lung metastases are presented as unilateral for simplicity.

The more complex patterns for prostatic and breast cancer involve bone as another generalizing site and are considered in more detail later in this chapter. It may seem surprising that the cascade process in so many major primary sites can be represented in three relatively simple schematic diagrams, but this reflects the underlying mechanisms of generalization (Viadana et al. 1978). Solid tumors show three principal patterns, depending on whether the drainage of the venous blood from the primary is to the lungs, the liver, or both organs. Two primary cancers, breast and prostate, differ from the other solid tumors in that often the vertebral or pelvic bones are the first generalizing site. The fact that there are these basic patterns suggest the following scientific point: Whatever role the lymphatic system may play in the early stages of dissemination of cancer, the eventual generalizing of the disease is through the blood system.

IMPLICATIONS OF THE ROLE OF PULMONARY METASTASES

The role of pulmonary metastases in the cascade processes shown in figures 4.1, 4.2, and 4.3 is somewhat different in each instance. In figure 4.1, the lung is the only generalizing site. In figure 4.2, the lung is the site which is primarily responsible for the generalized disease, but it is the second metastatic site in the cascade process. The distinction can be clarified by supposing that it is possible to determine very accurately whether or not there are lung metastases. Then for the primary sites in figure 4.1, the absence of lung metastases implies that the disease was still localized in the primary or adjacent lymph glands. Localized therapy could still cure the patient. In figure 4.2, however, the absence of lung metastases does not have the same force because there still could be liver metastases. For both figures, the presence of pulmonary metastases indicates that generalized metastasis has occurred or will occur.

In figure 4.3, the implications from the absence of pulmonary metastases are similar to those of figure 4.2, but there are different implications in these two cases if lung metastases are present. For figure 4.2 this implies that liver metastases are also present; this is not true for figure 4.3. The main purpose of distinguishing the role of pulmonary metastases in the different situations represented by the three figures is to illustrate an important point: the clinical implications of positive or negative findings in the lung depend on the location of the primary site.

What is clear from all the figures (and what applies also for the breast and prostate primaries) is that the lung is the site that is primarily responsible for the actual generalization of the great majority of all human cancers. In this sense, then, the information about the status of a patient with respect to pulmonary metastases is the most important single item of information for decision-making on clinical management of a cancer patient. If there is no pulmonary metastasis, then there is justification for directing the medical effort toward curative surgery or other localized therapy. It is sensible to allocate the medical resources necessary to achieve a cure, and there is much to gain.

On the other hand, if there is evidence of pulmonary metastases, localized therapy offers little or no prospect of achieving a cure. The allocation of medical resources in a situation where the only likely effect is to prolong the agony of the patient becomes open to serious question. The only real prospect for cure is a very unlikely one at present—the hope that the generalization has not yet occurred and that the lung metastases can be destroyed before the generalization takes place (Slack and Bross, 1975). There is no other rational basis for therapy aimed at a cure in this situation.

TWO SPECIAL PRIMARIES: BREAST AND PROSTATE CANCER

The implications of a cascade process of metastasis can be confirmed directly by analysis of the results of surgical or radiologic intervention. For example, some of the largest collaborative clinical studies have been carried out on breast cancer patients and have involved various methods and modalities for eliminating local spread to the lymphatics. The results are similar for all variants (Fisher at al. 1970). The erroneous traditional picture of the process of metastasis is one of the main reasons for the lack of therapeutic progress in breast cancer in the past 75 years.

The clinically disappointing results for breast cancer and other disease are hardly surprising once the metastatic patterns are understood. Figure 4.4 shows the spread of primary adenocarcinomas of the breast. Metastases spread directly from the primary cancer to the lungs, vertebrae and liver. The lungs may also seed the liver, bones (except vertebrae), central nervous system, and endocrine glands. The vertebrae disseminate metastases to other bones. The lungs seed the liver. The same sequence holds true in the absence of vertebral metastases, probably an early stage of the disease. Metastatic spread between the lungs and liver is not detectable when the vertebrae are seeded, probably because this takes place in a later stage of the disease.

In breast cancer and most other cancers, an understanding of the cascade process clarifies why the focus on localized lymphatic spread which has received so much attention in the past was a serious strategic mistake. As Dr. Bernard Fisher, reporting the results of the current National Surgical Adjuvant Breast Cancer Project, has pointed out, the study strongly indicates that positive axillary nodes are not predecessors of distant metastasis but represent "one more manifestation of disseminated disease" (Fisher et al. 1975). This point was also evident in previous collaborative breast studies and was embodied in our 1966 mathematical model for the growth and spread of breast cancer (Blumenson and Bross 1969; Bross and Blumenson 1968).

Prostate cancer is another situation in which the bones are a key site in the cascade process (fig. 4.5). Note that the bones are usually the first

Figure 4.4.

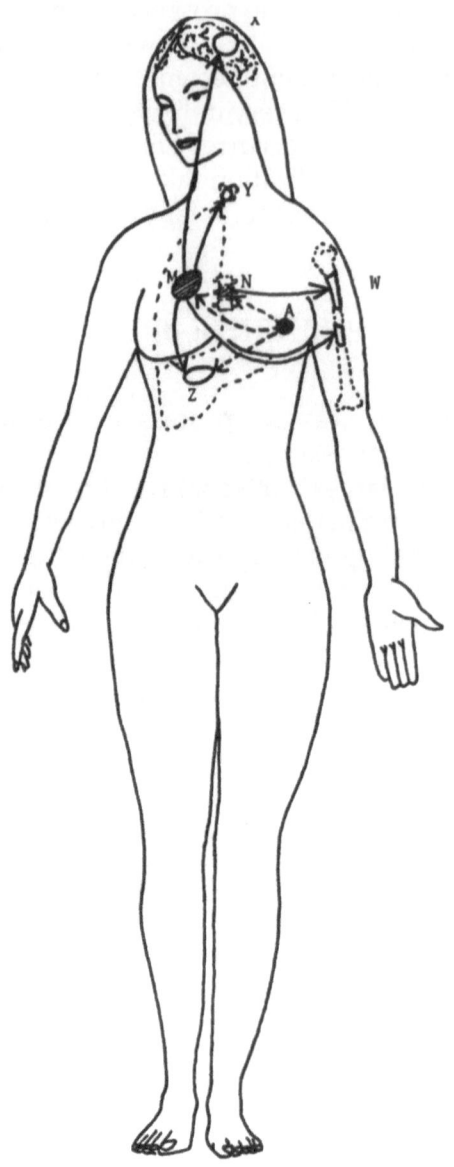

Breast cancer generalized either by vertebrae or lung metastases with dissemination to the liver, bones, endocrine glands, and central nervous system. Dark
areas indicate primary cancers. A = primary cancer of breast (nipple area).
Cross-hatched areas indicate key disseminating organs. M = lung as key disseminating site; N = vertebrae as key disseminating site. Unshaded areas identify generalized metastases. W = bone (except vertebrae) metastases; X = central nervous system metastases; Y = endocrine system metastases; Z = liver
metastases. Lung metastases are presented as unilateral for simplicity in the
drawing.

Figure 4.5.

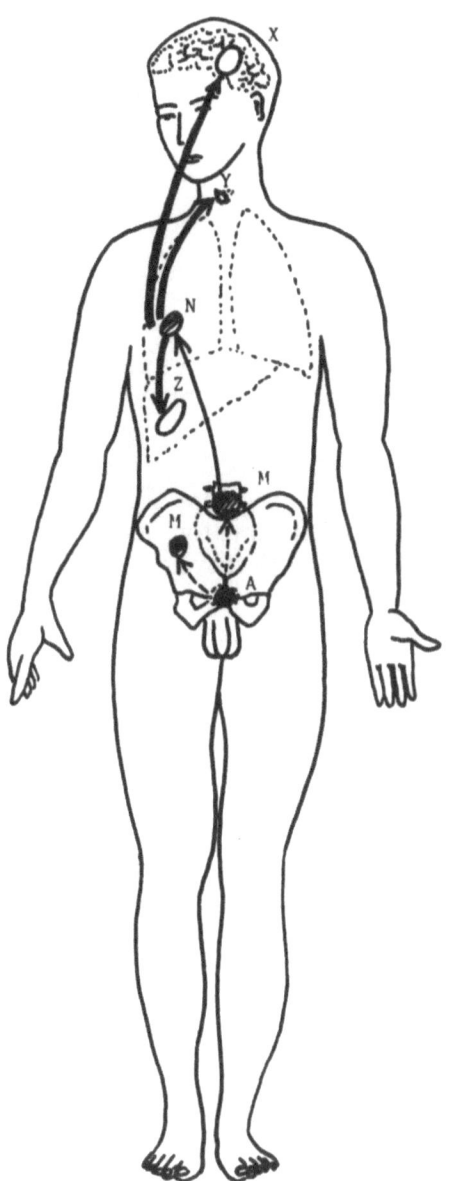

*Prostate cancer generalized by bone metastases through the lung with dissemi-
nation to the liver, endocrine glands, and central nervous system. Dark areas
indicate primary cancers. A = primary carcinoma of prostate. Cross-hatched
areas indicate the key disseminating organs. M = pelvis and vertebrae as first
key disseminating site; N = lung as the second key disseminating site. Unshaded areas identify generalized metastases. X = central nervous system
metastases; Y = endocrine system metastases; Z = liver metastases. Lung
metastases are presented as unilateral for simplicity in the drawing.*

generalizing site in the cascade sequence and therefore are crucial to staging prostate cancer. Note also that the pulmonary metastases once again play their usual key role in the generalization of the cancer: for both breast and prostatic cancer, the brain is seeded from pulmonary metastases.

IMPLICATIONS OF THE CASCADE HYPOTHESIS FOR BRAIN METASTASES

Although many implications of the cascade hypothesis for brain metastases are fairly evident from the preceding text, it is perhaps worthwhile to review them explicitly. In setting research and therapeutic policies in the management of human cancer, there has been a strong tendency in the past to act on implicit or ambiguously expressed opinions about the natural history of cancer. When physicians are forced to express their views clearly and explicitly, some apparent agreements turn out to be concealed disagreements and vice versa. Failure to make plain statements about the underlying presumptions for various treatments or lines of research has resulted in lack of effectiveness persisting for many years because it is so hard to see where the reasoning went wrong. In breast cancer there has been little progress for most of this century because the picture of the natural history of this disease which had been and still is taught in medical schools is simply wrong.

The first obvious point about brain metastases which is clear from the cascade analyses is that in most cases brain metastases come at the tail end of the cascade process. Even if the systemic spread of the cancer is not entirely evident clinically, it is very likely that the disease has generalized. The one feature of metastatic cancer to the brain that is very different from corresponding spread to other organs such as the liver is that a very small lesion (and relatively small number of cancer cells) in the brain can produce effects which are not likely to be missed by the clinician (see Chapter 1). At other sites, even fairly large lesions may not produce clinical signs that are easily recognized. This may result in an erroneous impression of the time sequence because a metastasis seeded earlier at some other site may only be detected later or at autopsy. The cascade analysis serves to make the situation clearer in this respect.

The second point concerns the probable site of cancer that has produced the brain metastasis. Again, the site may not be entirely evident clinically or there may seem to be a number of possibilities. Here again the cascade analysis helps to clarify the picture. For all of the major sites of solid tumor that have been studied, the generalizing site that seeds the brain is nearly always the lung. There may be sites of generalized disease that develop before the lung metastasis, but they seem to seed the lung rather than to seed the brain. So it is a reliable inference, as medical inferences go, that if a brain metastasis has occurred, there are very likely to be lung metastases. The probability is higher than for most clinical inferences.

Although it may or may not be important in therapy, backtracking along the cascade to locate the primary lesion can also be guided to some extent by the findings of cascade analysis. For example, if there is evidence that the sequence of generalizing sites has involved the bones, then the likely primary is breast cancer for women or prostatic cancer for men. Similarly, if it is known that there are liver metastases, some primaries are more probable and others less probable, although the possibilities are too numerous to draw any firm conclusions about the primary on this basis alone. The process can only suggest priorities in the search for the primary.

As a cautionary note in interpretation of the diagrammatic representations, the choice of the single site in the brain as a representative for the central nervous system metastases only simplifies the representation. Strictly speaking, the combination of sites into the central nervous system obscures the differential patterns in the dissemination to these sites. The analytic decision here is always a hard one. There is the trade-off between the inevitable loss of specificity involved in the grouping of sites and the gain from more stable patterns when the number of observations is greater. We are not likely to reanalyse the data more specifically but this would be worth doing. Such a reanalysis is not likely to change the general statements that have been made here because the brain metastases are the largest category in the grouping, but there may be some specific patterns of interest that we may be missing.

The fact that brain metastases occur at the tail end of the cascade process and that their capability for producing unmistakable clinical signs has specific implications for the use of invasive diagnostic technology. The advent of more sophisticated radiologic scanning equipment such as computed tomography (CT) and related hardware makes it particularly important to set policies for use of this technology so that the benefits outweigh the risks. The current dosage of radiation delivered in CT scans of the trunk are about the same as the doubling dose for leukemia (Bross et al. 1979). This poses a serious hazard to the patient: doubling the risk of leukemia is not something to be lightly inflicted on a patient who does not have malignant disease. On the other hand, if a CT scan identifies a brain lesion, there may be a strong incentive to do further scans to locate the primary lesion. The balancing of benefits and risks, the calculation of what is called a *benefit-to-cost ratio*, is not easy here, but this is the rational way to make the difficult decisions.

Without attempting to get into the numerical details (which are an article in their own right), the factors in this balance can be briefly stated. If the lesion in the brain CT scan is not cancerous, then the body CT scan can double the risk of leukemia and a false-positive diagnosis has a very serious cost. If there is a brain cancer, then the question is: "How much offsetting medical advantage accrues to the patient?" If the disease is (as is likely) already generalized, then the chances of curing the patient are near zero. Palliation, as is clear from the discussion elsewhere in this monograph, is about all that can be expected, and the benefits to the patient are limited.

In Section III, that deals extensively with the treatment, there is a question that might seem strange to professionals but which is crucial from the standpoint of the public and public health: Should costly sophisticated therapeutic technology be used on very many of these patients? If, as is generally the case, the patients are terminal or nearly so, should alternative kinds of care (such as represented by the Hospice Movement) be provided instead of the kinds of treatment discussed here?

The statement in the original text put the issue bluntly but the editors of this monograph felt it might be misunderstood and asked me to clarify my position. What I has said was: "The public is no longer convinced, as many doctors are, that prolonging the agony of a cancer patient is a benefit to the individual or to society. When it may cost about $30 billion a year to keep near terminal patients alive for a few months, the issue may look different depending on who is paying and who is getting the money."*

Perhaps this sounds unfair to the medical profession because it is curt and cryptic, but the issue here is one that needs to be faced fairly and squarely. It may not be tactful to say "prolonging the agony" instead of "prolonging life," but for a terminal cancer patient it is not easy to separate pain and life. According to government figures on federally funded health care programs, approximately a quarter of the entire budget is spent on the care of persons in their last year of life. With the American Medical Association estimating $188 billion spent last year and predictions of a trillion dollars a year in the not-so-distant future, we are talking about an enormous commitment of both dollars and health resources to keeping persons alive for a relatively short time. The question, then, is whether this is a sensible policy or whether the resources would accomplish far more if spent on primary prevention of disease at a much earlier point in life or in other ways.

The question is particularly pertinent in a book on brain metastases because treatment in this context is a very good example of the heavy investment of resources for persons who are probably in their last year of life. There is no dodging the thorny issue: Who should make these decisions and how should they be made? At present such decisions are generally made (or heavily influenced) by physicians. As the Hospice Movement has shown, when the patients have a choice in these matters, they do not necessarily make the same choice as radiotherapists or chemotherapists might make. They often do choose to forego further therapy. In my opinion, decisions at this terminal stage should be made with informed consent of the patient. Many readers may disagree with this or with my position that medical resources can better be used for other purposes than prolonging life at the very end, but it is nonetheless appropriate that these issues be explicitly raised.

_____

Editors' note: It was made clear by all of the clinicians participating in the workshop and contributing to this monograph that they are well aware of the differences between merely prolonging life and improving its quality.

SUMMARY AND STRATEGIC IMPLICATIONS

What emerges from the cascade analyses is a picture of the metastatic process that is strikingly different from the traditional pictures. They should elicit an agonizing reappraisal of the current strategies for treatment and research that are based on outdated ideas about dissemination. A drastic change in focus is needed. The traditional focus in treatment has been the primary tumor even though in most cases the physician is actually treating metastatic disease. It has been shown that the response to therapy depends more on the location of the metastases than on the location of the primary (Slack and Bross 1975).

Perhaps the main reason for focus on the primary is administrative. At many cancer hospitals the anatomic location of the primary provides a way of allocating patients to services which is acceptable to the staff. The usual rationale, however, is based on the traditional picture of dissemination and is invalid. The new concepts of dissemination suggest that neither anatomy nor modality is an appropriate basis for allocating patients with metastatic disease.

The new findings shift the focus from the primary to the generalizing site. They indicate that generalized disease is a more homogeneous entity than is currently recognized and that it should be treated as such. Most of the unique characteristics of primary cancer cells are much less evident after the passage through the generalizing site. The subsequent patterns of metastasis, for instance, tend to be similar for the different primaries. By the end of the cascade process, by the time there are brain metastases, many or most of the original cell characteristics are probably lost.

Traditional chemotherapeutic strategies are therefore open to serious question. Thus when new agents are tested using objective assessment of the response, the measured sites are usually metastatic. Although it is customary to make the tests and report the results by primary site, this factor is usually less important to the response than other factors. This focus on the primary has hampered and delayed the development of more effective therapies for the generalized form of cancer.

The traditional therapeutic strategies of the surgeon and radiologist are as open to question as those of the chemotherapist. The generalizing sites are clearly the primary route of dissemination. Apart from localized spread, adjacent lymph nodes tend to be involved only in a secondary or tertiary role. The traditional surgical and radiologic emphasis on the local lymph nodes in both treatment and research thus lacks a valid rationale.

REFERENCES

Blumenson, L. E., and Bross, I. D. J. A mathematical analysis of the growth and spread of breast cancer. *Biometrics* 25:95–109, 1969.

Bross, I. D. J., and Blumenson, L. E. Statistical testing of a deep mathematical model for human breast cancer. *J. Chronic Dis.* 21:493–506, 1968.

Bross, I. D. J.; Viadana, E.; and Pickren, J. W. The metastatic spread of myelomas and leukemias in men. Virchows arch. [Pathol. Anat.] 365:91–101, 1975a.

Bross, I. D. J.; Viadana, E.; and Pickren, J. W. Does generalized metastasis occur directly from the primary? *J. Chronic Dis.* 28:149–159, 1975b.

Bross, I. D. J., and Blumenson, L. E. Metastatic sites that produce generalized cancer: identification and kinetics of generalizing sites. In *Fundamental Aspects of Metastasis*, ed. L. Weiss. Amsterdam: North-Holland Publishing Co., 1976.

Bross, I. D. J.; Ball, M.; and Falen, S. A dosage response curve for the one rad range: adult risks from diagnostic radiation. Am. J. Public H. 69:130–136, 1979.

Fisher, B. A. et al. Postoperative radiotherapy in the treatment of breast cancer: results of the NSABP clinical trial. *Ann. Surg.* 172:711–732, 1970.

Fisher, B. A., et al. Ten-year follow-up of breast cancer patients in a cooperative clinical trial evaluating surgical adjuvants chemotherapy. *Surg. Gynecol. Obstet.* 140:528–534, 1975.

Slack, N. H., and Bross, I. D. J. The influence of site of metastasis on tumor growth and response to chemotherapy. *Br. J. Cancer* 32:71, 1975.

Viadana, E. The metastatic spread of head and neck tumors in man (an autopsy study of 371 cases). Z. Krebsforsch. 83:293–304, 1973.

Viadana, E.; Bross, I. D. J.; and Pickren, J. W. An autopsy study of some routes of dissemination of cancer of the breast. *Br. J. Cancer* 27:336–340, 1973.

Viadana, E.; Bross, I. D. J.; and Pickren, J. W. The metastatic spread of kidney and prostate cancers in man. *Neoplasma* 23:323–333, 1976a.

Viadana, E.; Bross, I. D. J.; and Pickren, J. W. The spread of blood-borne metastases in malignant lymphomas of man. *Oncology* 33:123–131, 1976b.

Viadana, E.; Bross, I. D. J.; and Pickren, J. W. Cascade spread of blood-borne metastases in solid and non-solid cancers of man. In *Pulmonary Metastasis*, ed. L. Weiss and H. A. Gilbert. Boston: G.K. Hall & Co., 1978.

5

Arrest and Extravasation of Cancer Cells with Special Reference to Brain Metastases and the Microinjury Hypothesis

B. A. Warren

METASTASES IN THE BRAIN IN HUMANS

Metastatic neoplasms of the brain and spinal cord from primary visceral malignancies may comprise the commonest tumors of the central nervous system (Escourolle and Poirier 1973). Although as Rubinstein (1972) points out, the incidence varies depending upon whether the figures reflect data from neurosurgical or from autopsy sources. The incidence of metastatic tumors as a percentage of total intracranial tumors has a range of 4.2–37%. For pathologic data, Rubinstein states a figure of 15–25%. Metastases in the central nervous system may occur in any location, vary in size, in number and in the site of origin of the primary tumor.

The sites most frequently involved are the cerebral hemispheres, cerebellum, brainstem, spinal cord, and least common, the nerve roots (Escourolle and Poirier 1973). The primary cancers which are the commonest sites of origin for brain metastatic cancer are carcinoma of the lung in males and mammary carcinoma in females (Escourolle and Poirier 1973; Richards and McKissock 1963). Overall, mammary adenocarcinoma is second in importance, being only about half as common as lung cancer as the primary site in patients with metastatic brain cancer (Rubinstein 1972). Malignant melanoma may provide 15% of metastatic malignancies. In diminishing frequency and variable in their order of importance are primary tumors of kidney, alimentary canal, pancreas, prostate and testis.

In some patients the presenting signs of neoplastic disease are due to the effects of a cerebral metastatic deposit from a small asymptomatic primary carcinoma, such as bronchial carcinoma (Rubinstein 1972). In other patients there may be a long latent period between the occurrence and removal of the primary cancer and the development of a significant metastatic cerebral deposit. In some cases of renal adenocarcinoma, 9–13 years have elapsed between removal of the primary and the clinical effects of a secondary deposit in the brain (Rubinstein 1972). In addition to blood-borne tumor spread, there may also be contiguous spread from deposits which initially colonized the skull and vertebrae. Such spread may form subdural deposits, and eventually subarachnoid metastases can ensue. Highly diffuse infiltration of the leptomeninges may result in the appearance of meningeal carcinomatosis, but parenchymatous involvement of the brain is the commonest form of metastatic colonization by cancer cells.

The cells of the metastatic cancer reproduce the histologic picture found in the primary tumor in most instances, but atypical features are not uncommon (Escourolle and Poirier 1973). Because of the frequency of the lung as a primary site, some reports recommend particular reference to the bronchial tree during followup if the origin of metastasis is uncertain (Richards and McKissock 1963). The natural history in some patients is such that after the development of clinically evident metastasis, the chest film, bronchoscopy and exfoliative cytology are all negative and only later reveal an enlarging primary tumor. The metastatic cycle starts with the source of the embolic tumor cells, which in advanced neoplastic disease can already be a metastatic deposit. Theoretically each turn of the cycle may alter the optimum growth characteristics of the clone of cells that are successful. The histologic types of tumors that predominate in cerebral metastases are therefore epidermoid carcinoma (of lung), adenocarcinoma (of lung, breast, kidney, pancreas and alimentary canal), small- and large-cell anaplastic carcinoma (of lung), and malignant melanoma (fig. 5.1).

In one series of 254 patients who received curative-style surgical resections for lung cancer, the incidence of persistent disease and distant metastases was assessed at autopsy (Matthews et al. 1977). Distant metastases were found in 15% of the epidermoid carcinomas (26 of 171 patients), 54% of the small-cell carcinomas (13 of 24 patients), 40% of the adenocarcinomas (13 of 32 patients), and 16% of the large-cell anaplastic carcinomas

Some types of malignant cells commonly involved in brain metastases. The photomicrographs show malignant cells exfoliated into secretions and fluid from human tumors. A and B. These malignant cells are from an adenocarcinoma of the lung. The typical appearance in the sputum is illustrated in fig. 5.1A (X 1,600), in which the cytoplasm is finely foamy. The cell group in fig. 5.1B (X 1,600) is from the pleural effusion present in the same patient. One of the cells is much larger than the others and contains accumulations of mucus (M). C and D. Epidermoid carcinoma of the lung frequently exfoliates malignant cells into the sputum, (C, X 1,600). The surfaces of these cells possess stubby microvilli on examination by scanning electron microscopy (D, X 2,500). E. Cells exfoliated from small-cell anaplastic carcinoma often occur in the sputum in strands and possess only a small amount of cytoplasm (X 1,600). F. Cells from large-cell anaplastic carcinoma are large and contain large bizarre nuclei (X 1,600).

Figure 5.1.

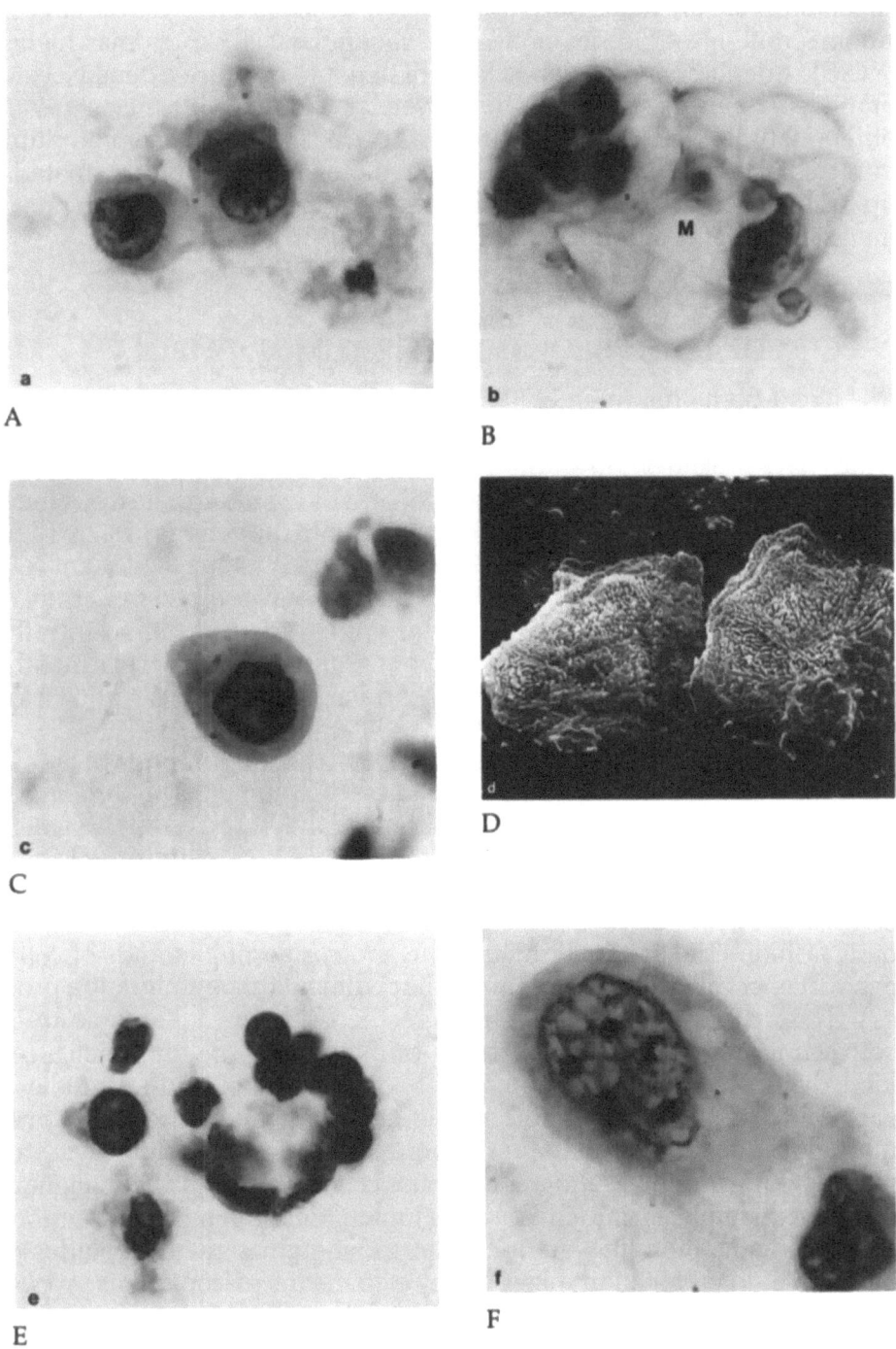

A

B

C

D

E

F

(4 of 25 patients). In another series, the principal cell types which metas-tasized were found to be the undifferentiated (small- and large-cell) types and adenocarcinomas (Jacobs et al. 1977). These authors noted that squamous-cell carcinoma had less tendency to metastasize than adenocar-cinoma, and in their series none of 13 squamous-cell carcinomas metas-tasized. Adenocarcinoma deposits were noted to produce extensive cere-bral edema and mass effects which were not found with metastases of other cell types. In their series there was not a single instance of multiple intracranial lesions, and other studies have shown that in autopsy material up to about a third of patients with pulmonary cancer have only one brain metastasis (Meyer and Rech 1953; Anuigbo 1958).

CIRCULATING BLOOD-BORNE TUMOR EMBOLI

Blood-borne tumor emboli are usually tumor cells which have emi-grated into the vascular compartment or fragments of cords of tumor cells which have broken off. In addition, lymphaticovenous communications in the lymph nodes and in the thoracic duct provide routes for the movement of tumor cells from involved lymphatic nodes into the venous system (Carr 1980). Although the capacity for active movement by some malignant cells has been questioned (Berenblum 1970), the profiles observed in a study of transplantable melanoma are consistent with active movement into the vascular lumen (Warren et al. 1978). This emigration of tumor cells into the lumen was observed at three days after transplantation of a tumor frag-ment into the hamster cheek pouch.

In human gliomas Kung and others (1969) examined various phases in the emigration of the tumor cells into the vascular lumen. The tumor cells first took up a perivascular position, indented, and ruptured the basement membrane of the endothelial cells of the vessel wall. The tumor cells then moved through the spaces and into the vascular lumen. In the transplant-able hamster melanoma, the cancer cells conducted themselves in a similar basic fashion. The basement membrane and supporting strands of colla-gen that ensheath some vessels are an impediment to the emigration proc-ess. The malignant cell breaks through the basement membrane to lie between it and the endothelial lining of the vessel. The endothelial cell immediately overlying the tumor cell becomes thinner and eventually a gap is produced in the endothelial lining. The emigrating cell moves through the space to exhibit a ruffle border in the vascular lumen. Cyto-plasmic flow into the leading edge of the cell ensues, and the malignant cell moves completely into the vascular lumen. Cells can be seen in various stages of emigration into the lumen of the marginal giant capillaries of melanomas in preparations observed by electron microscopy. This process is similar to that described by Marchesi and Florey (1960) for the emigration of leukocytes through vessel walls although in this case it is emigration out from the tumor into the blood vessels.

Initially the tumor-cell embolus is only one cell in size. The embolus may increase in size due to multiplication in the vascular lumen. Cells in mitosis have been observed repeatedly in tumor cell emboli, and it is probable that the cells in most tumor emboli continue to undergo mitotic divisions. Willis (1973) examined arrested emboli in pulmonary capillaries of humans and concluded that the size range which contained the greatest number of emboli was between 20–200 microns in diameter. Tumor-cell masses growing into major veins can be much larger, and fatal pulmonary embolism has occurred from such masses (Willis 1973).

In addition to active emigration from the tumor into the vascular lumen, the coagulation and fibrinolytic systems influence tumor shedding into the circulation. This is particularly true in those tumors which have blood channels with a partially or completely deficient endothelial lining, such as some melanomas (Warren and Shubik 1966) and sarcomas. Griffiths and Salsbury (1965) found that when plasmin was added to the fluid perfusate of carcinomas of the gut, increased numbers of malignant cells were noted in the issuing fluid. After studies of a spontaneous mammary carcinoma and a 20-methylcholanthrene-induced sarcoma in mice, Peterson and coworkers concluded that alteration of fibrinolytic levels in animals with tumors had a greater effect on the shedding of cells from the primary tumors than on the fate of the malignant cells (Peterson 1968; Peterson et al. 1969). Removal of a malignant tumor or any form of manipulation of a malignant tumor also increases the numbers of cells shed into the circulation (Roberts 1961). Since the pattern of necrosis in some tumors is distinctive, the influence of tumor necrosis on tumor shedding has some importance. By removing cores of tumor tissue and using a standardized shaking procedure in vitro, Weiss (1977) concluded that the volume of cells detached in this way from tumors of similar size was independent of the location of Walker 256 carcinoma in the sites examined (spleen, liver, muscle, and subcutaneous sites).

The actual significance of circulating tumor cells for patient management and prognosis has been the subject of a number of reviews (such as Goldblatt and Nadel 1963, 1965; Christopherson 1973). The occurrence of tumor cells in blood was demonstrated in 1955 by Engell, who found malignant cells, sometimes in large numbers, in the blood of patients who possessed malignancies in the curable and incurable stages. Ritchie and Webster (1961) reported that the great majority of patients with carcinoma of the breast have malignant cells in their blood at some time in the progression of the disease. Technical difficulties in interpretation of the morphology of the cells, however, together with the presence of normal megakaryocytes, which may be confused with malignant cells, necessitate strict criteria for correct diagnosis (Christopherson 1973).

At the present time, determining the presence of circulating tumor cells in humans has little value in routine workup of patients. Such investigations do not yield clearcut markers for prognostic and therapeutic guidance because approximately 20% of curable cancer patients and 30% of terminal cancer patients have cancer cells in their peripheral venous blood (Goldblatt and Nadel 1963). Goldblatt and Nadel (1965), summarizing the experience over a decade, concluded from a study of over 5,000 cancer patients by 40 groups of investigators using at least 20 methods that there was "no unifying concept or understanding of the biological significance of this phenomenon." Christopherson (1973) also concluded that examination of the peripheral blood for tumor cells is not warranted for diagnosis or patient management in general.

THE MICROINJURY HYPOTHESIS

Standard terminology is inadequate for detailing the microinjury hypothesis for arrest of tumor emboli and the development of micrometastases. I use the term *micrometastasis* to indicate living active tumor cells present in an extravascular position before the development of an intrinsic tumor vasculature. The fact that tumor embolism is not tumor metastasis has been shown in a number of experimental situations (Baserga and Saffiotti 1955) and can be inferred from the lack of correlation in human studies of the presence of cancer cells in the blood and subsequent metastatic development. This is true for tumor cells in intact, uninjured vascular bed including the smallest unit, the microcirculatory module. Blood-borne tumor emboli can and do produce metastatic deposits of tumor cells, however, and there is a dose relationship in that a certain number of neoplastic cells needs to be injected before tumor metastases will occur (Wallace 1961).

In the Walker 256 carcinoma 11,000 cells must be injected intramuscularly to get 100% takes; between 110 and 1,100 cells are required for 50% takes; and for any takes at all, at least 11 cells must be injected (Wallace 1961). Similarly in sarcoma, more than 500,000 cells had to be injected intravenously for 100% takes, and for any takes at all the number of cells required ranged from a lower level of 4,000–20,000 to a higher level of 100,000–500,000. From this work Wallace (1961) concluded that the transplantability of the malignant cells released into the bloodstream determined the outcome of the effect of circulating tumor cells. Thus, if enormous numbers of certain malignant cells were required in the circulation before metastases developed, then metastases might never occur; whereas if only a few cells allowed transplantation, then metastatic development would be almost certain to occur. Wallace attributed the variation in dose required by different neoplasms to a variety of factors including the necessity of overcoming immunologic host resistance and differing capabilities for survival and multiplication among tumor cells in the emboli. In a further study with rats, inoculation with 1,000 Walker 256 tumor cells produced no tumors in 8 animals; after inoculation with 10,000 cells, 3 of 8 rats developed tumors; and after inoculation with 100,000 cells, 9 of 10 rats developed tumors (Wallace and Hollenberg 1965).

Injury to tissues will result in preferential development of metastases from circulating tumor cells in those injured tissues. Localized conversion of tumor embolism to tumor metastasis has been shown to occur after local mechanical trauma (Fisher et al. 1967; Robinson and Hoppe 1962), turpentine injection (Agostino and Cliffton 1965), local ischemia (Robinson and Hoppe 1962; Alexander and Altemeier 1964), intravenous nitrogen mustard injection (Alexander and Altemeier 1964), and irradiation (Berkovich and Chernukh, 1967). A review of studies on the relationship between trauma and metastasis formation has been published by Rudenstam (1968).

The converse (that is, in one sense) is trans-organ passage of tumor cells. In one series of studies Zeidman and others examined the passage of tumor cells through capillaries in vivo (Zeidman 1961, 1965; Zeidman and Buss 1952; Zeidman et al. 1956). Suspensions of the transplantable V2 carcinoma and Brown-Pearce carcinoma were injected into the mesenteric artery of rabbits while the arteriocapillary junctions of the mesentery were observed and photographed by cinephotomicrography. In each type of tumor suspension, most of the cells passed through the capillaries into the venous circulation (Zeidman 1961). Cells of the V2 carcinoma arrested more frequently than those of the Brown-Pearce carcinoma. Zeidman's direct observations were that many tumor cells are sufficiently deformable that passage through the capillaries readily occurs and that arrested cells are too rigid to perform the transit of the capillary bed. In similar experiments testing the microcirculation of the lung, liver and kidney, the passage of tumor cells was found again (Zeidman and Buss 1952; Zeidman et al. 1956). Tumor cells readily adhere to the basement membrane underlying endothelium in vitro in human specimens such as HeLa cells and human vein wall (Warren and Güldner 1969) and to damaged vessel walls in vivo in the rat and mouse (Warren and Vales 1972). It is likely that the preferential location of metastasis in injured animals is mediated through injury to the vascular system.

Kawaguchi and Nakamura (1977) examined transcerebral passage of tumor cells and its relationship to brain metastases using Yoshida sarcoma and six strains of rat ascites hepatoma. These tumors could be divided into so-called island-forming strains (AH-130, AH-272, and AH-7974) and single-cell strains (Yoshida sarcoma, AH-7974F, AH-66F and AH-13). The island-forming strains, in which the tumor emboli were large, showed a low passage rate through the cerebral capillaries and readily produced metastases. The tumors which produced emboli of single cells possessed a high passage rate through the cerebral capillaries. Tumor cells are readily detected in the cerebral substance, and they found that the incidence of arrested tumor cells corresponded directly to the frequency of developing tumors. From their studies Kawaguchi and Nakamura (1977) suggested that many foci of microinjury could be produced by the larger emboli of the island-forming strains. Rapid passage through the brain would result in minimal injury. This would be one answer to the conundrum of characteristics of the environment of the successful tumor embolus that lead to micrometastasis. Another suggestion has been the development of a mutant tumor strain which is particularly liable to retention in the circulation (Zeidman 1965) and variability in transplantability has already been mentioned.

We have, then, the following information: (1) tumor cells can pass through intact circulatory beds without arrest and without producing metastases; (2) the development of metastases is dose-dependent: below a certain number of tumor cells, metastases will not occur and this number varies for each individual tumor; and (3) circulating tumor cells preferentially produce metastases in injured tissues.

The microinjury concept of the location and development of micrometastases (suggested by Kawaguchi and Nakamura 1977) unites this information in the following way (fig. 5.2). The first microcirculatory bed downstream from the tumor is showered by tumor cells. The standard pattern for a microcirculatory unit or module, the smallest unit of the circulation, is an arteriole which divides into a thoroughfare channel and a segment of vessel leading into the capillary bed. The thoroughfare channel directly unites, without branching, the arteriole and the venule. The smooth-muscle cells of the arteriolar branch, which passes into the capillary network, become fewer in number and the last complete unit around the vessel is the precapillary sphincter. (For reviews of the microcirculatory module, see Zweifach 1961 and Frasher and Wayland 1972). The tone of the precapillary sphincter determines the proportion of blood that enters the capillary bed from the particular arteriole and by reduction, the proportion of flow through the direct channel to the venule. There are many different arrangements of these units in various tissues. The units are often in series so that a certain proportion are filled with flowing blood, a certain number are partially open, and some are closed. Depending on the local tissue needs, any particular precapillary sphincter opens and closes. At any one time only a certain proportion of all the precapillary sphincters would be open. Into this arrangement is showered numbers of tumor cells. In many of the microcirculatory modules observed in vivo (that is, in the rabbit ear and hamster cheek pouch membrane), leukocytes can stick in the precapillary sphincter or branches of the unit and block the further flow in such a unit. The leukocyte frequently changes shape at this time and either passes through the unit or out of the branch, remaining in the larger vessel.

Epidermoid carcinoma cells and adenocarcinoma cells are, in the great majority of instances, much larger than the leukocyte when they are observed in tissue secretions and fluids. Even allowing for such factors as considerable deformability and even sheet flow in the capillary bed (this is suggested for flow in the lungs of some species), blockage of the microcirculatory units for varying periods of time much longer than the blockage time for a single leukocyte is liable to occur during the passage of a shower of tumor cell emboli through an organ. During this enforced deprivation of blood, if it is sufficiently long or repeated for a sufficient number of times, microinjury may occur within the unit. Exfoliation of endothelial cells from their basement membrane and the exposure of this surface to circulating tumor cells and the blood is liable to occur. There may not be a great buildup of platelets on such surfaces. A single layer of platelets together with some fibrin deposition may be the only reaction.

Looking at the tissue as a whole, the status of the different units in the tissue will differ markedly at the time of peak showering with tumor emboli. Some will have just closed down as part of their normal cycle; others will need blood and will have just opened. Still others will be beginning to

Figure 5.2.

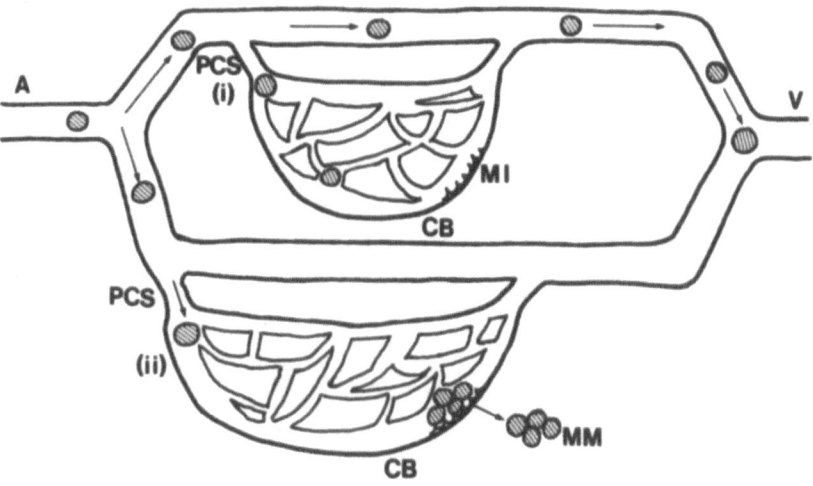

The microinjury hypothesis of organ retention of malignant cells. This is a diagrammatic representation of an artery (A) which breaks up into two microcirculatory units in series (i) and (ii), each containing a thoroughfare channel. The tumor cells are represented by shaded circles. The precapillary sphincter (PCS) in unit (i) is occluded by a tumor cell, which results in a microinjury (MI) to the capillary bed (CB) of the unit. When the tumor cell which had occluded the capillary bed moves onward, as illustrated in (ii), blood flows over the injured site and tumor cells adhere to the injured tissues. Because of the injury, transit through the vessel wall is easier and a micrometastasis (MM) is thereby seeded. The capillary beds are drained by the venule (V).

close down, and others beginning to open up. There will be a considerable variation in the vulnerability of the capillary beds to injury due to microembolism. Equally, the composition of the tumor-cell emboli will be diverse. Some cells will be more capable of invasion and multiplication in the tissues than others.

This theory proposes that showering the microcirculation with tumor emboli and repeated blockage of microcirculatory units results in microinjury to the capillary beds involved. The theory explains the necessity for a certain number of tumor cells to be injected before a unit is hit in the particular stage of cyclic opening and closing of the sphincter when it is most vulnerable. It also furnishes an explanation of the dose dependency. The microinjury prepares the sites for the arrest of tumor emboli. The injured site provides a window through the vascular system through which tumor cells can invade to form micrometastases in the extravascular tissues. Intravascular thrombi may allow the growth of adherent cancer cells and their subsequent migration through the vessel wall (Wood et al. 1961).

MICROCIRCULATORY UNITS OF THE BRAIN

If tumor-cell arrest and extravasation are regarded as specific examples of the microembolism syndrome, then the nature of the microcirculatory units of the organ under consideration represent the other half of the process to the tumor-cell embolus itself. Hardman (1940) described the normal capillary network which is found in humans in radiographs of brain slices with the arteries injected with barium. He recognized two main types of end-arteries, the long and short "perforating" types. The short perforators were confined to the gray matter, and the long perforators ran a straight or spiral course toward the center of the hemisphere, were fewer in number, and were uninfluenced by the tracts in the white matter. The short perforators were found to break up rapidly into a fine mesh of dense capillary network. The long perforating vessels were often parallel and linked by interlacing short capillaries. Hardman noted some variation from one part of the brain to another. In gray matter (both cortical and basal), he found a fine meshwork, while in the white matter the network was more open.

Romanul (1970) in Tedeschi's neuropathology text described a further type, the medium "penetrators" (equivalent to the "perforators" discussed by Hardman). This investigator proposed that the cerebral cortex and the white matter were supplied from vessels arising from an arterial network (pial network) formed by each major cerebral artery. These so-called pial penetrators branched at different depths in the tissue. The short vessels branched in the third cortical layer whereas the medium penetrators progressed to the fifth cortical layer and the long penetrators progressed to the junction of the cortex and subcortical white matter. The white matter was found to be supplied by long vessels which did not branch while they passed through the cortex. Penetrator vessels arising from the proximal portions of the large cerebral arteries supplied the gray matter structures at the base of the brain and the internal capsule. The pial and basal penetrators form a capillary network that is continuous throughout the brain. Pial penetrators supply the cerebellum, and basal penetrators supply the brainstem (Romanul 1970). The initial venules which drain blood from the cerebral hemispheres (both the white and gray matter) run parallel to the pial penetrator arteries. The territory of each intracerebral vein is larger than that of a pial penetrator artery since there are more arteries than veins.

In a similar though not identical fashion to the distribution of the arteries, the cortex is drained by short cortical veins and by the long veins during their passage through the cortex. The veins which emerge on the surface merge to form the superficial venous system. A deep venous system drains blood from the basal nuclei and the two systems are connected by direct anastomoses.

On electron microscopy the capillaries of the brain show some unique features (fig. 5.3). They possess a basically similar morphology to the non-fenestrated capillaries of other organs and have relatively few pinocytotic vesicles in the endothelial cells (Hirano and Matsui 1975). The junctions between endothelial cells are of the five-layer tight-junction type. Horse-radish peroxidase, which passes through the endothelial barrier in capil-laries in most other organs, will not penetrate the endothelial barrier of cerebral capillaries (Hirano and Matsui 1975). A thick basal lamina or basement membrane lies external to the endothelial lining of the vessel (Matthews and Martin 1971). The end-feet of astrocytes extend to the sur-face of the vessel and occasionally the cell bodies of astrocytes lie next to the vessels and support them (Matthews and Martin 1971). The endothelial basement membrane nearly touches the basement membrane associated with the vascular feet of the astrocytes. These cells surround the capillary and separate it from the rest of the neural parenchyma (Hirano and Matsui 1975). Most cerebral capillaries have only a narrow perivascular space and in it no collagen fibers or fibroblasts are found.

According to the classification of Bennett et al. (1959) cerebral capil-laries would be described as nonfenestrated with a complete basement

Figure 5.3.

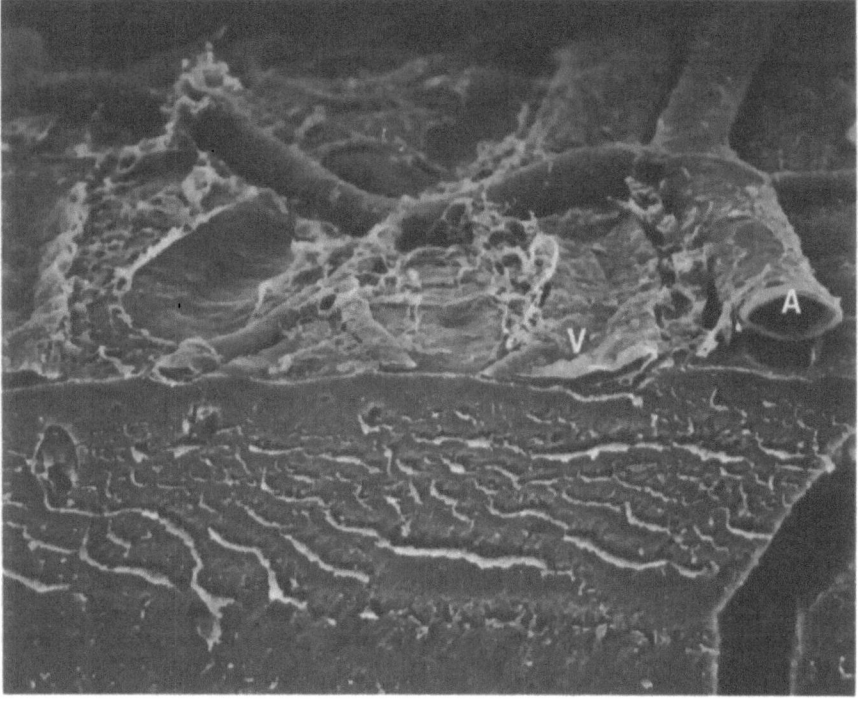

Vessels on the surface of a rabbit brain as shown by scanning electron mi-croscopy. The photomicrograph shows the edge of the cut surface and the natural surface of the brain. The venous system is collapsed while the arterial network, because of the wall structure, does not collapse and is more obvious. An artery (A) and a vein (V) run parallel on the brain surface. (X 150.)

membrane and with a complete pericapillary investment interposed between the endothelial cells and the parenchymal cells. Apart from the more obvious localized differences in the microcirculation, such as the portal system associated with the pituitary gland, there are likely to be more subtle changes in the microcirculatory beds throughout the brain.

It is tempting to speculate, for example, whether the location of cerebral metastases of mammary adenocarcinoma in the brainstem is due to some unique variation of the microcirculation in this site. In one retrospective statistical survey of the frequency and topographic distribution of brain metastases, data from 10,123 autopsies on patients over 15 years served as the study sample (Kane et al. 1976). In this series, metastases in men arose most often from the lung (61%) and stomach (13%). In women, the commonest primary tumors were found in the breast (39%) and lung (22%). Topographic analysis in patients with mammary adenocarcinoma showed a disproportionate involvement of the brainstem, especially the pons (27% for breast, 12% for lung). Dural and leptomeningeal involvement occurred frequently in females with breast cancer or lung cancer. Otherwise topographic analysis yielded a random pattern similar to that found in encephalomalacia of emboli origin. This investigation suggests that the sex of the patient may influence the topographic distribution of brain metastases.

MIGRATION OF TUMOR CELLS AND EXTRAVASCULAR MULTIPLICATION

Walker 256 carcinosarcoma arose spontaneously in the region of the mammary gland of a pregnant rat and has been used extensively in a number of laboratories. (For review of the nature of the tumor, see Stewart et al. 1959.) The appearance of the surface of these cells is illustrated in figure 5.4.

Josephson (1974) injected 1×10^6 Walker 256 cells into the left external carotid artery of rats using 78 animals in a study of metastases in the brain. The capillaries near the junction of the gray and white matter of the cerebrum and cerebellum contained most of the tumor cells. At 5 minutes after tumor-cell injection, the malignant cells were found in the superficial layers of the cortices of the cerebrum and cerebellum. Only very occasionally were they noted in the meningeal arteries. Cells in mitosis were found frequently. At 5 minutes some of the tumor cells were associated with platelets and fibrin while others were free of such encrustation. Cells both loosely within vascular channels and occluding the lumen were noted. After 15–30 minutes the tumor cells were often associated with platelets. With tumor cell-platelet emboli, endothelial cell-platelet-tumor cell contacts were often noted. Swollen astrocytic foot processes occurred at this stage. At 1–6 hours after injection, tumor cells were hard to find. Those found were often associated with platelets and indeed some appeared to be phagocytosing platelet aggregates. Tumor cells at 12 hours after injection were sometimes associated with degranulating platelet masses and

Figure 5.4.

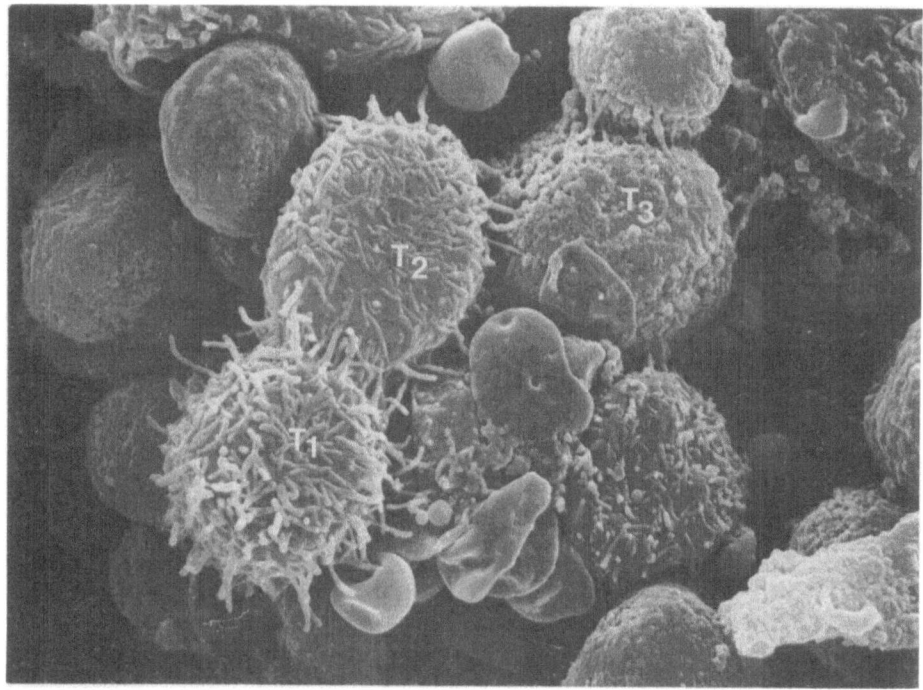

Detail of malignant cells and red cells in a section of a Walker 256 carcinoma growing in the thigh of a rat by scanning electron microscopy. Some of the tumor cells (T₁ and T₂) show multiple microvilli on their surfaces, while others (for example, T₃) appear to be undergoing degeneration. (X 2,250.)

sometimes were flattened along the endothelium. The malignant cells occasionally possessed complex pseudopodial extensions at this time. Tumor-cell contact with the basement membrane was first noted 24 hours after injection. An appearance of attrition and thinning of the endothelium occurred, similar to that described earlier for intravasation. Although at 48 hours most tumor cells were still totally within the lumen of blood vessels, the first extravascular tumor cells were noted. They remained intimately associated with the blood vessels. Josephson (1974) did not observe the process by which the cells passed through the vessel wall.

At 4 days after the tumor-cell injection, a process of tumor destruction of the vessel wall was frequently found. The expansile growth of tumor cells fragmented the endothelium and eventually caused complete rupture of the vessel wall. Tumor microvilli and cytoplasmic processes extended into the remains of the endothelium and into the parenchyma. Metastatic deposits were always found around capillaries in the cortices of the cerebrum and cerebellum in the later periods (8–12 days after injection). The choroid plexus was often involved. In the late stages tumor foci were found in all areas of the cortex and sometimes along the meninges. Occasional ventricular carcinomatosis occurred due to penetration by tumor cells of the surface of the choroid plexus. The tumor nodules grew around capillaries initially in a concentric fashion but later extended irregularly into the cerebral parenchyma. Malignant cells were not found in the vessels of the neurohypophysis even in the later stages. In the adenohypophysis tumor cells were noted in the sinusoids, which in some instances passed through the basement membrane by pseudopodial extensions. At 6 days after the tumor injection, gross metastatic nodules were visible (Chew et al. 1976).

Ballinger and Schimpff (1977) examined the induction of cerebral metastases after intracarotid injection of suspensions of C57Bl/6 methylcholanthrene-induced fibrosarcoma and B16 melanoma cells. At a level of 1.5×10^5 tumor cells, they noted malignant cells in the capillary bed and penetrating the vessel walls. Malignant cells also may pass through the endothelium by way of the cell junctions, expanding and opening them (Warren 1976). In studies on the adhesion of mouse lymphoma cells to damaged vein walls, the progression of malignant cells was traced from the lumen into the vessel wall. The cells passed to a position beneath the endothelial layer, which on section appeared intact. The malignant cells were held up at the level of the basement membrane.

The development of radioactive labeling of living cells has permitted a closer study of the arrest and subsequent development of tumor cell emboli (Fidler 1976). In studies with B16 lines of a melanoma, Fidler found that tumors which yield high numbers of metastases tended to clump with the lymphocytes in the blood and also to cause aggregation of platelets both in vivo and in vitro. He concluded that the increased metastatic capability of this tumor line was directly related to the degree of their initial arrest in the pulmonary capillary bed.

Variation is the benchmark of malignancy so it is not surprising to find that the thrombogenic activities of both mouse and human tumors vary remarkably. What is unexpected is that considerable variation even extends to tumors of the same histologic type. Gasic and others (1976) examined 12 mouse tumors and 29 human malignancies for their ability to aggregate platelets, to induce the release of radiolabeled serotonin, to coagulate plasma, and to lyse fibrin. No correlation was found between these properties. The platelet aggregating activity of 11 human breast carcinomas ranged from a low of 4% to a high of 87%. Sites other than the vascular compartment appear to be more beneficial for the survival and multiplication of tumor cells. For example, 1,000 Walker 256 carcinoma cells injected intravenously gave no tumors in 8 rats whereas the same number of cells injected into lymphatics gave rise to tumors in 7 of 8 rats (Wallace and Hollenberg 1965). The factors which determine continued prosperity of the micrometastasis outside the vessel wall are largely unknown. Continued growth beyond a certain size becomes dependent upon the induction of new blood vessels from the host microcirculation.

Around a growing tumor transplant there usually occurs initially a considerable inflammatory exudate as well as the fibrovascular stromal

Figure 5.5.

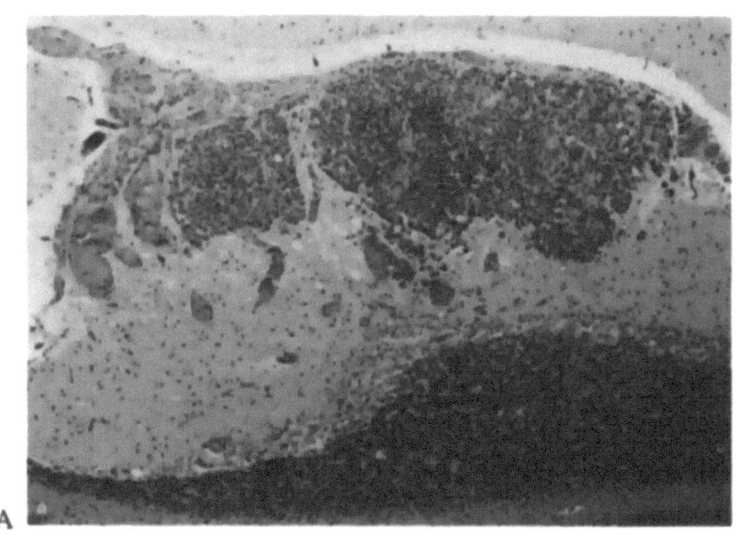

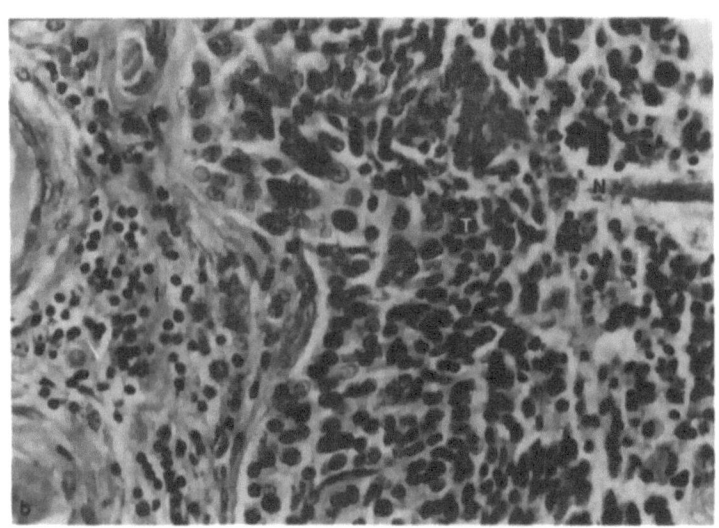

Small metastasis in the cerebellum. These photomicrographs show an established metastasis from an invasive intraductal carcinoma of the breast in a woman aged 60 years. At autopsy she was found to have widespread dissemination of the neoplasm with metastases to the liver and bone marrow. A. This metastasis could be contained in a rectangle 1 mm by 2 mm in the sections prepared from parafin-embedded tissue. The tumor involves the meninges and the molecular layer of the cerebellum, and there are a number of dilated vessels at its periphery. (Hematoxylin and eosin, X 75.) B. Higher-power view of a serial section. A round-cell infiltration (I) is visible near the dilated vessels at the periphery of the tumor. The tumor tissue itself (T) and some necrosis (N) are apparent. (Periodic acid Schiff, X 500.) Courtesy of Dr. J. C. E. Kaufmann. Courtesy of Dr. J. C. E. Kaufmann.

reaction induced by the tumor cells. Figure 5.5 illustrates a small established metastasis in the cerebellum of a woman who died due to metastases from an intraductal mammary adenocarcinoma (A). As mentioned above, leptomeningeal involvement was a frequent occurrence in brain metastases due to mammary adenocarcinoma in the series studied by Kane and others (1976). At higher power (B) the region of the host reaction to the metastasis, the tumor itself, and an area of necrosis can be observed even in this small metastasis.

REFERENCES

Agostino, D., and Cliffton, E. E. Trauma as a cause of localization of blood borne metastases: preventive effect of heparin and fibrinolysin. *Ann. Surg.* 161:97–102, 1965.

Alexander, J. W., and Altemeier, W. A. Susceptibility of injured tissues to hematogenous metastases—an experimental study. *Ann. Surg.* 159:933–943, 1964.

Anuigbo, W. I. B. Spread of cancer to the brain. *Br. J. Tuberc.* 52:141–148, 1958.

Ballinger, W. E., and Schimpff, R. D. Electron microscopic study of the development of experimentally induced cerebral metastases. *Fed. Proc.* 36:1086, 1977.

Baserga, R., and Saffiotti, U. Experimental studies on histogenesis of blood borne metastases. *Arch. Pathol.* 59:26–34, 1955.

Bennett, H. S.; Luft, J. H.; and Hampton, J. C. Morphological classification of vertebrate blood capillaries. *Am. J. Physiol.* 196:381–390, 1959.

Berenblum, I. The nature of tumor growth. Chapter 21 in *General pathology*, ed. H. Florey, 4th ed. Philadelphia: W. B. Saunders Co., 1970.

Berkovich, M. L., and Chernukh, A. M. Effect of irradiation and cortisone on spread of metastases of Ehrlich's carcinoma. Byulleten' Eksperimentol' noi Biologii, i Meditsiny 64:89–92, 1967 (in Russian). English translation, *Bull. Exp. Biol. Med.* 64:768–771, 1967.

Carr, I. The mechanism of tumor spread by lymphatics. In *Companion to the life sciences*, vol. 2, ed. S. Day. New York: Van Nostrand Reinhold, in press.

Chew, E. C.; Josephson, R. L.; and Wallace, A. C. Morphologic aspects of the arrest of circulating cancer cells. Pp. 121–150 in *Fundamental aspects of metastasis*, ed. L. Weiss. Amsterdam: North-Holland Publishing Co., 1976.

Christopherson, W. M. A re-evaluation of the significance of circulating cancer cells in the peripheral blood. Pp. 140–145 in *Recent advances in the diagnosis of cancer*, eds. R. W. Cumley, J. McCay, D. Aldridge-Beane, and W. White. Chicago: Year Book Medical Publishers Inc., 1973.

Engell, H. C. Cancer cells in the circulating blood. *Acta Chir. Scand.* 201:1–70, 1955.

Escourolle, R., and Poirier, J. *Manual of basic neuropathology*. Trans. by L. J. Rubinstein. Philadelphia: W. B. Saunders Co., 1973.

Fidler, I. J. Patterns of tumor cell arrest and development. Pp. 275–289 in *Fundamental aspects of metastasis*, ed. L. Weiss. Amsterdam: North-Holland Publishing Co., 1976.

Fisher, B.; Fisher, E. R.; and Feduska, N. Trauma and the localization of tumor cells. *Cancer* 20:23–30, 1967.

Frasher, W. G., and Wayland, H. A repeating modular organization of the microcirculation of cat mesentery. *Microvasc. Res.* 4:62, 1972.

Gasic, G. J. et al. Thrombogenic activity of mouse and human tumors: effects on platelets, coagulation and fibrinolysis and possible significance for metastasis. *Z. Krebsforsch.* 86:263–277, 1976.

Goldblatt, S. A., and Nadel, E. M. Cancer cells in the circulating blood. Pp. 119–140 in *Cancer progress*, ed. R. W. Raven. London: Butterworths and Co., 1963.

Goldblatt, S. A., and Nadel, E. M. Cancer cells in the circulating blood. A critical review II. *Acta Cytol.* (Baltimore) 9:6–20, 1965.

Griffiths, J. D., and Salsbury, A. J. *Circulating cancer cells*. Springfield, Ill.: Charles C Thomas, 1965.

Hardman, J. The angioarchitecture of the gliomata. *Brain* 63:91–118, 1940.

Hirano, A., and Matsui, T. Vascular structures in brain tumors. *Hum. Pathol.* 6:611–621, 1975.

Jacobs, L.; Kinkel, W. R.; and Vincent, R. G. Silent brain metastasis from lung carcinoma determined by computerized tomography. *Arch. Neurol.* 34:690–693, 1977.

Josephson, R. L. Ultrastructural studies of experimental hematogenous and lymphogenous metastases. Ph.D. thesis, University of Western Ontario, London, Canada, 1974.

Kane, W.; Munoz, A.; and Sher, J. Patterns of metastasis to brain. *J. Neuropathol. Exp. Neurol.* 35:362, 1976.

Kawaguchi, T., and Nakamura, K. Relationship between transcerebral passage of tumor cells and brain metastasis. *Gann.* 68:65–71, 1977.

Kung, P. C.; Lee, J. C.; and Bakay, L. Vascular invasion by glioma cells in man: electron microscopic study. *J. Neurosurg.* 31:339–345, 1969.

Marchesi, V. T., and Florey, H. W. Electron microscopic observations on the emigration of leucocytes. *Quart. J. Exp. Physiol.* 45:343–348, 1960.

Matthews, J. L., and Martin, J. H. Pp. 136–137 in *Atlas of human histology and ultrastructure*. Philadelphia: Lea and Febiger, 1971.

Matthews, M. J.; Pickren, J.; and Kanhouwa, S. Who has occult metastases? Residual tumor in patients undergoing surgical resections for lung cancer. Pp. 9–70 in *Perspectives in lung cancer*, Frederick E. Jones Memorial Symposium in Thoracic Surgery, Columbus, Ohio. Basel: Karger, 1977.

Meyer, P. C., and Rech, T. C. Secondary neoplasms of the central nervous system. *Br. J. Cancer* 7:438–448, 1953.

Peterson, H.-I. Experimental studies on fibrinolysis in growth and spread of tumor. *Acta Chir. Scand.*, (Suppl.) 394, 1968.

Peterson, H.-I.; Appelgren, K. K.; and Rosengren, B. H. D. Fibrinogen metabolism in experimental tumors. *Eur. J. Cancer* 5:535–542, 1969.

Richards, P., and McKissock, W. Intracranial metastases. *Br. Med. J.* 1: 15–18, 1963.

Ritchie, A. C., and Webster, D. R. Tumor cells in the blood. Pp. 225–236 in *Canadian cancer conference 4*, eds. R. W. Begg et al. New York: Academic Press, 1961.

Robert, S. S. Spread by the vascular system. Pp. 61–222 in *Dissemination of cancer*, eds. W. H. Cole et al. New York: Appleton-Century-Crofts Inc., 1961.

Robinson, K. P., and Hoppe, E. The development of blood borne metastases: the effect of local trauma and ischemia. *Arch. Surg.* 85:720–724, 1962.

Romanul, F. C. A. Examination of the brain and spinal cord. Chapter 4 in *Neuropathology: methods and diagnosis*, ed. C. G. Tedeschi, Boston: Little, Brown and Co., 1970.

Rubinstein, L. J. Tumors of the central nervous system. In *Atlas of tumor pathology*, 2nd Series, Fasc 6. Washington, D.C.: Armed Forces Institute of Pathology, 1972.

Rudenstam, C.-M. Experimental studies on trauma and metastasis formation. *Acta Chir. Scand.* (Suppl.) 391:1–83, 1968.

Salsbury, A. J. The significance of the circulating cancer cell. *Cancer Treat. Rev.* 2:55–72, 1975.

Stewart, H. L. et al. Pp. 261–271 in *Transplantable and transmissible tumors of animals*. Washington, D.C.: Armed Forces Institute of Pathology, 1959.

Wallace, A. C. Metastasis as an aspect of cell behaviour. Pp. 139–165 in *Canadian cancer conference 4*, eds. R. W. Begg et al. New York: Academic Press, 1961.

Wallace, A. C., and Hollenberg, N. K. The transplantability of tumours by intravenous and intralymphatic routes. *Br. J. Cancer* 19:338–342, 1965.

Warren, B. A. Some aspects of blood-borne tumor emboli associated with thrombosis. *Z. Krebsforsch.* 87:1–15, 1976.

Warren, B. A., and Shubik, P. The growth of the blood supply to melanoma transplants in the hamster cheek pouch. *Lab. Invest.* 15:464–478, 1966.

Warren, B. A., and Güldner, F.-H. Ultrastructure of the adhesion of HeLa cells to human vein wall. *Angiologica* 6:32–53, 1969.

Warren, B. A., and Vales, O. The adhesion of thromboplastic tumor emboli to vessel walls *in vivo*. *Br. J. Exp. Path.* 53:301–313, 1972.

Warren, B. A.; Shubik, P.; and Feldman, R. Metastasis via the blood stream: the method of intravasation of tumor cells in a transplantable melanoma of the hamster. *Cancer Letters* 4:245–251, 1978.

Weiss, L. Tumor necrosis and cell detachment. *Int. J. Cancer* 20:87–92, 1977.

Willis, R. A. Metastasis via the blood stream. Chapter 4 in *The spread of tumors in the human body*. London: Butterworths and Co., 1973.

Wood, S., Jr.; Holyoke, E. D.; and Yardley, J. H. Mechanisms of metastasis production by blood-borne cancer cells. Pp. 167–223 in *Canadian cancer conference 4*, eds. R. W. Begg et al. New York: Academic Press, 1961.

Zeidman, I. The fate of circulating tumor cells. I. Passage through capillaries. *Cancer Res.* 21:38–39, 1961.

Zeidman, I. The fate of circulating tumor cells. *Acta Cytol.* (Baltimore) 9:136–138, 1965.

Zeidman, I., and Buss, J. M. Transpulmonary passage of tumor cell emboli. *Cancer Res.* 12:731–733, 1952.

Zeidman, I.; Gamble, W. J.; and Clovis, W. L. Immediate passage of tumor cell emboli through the liver and kidney. *Cancer Res.* 16:814–815, 1956.

Zweifach, B. W. *Functional behaviour of the microcirculation*. Springfield, Ill.: Charles C Thomas, 1961.

6

Quantitative Aspects of Osmotic Opening of the Blood-Brain Barrier

Stanley I. Rapoport

For some patients with intracerebral tumor, systemically administered chemotherapeutic agents may be ineffective because a blood-brain barrier at the cerebral vasculature prevents access of water-soluble drugs to growing regions of the tumor edge. A concentration gradient of systemically administered water-soluble drug may develop from the center to the edge of intracerebral tumors and into the surrounding brain (Tator 1972; Levin et al. 1975). At the center, the blood-brain barrier is defective (see Chapter 7), but at the edge of the tumor the vasculature may be partially intact and drug that does enter can diffuse into the surrounding parenchyma (the sink effect).

The chemotherapeutic effectiveness of water-soluble drugs to which a central neoplasm should in principle be sensitive might be enhanced by several measures designed to overcome the blood-brain barrier. The selective permeability of the barrier to lipid-soluble drugs could be exploited by converting water-soluble to lipid-soluble agents, provided antineoplastic activity was retained. This approach has been employed in synthesizing various esters of methotrexate (Johns et al. 1973). A water-soluble drug also can be administered intrathecally (Whiteside et al. 1958). Intrathecal administration is effective with cytosine arabinoside and methotrexate, to which cortical neurons are not particularly sensitive, but other agents often are neurotoxic when administered in the high concentrations necessary to produce significant diffusion into brain parenchyma. Intrathecal administration can be effective against meningeal neoplasms but may not be useful for intracerebral tumors because of limited transparenchymal diffusion (Whiteside et al. 1958; Patlak and Fenstermacher 1975). A third approach to brain chemotherapy, which remains at the experimental stage, involves reversible modification of cerebrovascular permeability.

Although many insults to the brain and cerebral vasculature can alter barrier permeability, most do so irreversibly by damaging cerebral or vascular structure (Rapoport 1976). Here I summarize recent results with an osmotic method to reversibly increase barrier permeability. The method has been applied with limited success to treat experimental intracerebral tumors with methotrexate (Hasegawa et al. 1979). The elements of increasing permeability detailed in this chapter are (1) normal blood-brain barrier structure and function, (2) physiologic and morphologic evidence for the mechanism of osmotic barrier opening, (3) brain changes associated with osmotic treatment, (4) quantification of threshold and time course of osmotic barrier opening, and (5) barrier opening to methotrexate.

BLOOD-BRAIN BARRIER STRUCTURE AND FUNCTION

The blood-brain barrier at the cerebral vasculature is due to a continuous lining of endothelial cells that are connected by tight junctions. The endothelial cells do not support transendothelial vesicular transport, and the tight junctions between them restrict intercellular diffusion (fig. 6.1). Thus, the barrier as a whole limits blood-brain exchange of water-soluble drugs, ions and proteins but allows passage of lipid-soluble agents that can permeate the lipoid membranes of the endothelial cells (Crone 1965; Reese and Karnovsky 1967; Rapoport 1976).

OSMOTIC BARRIER OPENING

In experimental animals, the cerebrovascular endothelium can be made permeable to normally excluded proteins and solutes by being exposed to a hypertonic solution of a water-soluble solute such as urea,

Figure 6.1.

NORMAL CAPILLARY

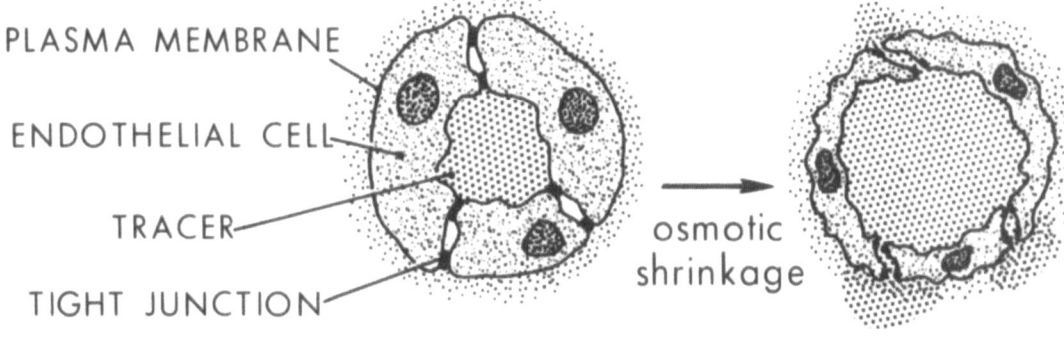

Normal capillary model for blood-brain barrier (left) and for barrier opening by widening of interendothelial tight junctions. When endothelial cells shrink in a hypertonic environment, their membranes stress and increase the permeability of the junctions to intravascular tracer. (Rapoport 1978a.)

mannitol, arabinose or lactamide (Rapoport 1970; Rapoport et al. 1972). Vessels at the pia-arachnoid can be reversibly opened to intravascular Evans blue dye (which is bound to plasma albumin) by applying a hypertonic solution of a water-soluble solute to the arachnoidal surface for 10 minutes, whereas a hypertonic solution of a lipid-soluble solute increases vessel permeability irreversibly. Furthermore, there is a negative relation between the threshold for reversible barrier opening by water-soluble solutes and their oil/water partition coefficient.

By comparing these relations with those obtained in studies of osmotically induced shrinkage of single cells (Overton 1895; Collander 1937; Rapoport 1976), my colleagues and I have suggested that reversible, osmotically induced barrier opening is mediated by shrinkage of cerebrovascular endothelial cells and consequent widening of interendothelial tight junctions (fig. 6.1). The model in figure 6.1 is supported by electron microscopic evidence of increased junctional permeability to intravascular horseradish peroxidase (fig. 6.2) as well as by evidence of occasional separation of vascular endothelial cells (fig. 6.3) in response to carotid infusion of hypertonic solutions (Brightman et al. 1973 and unpublished observations; Sterrett et al. 1976).

Figure 6.2.

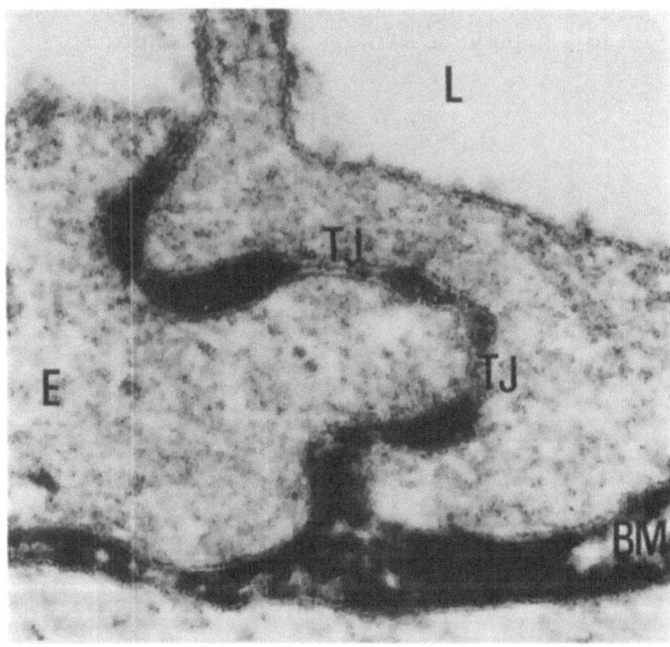

Opening of tight junctions between cerebrovascular endothelial cells to horseradish peroxidase tracer after intracarotid infusion of 3 M urea solution in rabbit. Peroxidase was administered intravenously before infusion, and the animal was killed 90 seconds after infusion. The tracer was washed from the capillary lumen (L) during fixation. Reaction product is present along the interface between endothelial cells (E), in the gaps between tight junctions (TJ), and in the basement membrane (BM). (X88,000.) (Brightman et al. 1973.)

Figure 6.3.

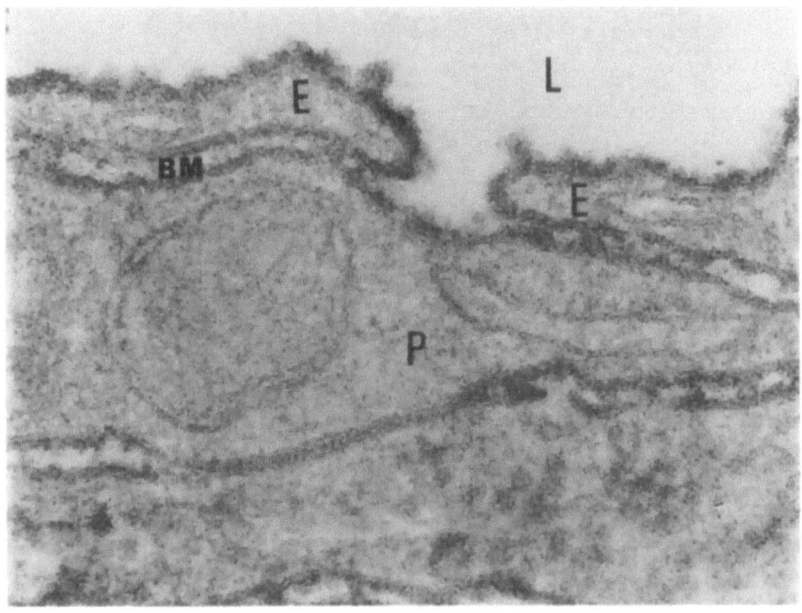

Separation of cerebrovascular endothelial cells after intracarotid infusion of 1.6 M arabinose solution in rat. Horseradish peroxidase was injected 1 hour after perfusion fixation of brain: E = endothelial cell; L = capillary lumen; BM = basement membrane; and P = brain parenchyma (Brightman, Sato, and Rappoport unpublished observations).

Figure 6.4 illustrates the procedure for osmotically opening the blood-brain barrier at the right cerebral hemisphere of the rat (Rapoport 1978a). A hypertonic solution is infused in a retrograde direction into the right external carotid artery at a rate of 0.12 ml/sec, which is sufficient to wash blood from the homolateral cerebral distribution of the anterior and middle cerebral arteries. Isotonic saline infused at this rate has no effect on cerebrovascular permeability.

Barrier opening by carotid infusion of a hypertonic solution of a water-soluble solute is reversible. As shown in figure 6.5, intravascular Evans blue dye (which is bound to plasma albumin) enters the brain if the dye is injected intravenously before or up to 2 hours after infusion of 1.6 M (Molal) arabinose solution but not if it is injected 4 hours after infusion (Chiueh et al. 1978).

BRAIN CHANGES

Although the osmotic effect is reversible with respect to cerebrovascular permeability and does not produce longterm gross neurologic changes (Rapoport and Thompson 1973), hypertonic infusion does result in transient changes in behavior, brain water content and brain metabolism. In

Figure 6.4.

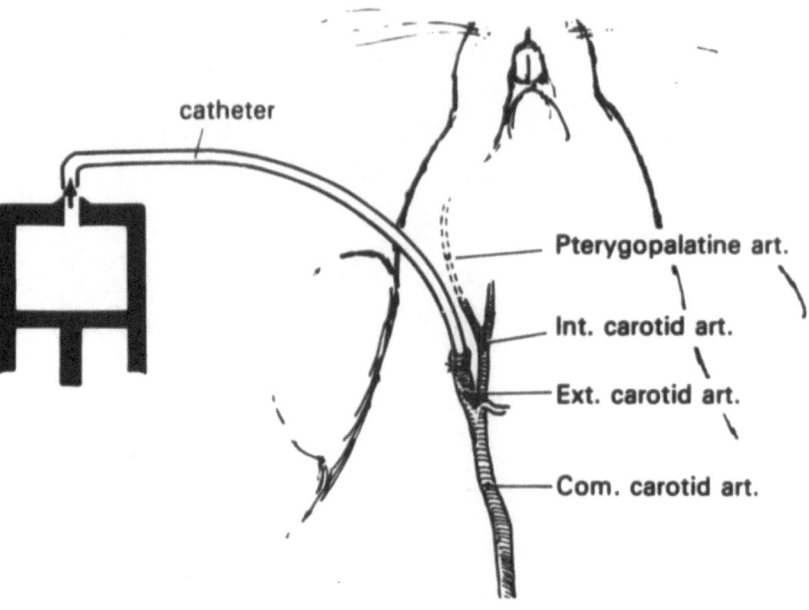

Infusion through a catheterized external carotid artery in a rat. (Rapoport 1978a.)

Figure 6.5.

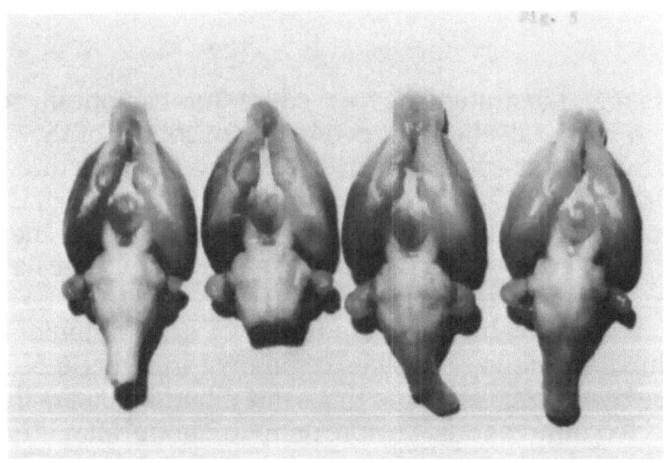

Reversibility of osmotic barrier opening to Evans blue albumin. The barrier was opened by 30 seconds of infusion of 1.6 M arabinose solution. Evans blue dye was injected before (left brain) and 30 minutes (next to left), 2 hours (third from left) and 4 hours (right) after barrier opening. Staining was absent at 4 hours. (From Chiueh et al. 1978.)

conscious rats, infusion of 1.4–1.6 M mannitol solution temporarily alters overt behavior and increases regional cerebral uptake of ^{14}C-2-deoxy-D-glucose, a marker of regional glucose consumption (Sokoloff et al. 1977; Pappius et al. 1979). Increased right-sided tracer uptake is illustrated by the autoradiograph of fig. 6.6, which was made from a section of brain from a rat administered ^{14}C-2-deoxy-D-glucose immediately after carotid infusion of 1.4 M mannitol solution. Uptake is not increased if the radiotracer is given 4 hours after osmotic treatment when barrier integrity is essentially reestablished.

Increased regional brain metabolism immediately after unilateral barrier opening is not accompanied by increased regional cerebral blood flow as measured with ^{14}C-iodoantipyrine; in fact, blood flow may fall (Pappius et al. 1979). Thus, osmotic treatment can interrupt the normally observed coupling in brain between regional metabolism and blood flow (Reivich and Sokoloff 1976). Uncoupling might be due to a direct longlasting action of hypertonic solutions on arteriolar smooth muscle in brain (Jonsson 1970) or to transient brain edema. Indeed, brain water rises by 1–1.5% in the first 2 hours after hypertonic infusion of arabinose in anesthetized rats (fig. 6.7). Edema is virtually absent 24 hours after treatment, however. The basis for transient brain edema is considered in detail elsewhere (Rapoport and others, unpublished observations; Rapoport 1978b, 1979).

Figure 6.6.

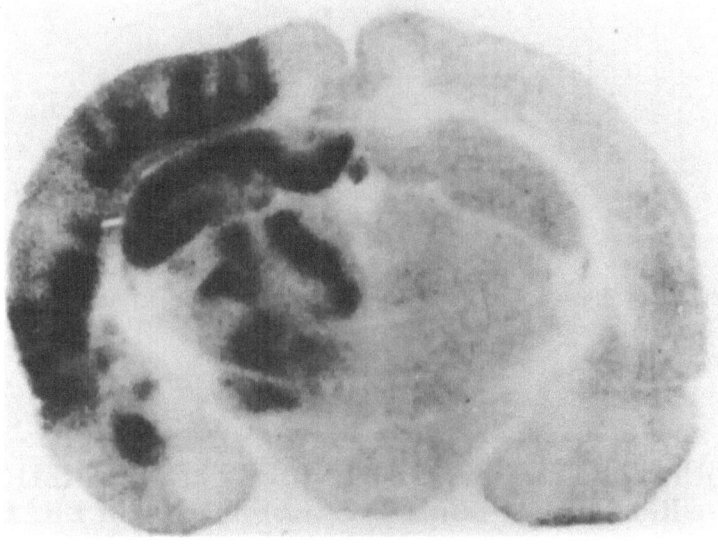

Autoradiograph of coronal brain section after right-sided carotid infusion of 1.4 M mannitol solution in rat and intravenous injection of 50 µCi of ^{14}C-2-deoxy-D-glucose. Animal was killed 45 minutes after tracer injection. Increased right-sided optical density indicates elevated uptake of ^{14}C tracer. (Pappius et al. 1979.)

Figure 6.7.

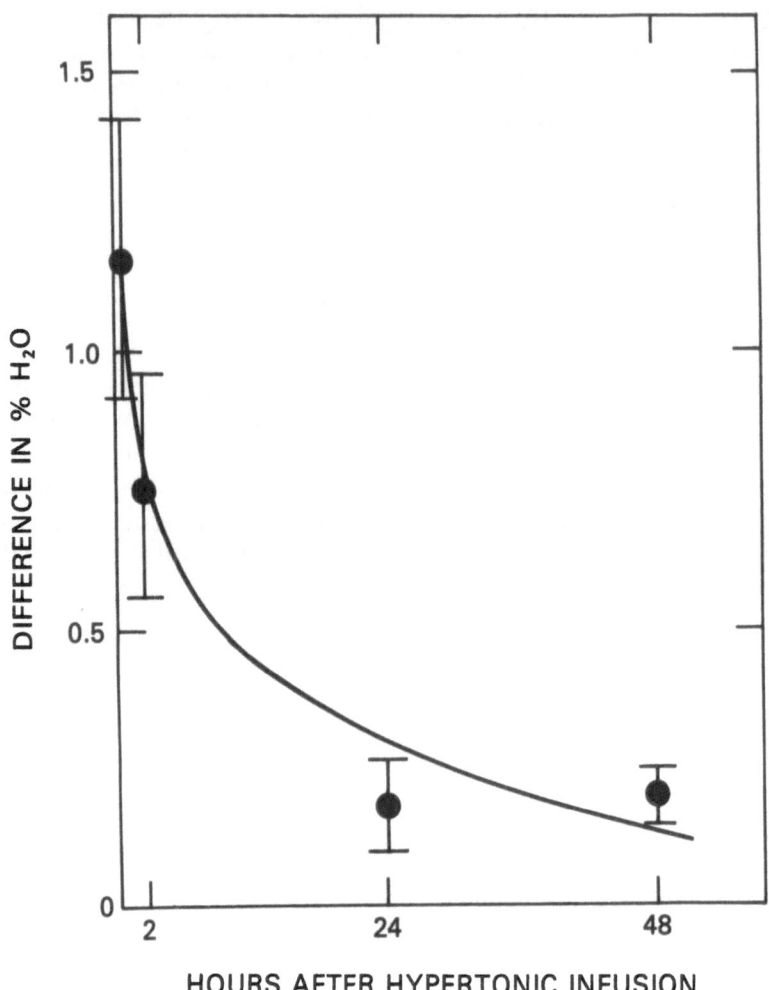

Right-left difference in percentage of water after 30 seconds of right-sided carotid infusion of 1.6–1.8 M arabinose solution in rat. All points are statistically significant (p < 0.05). (Rapoport 1979.)

QUANTIFICATION OF BARRIER PERMEABILITY IN NORMAL AND OSMOTICALLY TREATED BRAIN

In order to quantitatively predict cerebral accumulation of systemically administered, centrally acting drugs in normal and osmotically treated brains and to establish quantitative central dose-response relationships for such drugs, we developed a procedure to directly determine cerebrovascular permeability (Rapoport et al. 1978; Ohno et al. 1978). Commonly employed methods to measure permeability—the brain uptake index (BUI) technique and indicator dilution technique—cannot be used if cerebral blood flow is altered, as may be the case after hypertonic infusion (Raichle et al. 1976; Lassen and Crone 1970; Oldendorf 1970; Crone 1965). Furthermore, these other methods apply to whole brain rather than to brain regions. They are not sufficiently sensitive to measure PA (product of capillary permeability and surface area) below 10^{-4} sec^{-1}, whereas the PA of agents like ^{14}C–sucrose and ^{3}H-methotrexate is 0.7–4×10^{-5} sec^{-1} (table 6.1) (Rapoport et al. 1978 and unpublished observations; Ohno et al. 1978). The new method is not subject to these objections and can be used to measure regional permeabilities of very poorly penetrating substances independently of cerebral blood flow.

Indwelling catheters are placed in the femoral artery and vein of a rat, and ^{14}C-sucrose is injected intravenously as a bolus. Femoral artery plasma concentration is followed until the time of death (T = 10 minutes) when plasma concentration has fallen sufficiently to assure that possible errors in estimating intravascular radioactivity (product of measured regional blood volume and whole blood radioactivity) do not significantly affect the calculated brain parenchymal concentration of tracer, C_{brain} dpm/g (net minus intravascular radioactivity). Up to 10 minutes after injection of ^{14}C-sucrose, furthermore, the plasma concentration C_{plasma} dpm/ml markedly exceeds C_{brain}, so that back diffusion of tracer from brain to plasma is negligible. Tracer entry into brain then is given as follows in which P = cerebrovascular permeability (cm sec^{-1}), A = capillary surface area (cm^2 g^{-1}), and t = time:

$$dC_{brain}/dt = PAC_{plasma} \tag{1}$$

Integration of equation 1 provides an expression for PA in terms of C_{brain} at the time of death (T) and the integrated plasma concentration up to time T:

$$PA = \frac{C_{brain}(T)}{\int_0^T C_{plasma}\, dt} \tag{2}$$

$\int_0^T C_{plasma} dt$ is obtained graphically from the integrated plasma concentration curve, and $C_{brain}(T)$ is obtained by subtracting intravascular from net regional brain radioactivity.

Figure 6.8 illustrates a typical experiment in which ^{14}C-sucrose was injected 5 minutes after right-sided carotid infusion with 1.6 M arabinose solution for 30 seconds. Plasma radioactivity was followed and integrated over the 10 minutes after injection. Regional values of C_{brain} (10 minutes) are given in the figure in relation to the extent of brain staining by intravascular Evans blue dye. Staining was graded from 0 (no staining) to 3 + (dark staining).

For the experiment described by figure 6.8, PA at right-sided gray matter with grade 3 + staining equaled 21.6×10^{-5} seconds or 16435 dpm/g

Figure 6.8.

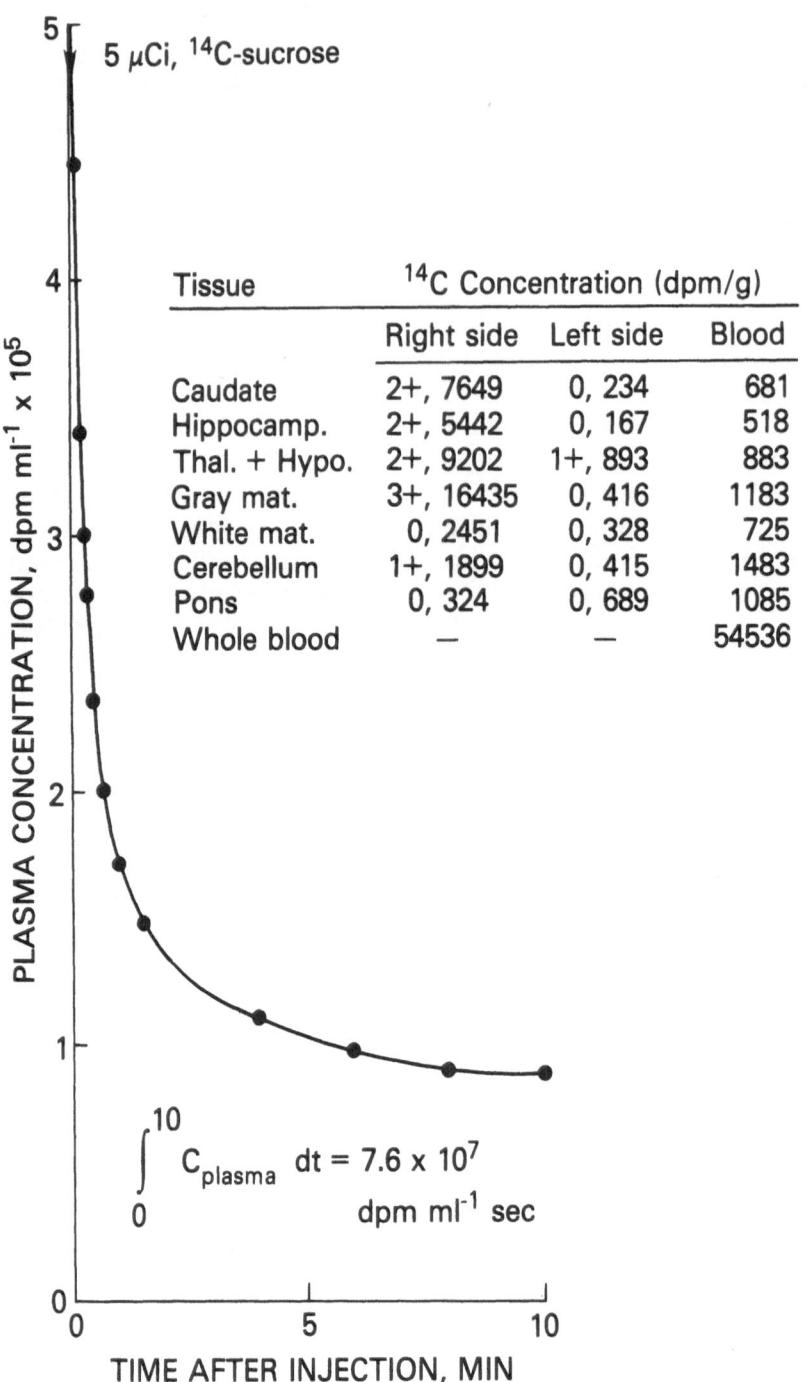

5 μCi, ^{14}C-sucrose

Tissue	^{14}C Concentration (dpm/g)		
	Right side	Left side	Blood
Caudate	2+, 7649	0, 234	681
Hippocamp.	2+, 5442	0, 167	518
Thal. + Hypo.	2+, 9202	1+, 893	883
Gray mat.	3+, 16435	0, 416	1183
White mat.	0, 2451	0, 328	725
Cerebellum	1+, 1899	0, 415	1483
Pons	0, 324	0, 689	1085
Whole blood	—	—	54536

$$\int_0^{10} C_{plasma}\ dt = 7.6 \times 10^7 \ \ dpm\ ml^{-1}\ sec$$

PLASMA CONCENTRATION, dpm ml^{-1} x 10^5

TIME AFTER INJECTION, MIN

Plasma and brain ^{14}C concentrations in rat after right-sided carotid infusion of 1.6 M arabinose solution and, 5 minutes later, intravenous injection of 5 μCi of ^{14}C-sucrose. Animal was killed 10 minutes after radiotracer was injected. Parenchymal brain concentrations are given (net − intravascular radioactivity). (Rapoport et al. 1978.)

divided by the plasma concentration integral. Table 6.1 presents mean values of PA for ^{14}C-sucrose derived in this way at right- and left-sided brain regions after right-sided carotid infusion of isotonic saline or hypertonic arabinose solution. PA was correlated with the grade of brain staining with Evans blue dye. Isotonic saline infusion did not produce brain staining nor elevate PA on the right side above PA on the left or above PA in unperfused brain. Hypertonic arabinose infusion increased PA from about 0.6–1×10^{-5} sec^{-1} to 17–22×10^{-5} sec^{-1} and occasionally affected the left side as well. Variability may have been due to variability in the cerebral distribution of infusate or to slight changes in regional blood volume (Rapoport et al. 1978).

In order to define threshold parameters for barrier opening by hypertonic arabinose in rats, we measured PA for ^{14}C-sucrose in relation to infusion duration and infusate concentration (Rapoport and others, unpublished observations). At an infusion duration of 30 seconds, PA rose by about 2-fold in some brain regions with 1.4 M arabinose infusate and by up to 20-fold in regions supplied by the right anterior and middle cerebral arteries with 1.6 M arabinose infusate. The 1.8 M solution did not further elevate PA. Thus, the concentration threshold for barrier opening was very abrupt, between 1.4 and 1.6 M.

When arabinose concentration was fixed at 1.6 M, on the other hand, at least 20 seconds of infusion was required to significantly and abruptly elevate PA. Shorter times were ineffective, and 30 seconds of infusion did not further augment permeability. The absence of a barrier effect at short infusion times explains why radiographic contrast media, whose osmolality may approach 1.6 osmol, can be used for cerebral angiography in man without producing neurotoxic sequellae (Rapoport et al. 1974). The less than 5-second period of angiographic administration would not open the barrier to these potentially damaging agents (Hoppe 1959).

BARRIER OPENING TO ^{3}H-METHOTREXATE

Table 6.1 also presents PA of intravenously administered ^{3}H-methotrexate in control rats that did not have carotid infusion, in rats after 30 seconds of right-sided carotid infusion of isotonic saline, and in rats after a similar infusion of 1.6 M arabinose solution (Ohno and others, unpublished observations). As shown by Shapiro and his colleagues (see Chapter 22 and Hasegawa et al. 1979), hypertonic mannitol infusion gives comparable increases in brain uptake of methotrexate. PA for ^{3}H-methotrexate was about 3 times higher than PA for ^{14}C-sucrose in unperfused brain regions, but PA for both substances rose to about 20×10^{-5} sec^{-1} in right-sided regions after 1.6 M arabinose infusion.

For pharmacotherapeutic purposes, brain uptake of ^{3}H-methotrexate at a given administered dose (which is the determinant of peripheral toxicity) can be increased further by a factor of 5 by infusing the drug into the external carotid catheter (fig. 6.4) rather than intravenously (Ohno and

Table 6.1

THE PRODUCT OF CEREBROVASCULAR PERMEABILITY (P) TIMES THE AREA (A) FOR ^{14}C-SUCROSE AND ^{3}H-METHOTREXATE IN RATS, IN CONTROL ANIMALS AND AFTER RIGHT-SIDED CAROTID INFUSION OF ISOTONIC SALINE OR 1.6 M ARABINOSE SOLUTIONS

Brain Region	Grade of Brain Staining	No Infusion
	^{14}C-sucrose	
Caudate nucleus	0 – 1+ 2+ – 3+	
Hippocampus	0 – 1+ 2+ – 3+	
Thalamus + Hypothalamus	0 – 1+ 2+ – 3+	
Pons	0 – 1+	
	^{3}H-Methotrexate (3)	
Caudate nucleus		4.0 ± 0.8
Hippocampus		3.0 ± 1.0
Frontal lobe		3.4 ± 0.8
Pons		3.0 ± 0.2

*Mean $\pm$ S.E.M. (Number of samples in parentheses.)
†Differs from isotonic saline infusion mean on same side of brain ($p < 0.05$).
SOURCE: Rapoport et al., 1978 and Ohno et al., 1978.
NOTE: Radiotracer was injected intravenously in uninfused animals 5 minutes after carotid infusion. The animal was killed 10 minutes after tracer injection. PA was calculated by equation 2.

others, unpublished observations; Fenstermacher and Cowles 1977). Thus, osmotic treatment plus intracarotid infusion of drug should augment brain uptake by a factor of 50 above uptake obtained by infusing the drug intravenously into untreated animals.

Summary

The blood-brain barrier in rats can be opened reversibly by infusing a hypertonic solution of arabinose or mannitol into the carotid circulation.

	PA, $sec^{-1} \times 10^5$		
Isotonic Saline Infusion		**1.6 M Arabinose Infusion**	
Right Brain	**Left Brain**	**Right Brain**	**Left Brain**
^{14}C-sucrose			
1.3 ± 0.4 (5)*	0.7 ± 0.1 (5)	5.4 ± 4.8 (2) 17.3 ± 1.4 (8)†	2.2 ± 0.5 (10)†
1.4 ± 0.6 (5)	0.7 ± 0.3 (5)	1.8 (1) 18.0 ± 1.8 (9)†	1.8 ± 0.4 (10)
1.4 ± 0.3 (5)	0.8 ± 0.1 (5)	16.5 (1) 21.2 ± 1.8 (9)†	2.6 ± 0.4 (10)†
0.6 ± 0.1 (5)	0.8 ± 0.01 (5)	2.3 ± 0.5 (10)†	2.4 ± 0.5 (10)†
^3H-Methotrexate (3)			
5.5 ± 1.2	3.8 ± 0.4	20.2 ± 3.0†	4.4 ± 0.8
7.2 ± 1.3	3.6 ± 2.3	22.1 ± 3.2†	4.0 ± 2.3
4.9 ± 1.0	3.3 ± 0.6	26.7 ± 3.5†	3.5 ± 0.3
3.8 ± 0.1	4.0 ± 0.1	3.3 ± 0.4	3.7 ± 0.1

Such opening probably is mediated by a transient (2–4 hours) widening of tight junctions that connect cerebrovascular endothelial cells. It is accompanied by a transient brain edema (1–1.5% increase in brain water). At 30 seconds of carotid infusion of hypertonic arabinose solutions, there is a sharp concentration threshold (1.4–1.6 M) for barrier opening. With 1.6 M arabinose, the PA product (cerebrovascular permeability × surface area) for ^{14}C − sucrose is increased from a normal value of 1×10^{-5} sec^{-1} to more than 20×10^{-5} sec^{-1} in affected regions; and for ^3H-methotrexate, from 3×10^{-5} sec^{-1} to 20×10^{-5} sec^{-1}. Thus, osmotic treatment can increase cerebrovascular permeability to poorly diffusing agents by a factor of 10–20. Intracarotid infusion of the agent immediately after osmotic treatment can further augment brain uptake 5-fold. These studies show that the osmotic method can be used in a quantitatively predictable way to allow drugs of potential therapeutic value into the brain.

REFERENCES

Brightman, M. W. et al. Osmotic opening of tight junctions in cerebral endothelium. *J. Comp. Neurol.* 152:317–326, 1973.

Chiueh, C. C. et al. Entry of (^{3}H)norepinephrine, (^{125}I)albumin and Evans blue from blood into brain following unilateral osmotic opening of the blood-brain barrier. *Brain Res.* 145:291–301, 1978.

Collander, R. The permeability of plant protoplasts to nonelectrolytes. *Trans. Faraday Soc.* 33:985–990, 1937.

Crone, C. The permeability of brain capillaries to nonelectrolytes. *Acta Physiol. Scand.* 64:407–417, 1965.

Fenstermacher, J. D., and Cowles, A. L. Theoretic limitations of intracarotid infusions in brain tumor chemotherapy. *Cancer Treat. Rep.* 61:519–526, 1977.

Hasegawa, H. et al. The enhancement of CNS penetration of methotrexate by hyperosmolar intracarotid mannitol and carcinomatous meningitis. *Neurology (Minneap)* 29:1280–1286, 1979.

Hoppe, J. O. Some pharmacological aspects of radiopaque compounds. *Ann. N.Y. Acad. Sci.* 78:727–739, 1959.

Johns, D. G. et al. Dialkyl esters of methotrexate and 3′,5′–dichloromethotrexate synthesis and interaction with aldehyde oxidase and dihydrofolate reductase. *Drug Metab. Dispos.* 1:580–589, 1973.

Jonsson, O. Extracellular osmolality and vascular smooth muscle activity. *Acta Physiol. Scand. Suppl.* 359:1–48, 1970.

Lassen, N. A., and Crone, C. The extraction fraction of a capillary bed to hydrophilic molecules: theoretical considerations regarding the single injection technique with a discussion of the role of diffusion between laminar streams (Taylor's effect). In *Capillary permeability*, eds. C. Crone and N. A. Lassen. Copenhagen: Munksgaard, 1970.

Levin, V. A.; Freeman-Dove, M.; and Landahl, H. D. Permeability characteristics of brain adjacent to tumors in rats. *Arch. Neurol.* 32:785–791, 1975.

Ohno, K.; Pettigrew, K. D.; and Rapoport, S. I. Lower limits of cerebrovascular permeability to nonelectrolytes in the conscious rat. *Am. J. Physiol.* 235:H299–H307, 1978.

Oldendorf, W. H. Measurement of brain uptake of radiolabeled substances using a tritiated water internal standard. *Brain Res.* 24:372–376, 1970.

Overton, E. Uber die osmotischen Eigenschaften der lebenden Pflanzen und Tierzelle. *Vierteljahresschr Naturforsch Ges. Zur.* 40:159–201, 1895.

Pappius, H. M. et al. Osmotic opening of blood-brain barrier and local cerebral glucose utilization.*Ann. Neurol.* 5:211–219, 1979.

Patlak, C. S., and Fenstermacher, J. D. Measurements of dog blood-brain transfer constants by ventriculocisternal perfusion. *Am. J. Physiol.* 229:877–884, 1975.

Raichle, M. E. et al. Blood-brain barrier permeability of ^{11}C-labeled alcohols and ^{15}O-labeled water. *Am. J. Physiol.* 230:543–552, 1976.

Rapoport, S. I. Effect of concentrated solutions on blood-brain barrier. *Am. J. Physiol.* 219:270–274, 1970.

Rapoport, S. I. *Blood-brain barrier in physiology and medicine.* New York: Raven Press, 1976.

Rapoport, S. I. Osmotic opening of the blood-brain barrier. In *Cerebral vascular smooth muscle and its control.* Ciba Foundation Symposium (New Series), No. 56. Amsterdam: Elsevier, 1978a.

Rapoport, S. I. A mathematical model for vasogenic brain edema. *J. Theor. Biol.* 74:439–467, 1978b.

Rapoport, S. I. Roles of cerebrovascular permeability, brain compliance and brain hydraulic conductivity in vasogenic brain edema. Pp. 51–62 in *Neural trauma: seminars in neurological surgery*, ed. A. J. Popp et al. in *Proceedings of the Third Chicago Conference on Neural Trauma.* New York: Raven Press, 1979.

Rapoport, S. I.; Hori, M.; and Klatzo, I. Testing of a hypothesis for osmotic opening of the blood-brain barrier. *Am. J. Physiol.* 223:323–331, 1972.

Rapoport, S. I., and Thompson, H. K. Osmotic opening of the blood-brain barrier in the monkey without associated neurological deficits. *Science* 180:971, 1973.

Rapoport, S. I.; Thompson, H. K.; and Bidinger, J. M. Equi-osmolal opening of the blood-brain barrier in the rabbit by different contrast agents. *Acta Radiol.* [*Diagn.*] (*Stockh*) 15:21–32, 1974.

Rapoport, S. I. et al. Regional cerebrovascular permeability to ^{14}C-sucrose after osmotic opening of the blood-brain barrier. *Brain Res.* 150:653–657, 1978.

Reese, T. S., and Karnovsky, M. J. Fine structural localization of a blood-brain barrier to exogenous peroxidase. *J. Cell Biol.* 34:207–217, 1967.

Reivich, M., and Sokoloff, L. Application of the 2-deoxy-D-glucose method to the coupling of cerebral metabolism and blood flow. *Neurosci. Res. Program Bull.* 14:474–476, 1976.

Sokoloff, L. et al. The (^{14}C)deoxyglucose method for the measurement of local cerebral glucose utilization: theory, procedure, and normal values in the conscious and anesthetized albino rat. *J. Neurochem.* 28:897–916, 1977.

Sterrett, P. R. et al. Cerebrovasculature permeability changes following experimental angiography. A light- and electronmicroscopic study. *J. Neurol. Sci.* 30:385–403, 1976.

Tator, C. H. Chemotherapy of brain tumors. Uptake of tritiated methotrexate by a transplantable intracerebral ependymoblastoma in mice. *J. Neurosurg.* 37:1–8, 1972.

Whiteside, J. A. et al. Intrathecal amethopterin in neurological manifestations of leukemia. *Arch. Intern. Med.* 101:279–285, 1958.

7

Brain Tumor Microvasculature

Nicholas A. Vick

Nearly a decade ago Darell Bigner and I, working with Milton Brightman, used the electron microscope to observe endothelial defects in hamster brain tumors induced by intracerebral inoculation of avian sarcoma virus (Brightman et al. 1971). We were impressed with the possible biologic and clinical significance of these defects and extended our findings to experimental gliomas in the dog (Vick and Bigner 1972b) and the rat (Yung et al. 1976). Subsequent studies by others of spontaneous human brain tumors, both primary and metastatic (Hirano and Matsui 1975; Waggener and Biggs 1976), and of chemically induced experimental gliomas (Cox et al. 1976) have led us to believe that endothelial abnormalities are characteristic of brain tumors. Moreover, we have become convinced that they are the prime structural basis for the well-known hyperpermeability of brain tumors to constituents of the blood vascular compartment and that their occurrence may have direct relevance for methods of effective chemotherapy (Vick et al. 1977).

Despite advances in the chemotherapy of systemic cancer, progress has been painfully slow with brain tumors, and some of the most favored forms of chemotherapy, initially of promise, have not been shown to be effective (Walker and Brain Tumor Study Group 1978). We are at a juncture in time, in this field, during which all suppositions and concepts need to be reevaluated and perhaps may be radically altered. In our experimental brain tumors, studies with the extracellular tracers Evans blue and horseradish peroxidase have demonstrated qualitatively the functional significance of these endothelial defects; in humans, others have demonstrated the phenomenon indirectly in surgical biopsy specimens with colloidal lanthanum. The radionuclide brain scan and the infusion scans made with computed tomography (CT) are obvious clinical counterparts of these observations. The actual frequency of occurrence, anatomic distribution, and quantitative functional significance of brain-tumor endothelial defects is not known. Because the electron microscope is not well-suited for such studies, we have looked closely at our experimental tumors with the light microscope and autoradiograph.

In this chapter I attempt to summarize what is currently known about the structure of brain tumor microvasculature, synthesizing our work in the past years with our current studies and with the others' studies of spontaneous human brain tumors. My laboratory uses gliomas induced in

115

neonatal Fischer-344 rats by intracerebral inoculation of 0.002 ml (5×10^8 FFU/ml) of the Schmidt-Ruppin strain of avian sarcoma virus. The inoculum is delivered with a gas-tight Hamilton syringe attached to an automatic injecting device through a 27-gauge needle. Tumor yield is 100%, the same as we achieved earlier in the dog (Vick et al. 1971; Vick and Bigner 1972a; Bigner et al. 1972a,b) and in another rat model (Yung et al. 1976). We use standard perfusion-fixation techniques and process the tissue by a variety of histologic methods for transmitted and differential interference

Figure 7.1.

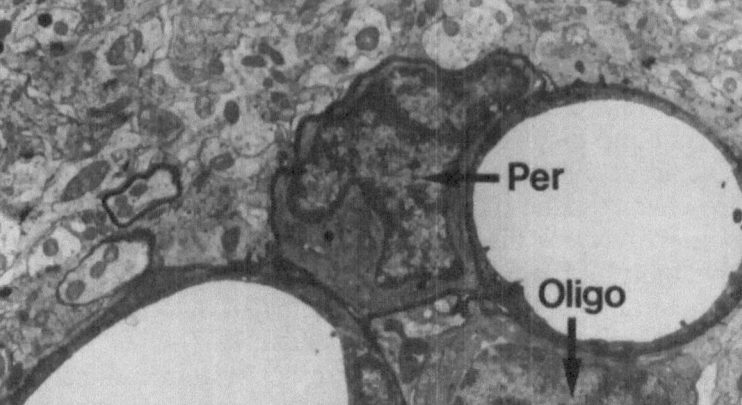

Low-magnification electronmicrograph of normal rat cerebral cortex. EN = endothelial cell; Per = pericyte; Oligo = oligodendrocyte. Note continuous endothelium with paucity of vesicles; the basal lamina encloses endothelial cell and pericyte. There is no pericapillary space.

light optics and electron microscopy. Our methods (Vick et al. 1971) and the general histopathologic characteristics of the model we now use (Wilfong et al. 1973; Copeland et al. 1976) have been described.

NORMAL BRAIN MICROVASCULATURE

Normal cerebral capillaries (fig. 7.1) are continuous, thin-walled and in many respects similar to those which occur elsewhere in the body (Peters et al. 1976). The endothelial cells are surrounded by a dense basal lamina approximately 35 mm thick. This basal lamina also encloses the ubiquitous pericytes whose processes are not usually distinguishable from the endothelium by light microscopy. Lying external to the basal lamina and tightly apposed to it without an intervening space is the neuropil of the subadjacent brain. The processes in this region usually can be identified with the electron microscope as astrocytic although now and then one may see a capillary immediately adjacent to a neuron. Except for a few special brain regions which contain heterotypical capillaries (discussed later in this chapter), the endothelium of normal mammalian brain is always continuous. In nearly ten years of study I have never seen a fenestrated or discontinuous parenchymal brain endothelial cell in the hamster, rat, dog or monkey.

Two other characteristics of normal brain endothelial cells are noteworthy: they have remarkably few pinocytotic vesicles (fig. 7.2), and as they form a lumen, they are joined one to the other by zonulae occludentes or so-called tight junctions (fig. 7.3). The former may be a morphologic marker of a specialized cytoplasmic microphysiology. The latter, about which considerably more is known, may be an even more distinctive feature of brain endothelium and it appears to be the basis for the unusual impermeability of brain endothelium to the contents of the blood vascular compartment (Brightman and Reese 1969; Brightman 1978; Brightman et al. 1970).

Zonulae occludentes are intercellular contacts in which the outer leaflets of the opposing plasma membranes seem to have fused, obliterating the intercellular space. The brain's zonulae occludentes appear in a single plane of section to be the same as those which occur elsewhere in the body and do not appear to be structurally unique. It is unique, however, that they occur in continuous belts around contiguous endothelial cells. The elegant studies of Brightman have shown these tight junctions to be the site, at least at the capillary level, where extracellular tracers such as horseradish peroxidase are impeded from entry into the substance of the brain from the blood vascular compartment (Brightman and Reese 1969; Brightman 1978; Brightman et al. 1970). Although certain experimental conditions may open the zonulae occludentes of brain endothelium (Rapoport et al. 1972; Westergaard 1977), they have been closed in the normal state whenever they have been observed in the proper plane of section.

Figure 7.2.

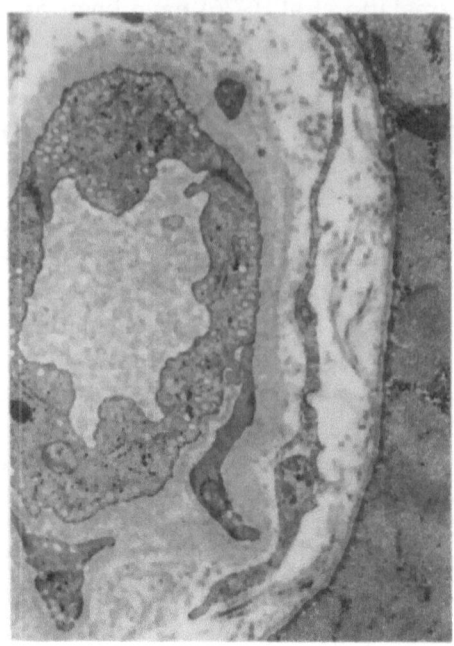

Normal skeletal muscle capillary in pericapillary space. The endothelial layer is continuous but contains abundant vesicles, unlike those of brain. (Compare to fig. 7.1.)

Figure 7.3.

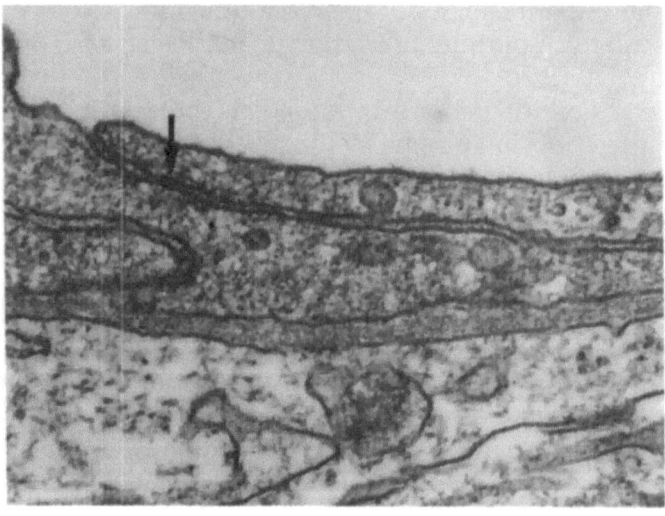

Endothelial tight junction (arrow) in normal dog cerebellum.

The regions of the brain which contain heterotypical endothelium (area postrema, choroid plexus, median eminence, epyphysis, subfornical organ, neurohypophysis and pineal) have been known for years to lie outside the blood-brain barrier. If one perfuses an experimental animal with one of the basic aniline dyes (such as Evans blue), the brain remains free of stain except for these specialized areas, which stain deeply. I have observed this in the living monkey. With proper exposure of the floor of the fourth ventricle and with the aid of the operating microscope, one can see virtually immediate blue coloration of the area postremae after intravenous injection of Evans blue in the living monkey. Area postrema and the other specialized structures have been shown in all species examined to be characterized by capillaries that are surrounded by a generous perivascular space containing collagen and fibroblasts (fig. 7.4). Of even greater interest, the endothelium in these structures is fenestrated (fig. 7.5) (Hashimoto 1966; Hashimoto and Hama 1968; Klara and Brizzee 1975, 1977). The fenestrated endothelium is virtually identical in all brain tumors.

Figure 7.4.

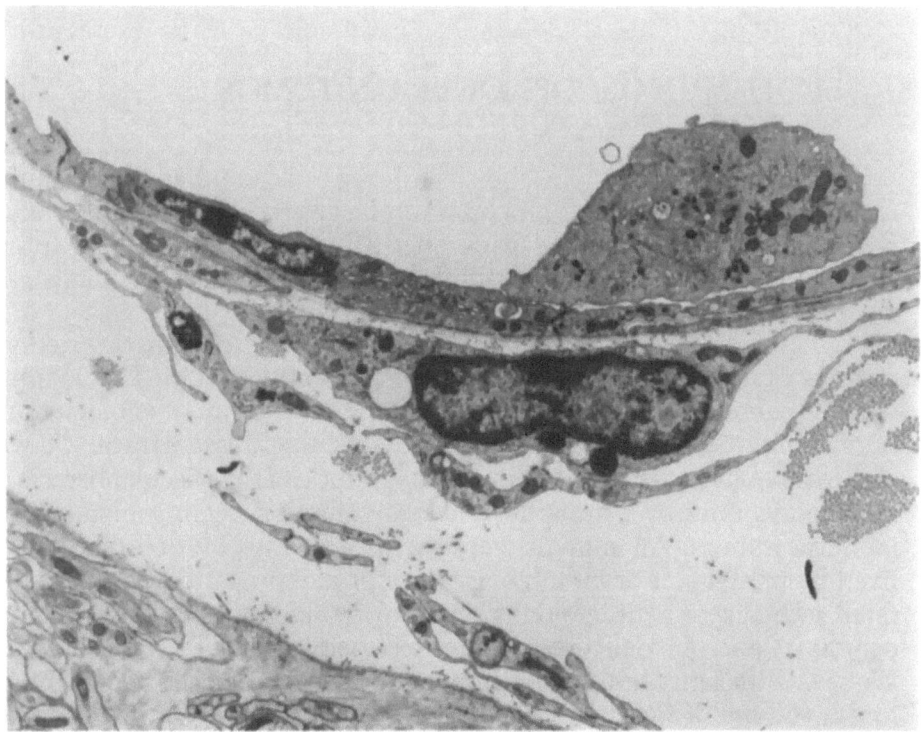

Area postrema (Rhesus monkey) with portion of a lymphocyte in the capillary lumen. Note the generous pericapillary space containing fibroblasts and collagen.

Figure 7.5.

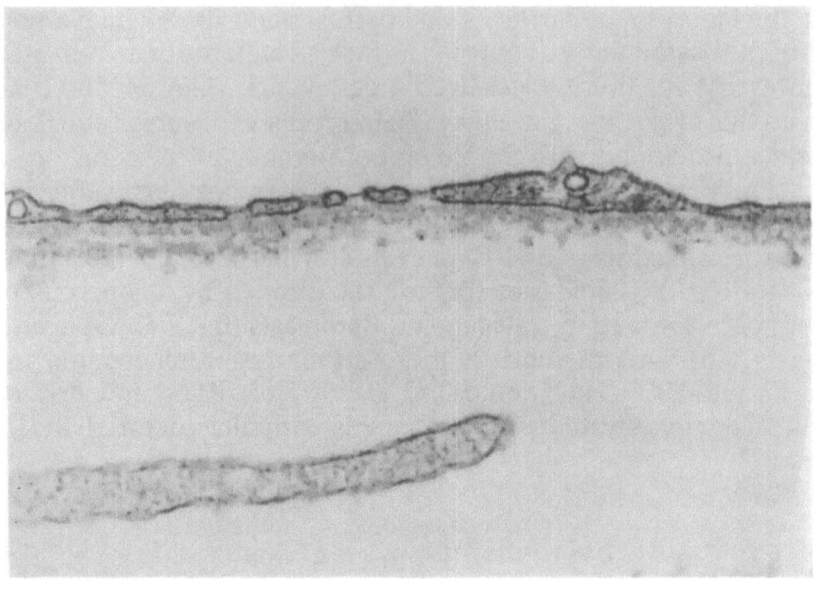

Fenestrated endothelium in the area postrema (dog).

LIGHT MICROSCOPY OF BRAIN TUMOR MICROVASCULATURE

Although it is only with the electron microscope that certain minute features of brain tumor endothelium can be appreciated, a number of important observations can be made about the capillaries of brain tumors with the light microscope. I can think of at least four of consequence, and doubtlessly there are others.

First, most histologic sections of brain tumors contain an excessive number of capillary profiles as compared to normal brain. This is not always apparent because immersion fixation, the usual manner of fixation in human brain tumors, invariably collapses the microvasculature. We were able to demonstrate for ourselves the magnitude of the vascular beds in *our* rat gliomas only by comparing a series of brains bearing histologically identical tumors. All animals were sacrificed either by decapitation and fixed by immersion or by intravascular perfusion-fixation with 10% buffered formalin or a gluteraldehyde-paraformaldehyde mixture of known osmolality and pH, delivered through a closed system at systolic pressure. We saw with clarity how misleading immersion fixation can be with regard to the volume of the tumor capillary beds (fig. 7.6). These experimental studies suggest that even the most avascular-appearing human brain tumors are abundantly endowed with completely collapsed capillaries whose endothelial cells cannot be distinguished from subadjacent tumor cells.

The second feature of the microvasculature of brain tumors apparent at the light microscopic level is the highly variable and generally increased cross-sectional diameter of the individual vessels (fig. 7.7). While thin-walled, with histologic characteristics typical of capillaries, the lumina as seen in the perfused state may be enormous.

Figure 7.6.

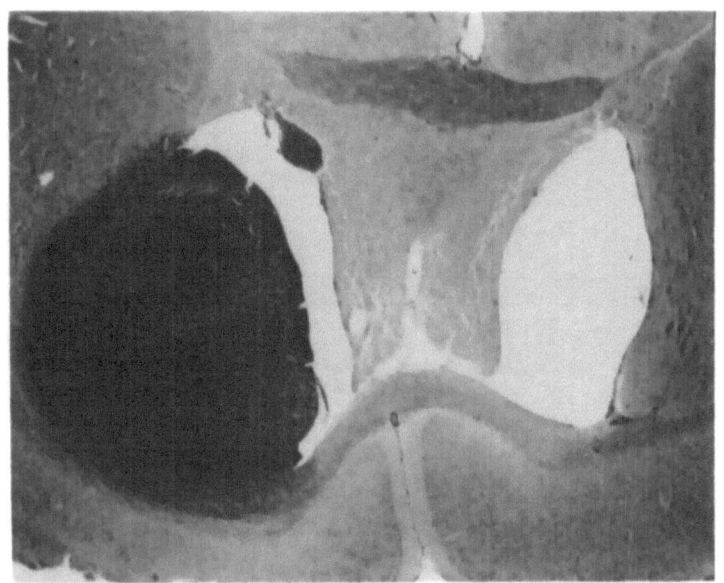

A

B

Rat gliomas induced with avian sarcoma virus. A. *An immersion-fixed specimen.* B. *A perfused specimen.*

Figure 7.7.

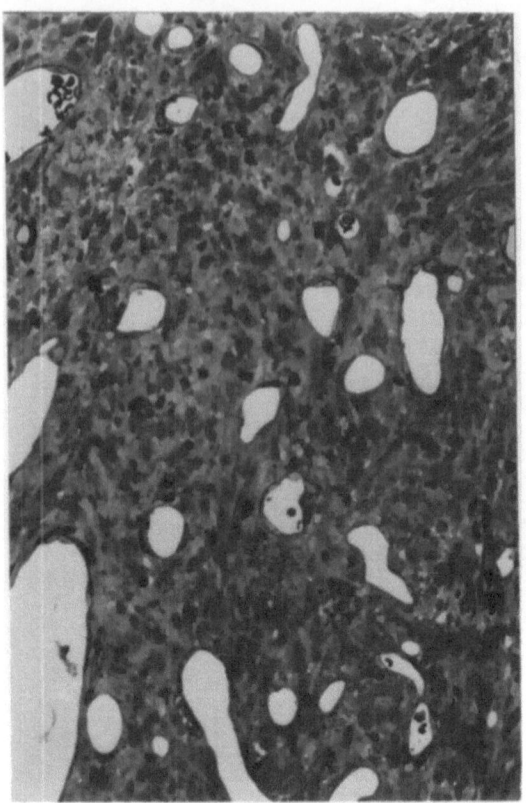

Rat glioma induced with avian sarcoma virus. Note the variable diameter of the vessels and abundance of the microvasculature.

The third feature worth noting is the excessive number of plump endothelial nuclei per circumference of vessel wall. Many of these nuclei are mitotic, but this has not been appreciated because of the artifactual effects of slow immersion fixation. In perfused specimens, one can see a greater number of mitotic endothelial cells than in immersion-fixed specimens. With autoradiographic techniques a surprisingly high percentage of the endothelial nuclei, 34% in some instances, are labeled after a single pulse of ^{3}H-thymidine (fig. 7.8). Whether this indicates that the endothelium of brain tumor vessels is neoplastic, in parallel with the parenchymal tumor-cell population, or that the vessels are multiplying to supply the tumor is an important but as yet not answerable question.

The fourth characteristic at the light microscopic level is one which has not often been appreciated because of the thickness of standard paraffin histologic sections. When one looks carefully with transmitted or differential interference light optics at thinly sectioned material embedded in plas-

Figure 7.8.

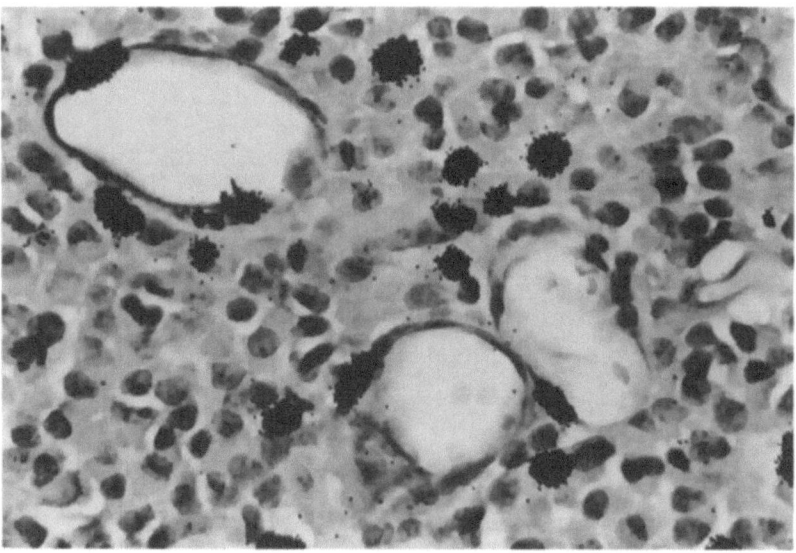

Rat glioma induced with avian sarcoma virus after single pulse of ³H-thymidine. Note labeling of endothelial nuclei as well as nuclei of parenchymal cells of the tumor.

tic, gross defects of the endothelial vascular wall within brain tumors can be seen (fig. 7.9*A*). The infrequency with which they have been seen is due to the problem of sampling and the small size of the defects. The great majority of thin-walled tumor capillaries, as seen in thinly sectioned plastic-embedded specimens, appear to have continuous walls (fig. 7.9*B*) in the beam of the light microscope, but many can be seen to be fenestrated with the electron microscope. It is only the apparently infrequent large gaps of endothelial continuity which can be appreciated with the light microscope.

ELECTRON MICROSCOPY OF BRAIN TUMOR MICROVASCULATURE

The transmission electron microscope truly opens one's eyes to the magnitude of endothelial defects which occur in brain tumors. One sees capillaries with endothelial cells so plump that the lumen they form is only a few microns in diameter (fig. 7.10). There are also many instances of completely occluded vessels (fig. 7.11), even in perfused material: the lumin are obliterated by either grossly hyperplastic endothelium or by so-called invasion of the lumen by parenchymal tumor cells with cytologic characteristics too ill-defined to be distinguished from hyperplastic endothelium. With the electron microscope, the fine structure of the plump

Figure 7.9.

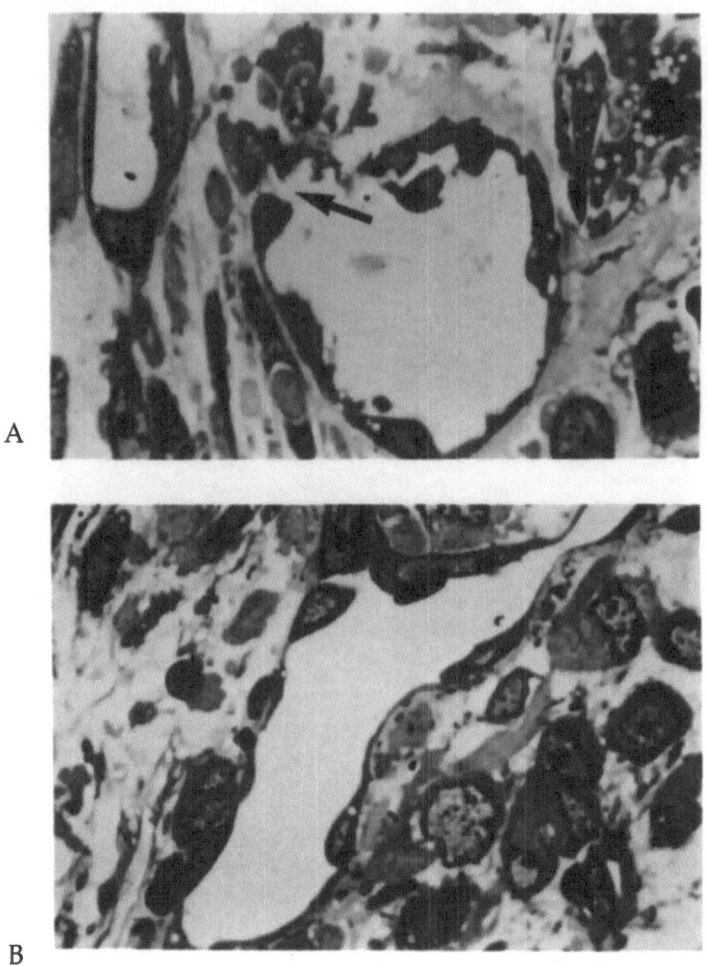

A

B

Dog gliomas induced with avian sarcoma virus. A. A gross defect in the endothelial wall at the light microscopic level (arrow). B. A typical thin-walled capillary. This vessel appeared continuous by light microscopy but was fenestrated when viewed with the electron microscope.

or mitotic endothelial cells which can also be seen at lower magnification with the light microscope can be appreciated (fig. 7.12). Many of these endothelial cells contain an excess of vesicles and dense bodies. The subcellular organelles have no specific alterations although occasionally there seems to be an excessive number of large mitochondria within cytoplasm of variable density. Our attempts to relate these general cytologic characteristics to embryonic or developing blood vessels do not suggest there is any important similarity. Others have arrived at the same conclusion in studies of human brain tumor endothelium (Waggener and Beggs

1976). The basal lamina of tumor vessels is more variable in width than in the normal brain. It is often remarkably reduplicated (fig. 7.11); at other times it is so wispy so as to appear nearly absent (figs. 7.13*B*, 7.13*C*, and 7.14*A*).

Figure 7.10.

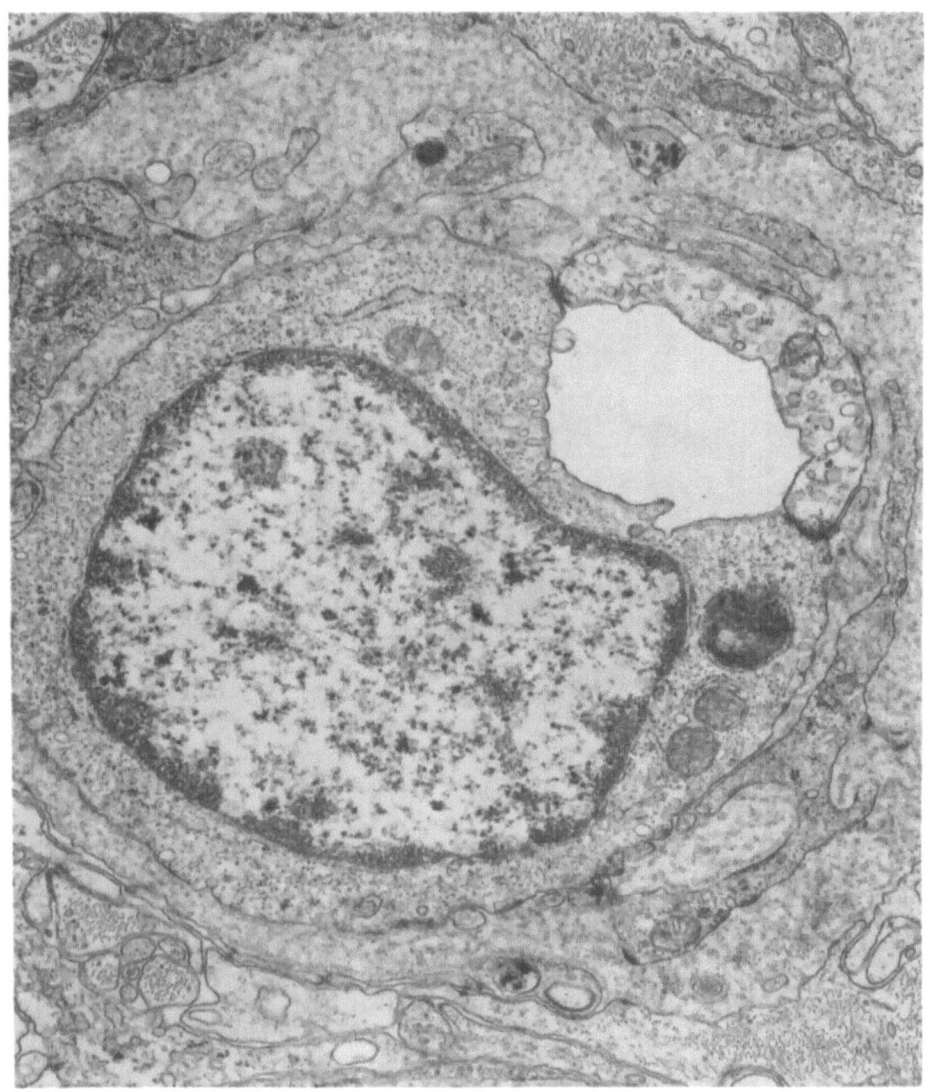

Plump tumor endothelium with small lumen in dog glioma induced with avian sarcoma virus.

Figure 7.11.

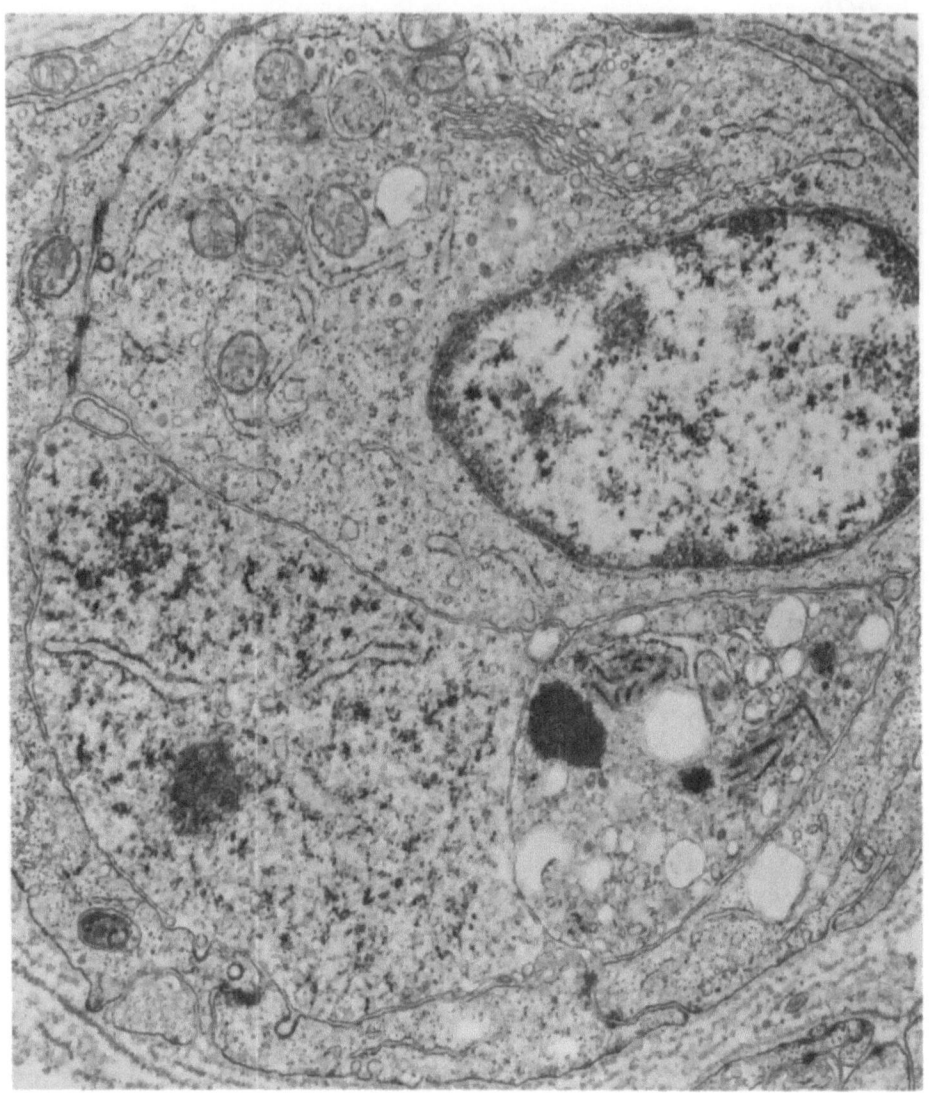

Occluded capillary in a rat glioma induced with avian sarcoma virus. Note the wispy, reduplicated basal lamina.

In the exceedingly vascular rat gliomas induced by intracerebral inoculation of the Kirsten strain of murine sarcoma virus 3, we found many vascular channels apparently devoid of endothelial cells. These channels appear to be formed by the primary tumor cell of neuroectodermal origin. In this tumor there were formed blood elements within the interstices between subadjacent tumor cells. This extreme example of absence of a blood-brain barrier apparently does not occur in the experimental gliomas induced by avian sarcoma virus in hamsters, rats, or dogs.

Figure 7.12.

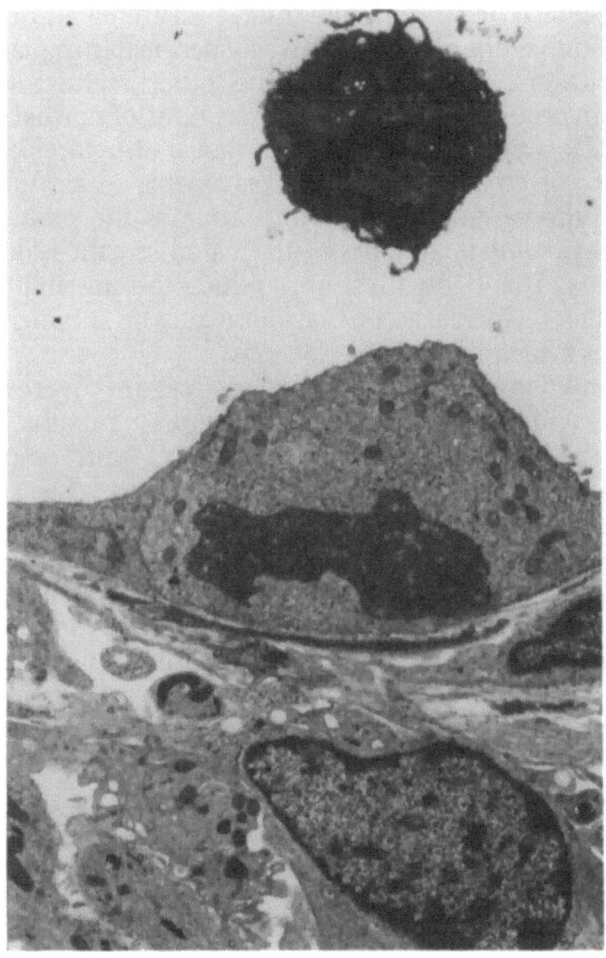

Electron micrograph of a hyperplastic endothelial cell in a rat glioma induced with avian sarcoma virus. Compare to those seen by light microscopy and labeled with ³H-thymidine in fig. 7.8.

We have never observed an unequivocally open intercellular junction between tumor endothelial cells. If one is rigid about the criteria for a tight intercellular junction, horseradish peroxidase must be used; even without this tracer, however, one can attempt to assess the appearance of the junctions at high magnification by electron microscopy. There are a plethora of problems in the effort, such as plane of section, but junctions are so plentiful that it seems reasonable to expect that if open junctions occurred with any frequency one would see one from time to time. Those that have been described by others in human biopsy specimens (Long 1970) may be due to imperfect fixation or to factors such as altered tonicity, which have been shown to open tight junctions in experimental studies (Rapoport et al. 1972; Westergaard 1977).

Perhaps the most important and most characteristic alteration in brain tumor capillaries is the occurrence of fenestrated and discontinuous endothelial cells. These fenestrations are structurally indistinguishable from those which occur normally in area postrema and other specialized regions of normal brain, which are freely permeable to plasma protein and histologic tracers. Since none of the other features of brain tumor endothelium occur in these specialized regions of normal brain, and since it is generally agreed that these endothelial structures are the basis for permeability of these regions, it is reasonable to assume that their occurrence in the vasculature of brain tumors is the primary morphologic mechanism by which contents of the blood stream leak into the tumor compartment. This belief does not exclude the possibility that vesicular transport may be increased or that there may be submicroscopic biologic mechanisms which play a role.

Fenestrations are round, by serial section, are covered by a 50-Å thick diaphragm, without an apparent substructure, and attached to the outer leaflet of the normal-appearing, bilaminar "unit" membrane of the neighboring endothelial cells (figs. 7.13, A and B). They occur only in the most attenuated portions of the endothelial cell wall and are usually single but may be seen in series. The subadjacent basal lamina is often wispy, and the extracellular space between the underlying parenchymal tumor cells is invariably expanded. We have learned to locate fenestrations by searching in those regions of tumor which appear loose. While the rationale is self-fulfilling—for example, one searches for leaky vessels in areas of tumor which appear to have been rendered excessively permeable to fluid—it affords an intuitively satisfying observation and suggests, a priori, that the fenestrations have functional significance.

Endothelial gaps (fig. 7.13C) occur less frequently than fenestrations. They are, perhaps, more questionable as actual in vivo structures than are fenestrations because they might be artificially induced by the pressure of perfusion-fixation. Gaps never occur in normal portions of brains of tumor-bearing animals, however, and they resemble normally occurring discontinuous endothelium which occurs elsewhere in the body (such as in the liver, spleen and bone marrow). Since fenestrations and gaps may occur in the same capillary profile, it is possible that they are related to each other in some fundamental way. The occasional occurrence of extremely attenuated but nonfenestrated zones of endothelium, covered with a nondescript "fuzz" (fig. 7.14A), and instances of totally bizarre structural abnormalities of an unclassified sort (fig. 7.14B) may be additional characteristics of brain tumor capillaries since they do not occur in normal brain.

THE MICROVASCULATURE OF HUMAN BRAIN TUMORS

Interest in the blood vessels of brain tumors did not begin with the electron microscope. A substantial volume of literature has dealt with the problem (Nystrom 1960), and as information accumulated about general aspects of the blood-brain barrier, many investigators recognized brain

Figure 7.13.

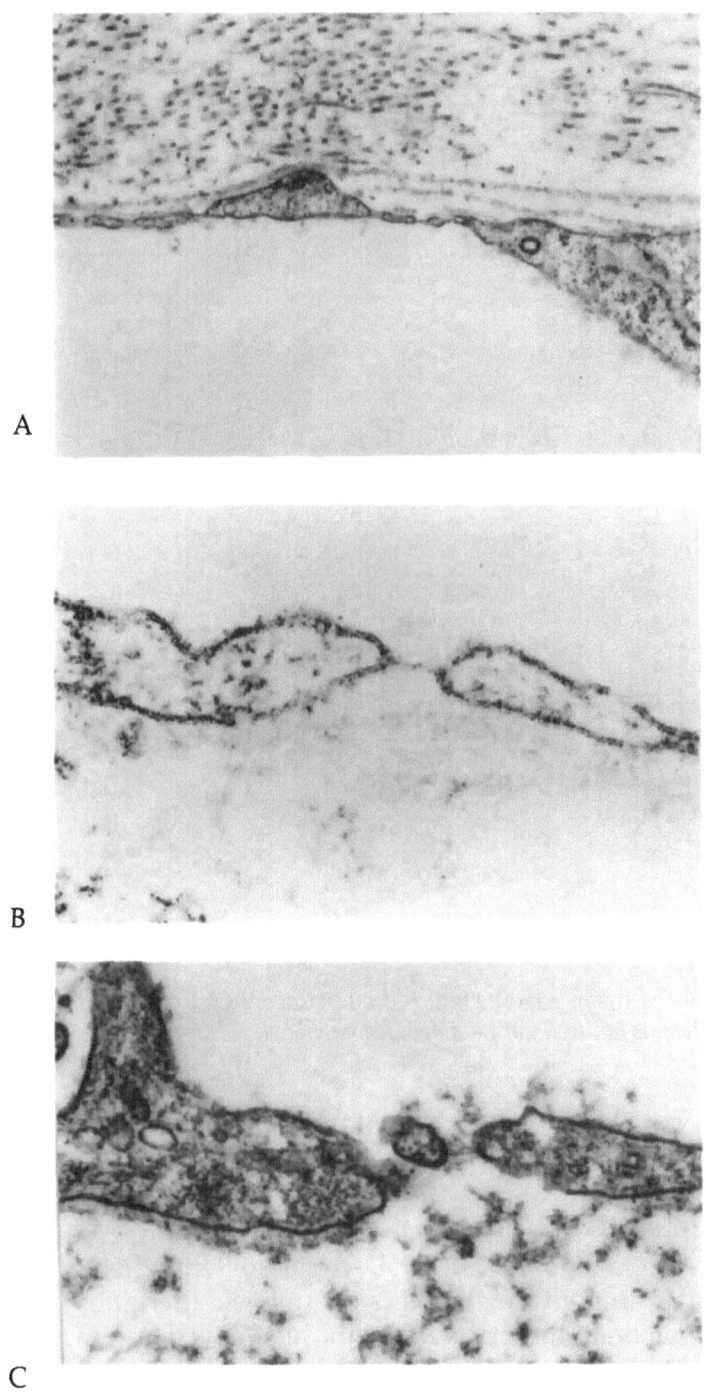

A

B

C

Endothelial fenestrations at low magnification (A) and at high magnification (B) with a discontinuous endothelium (C). All are from dog gliomas induced with avian sarcoma virus.

Figure 7.14.

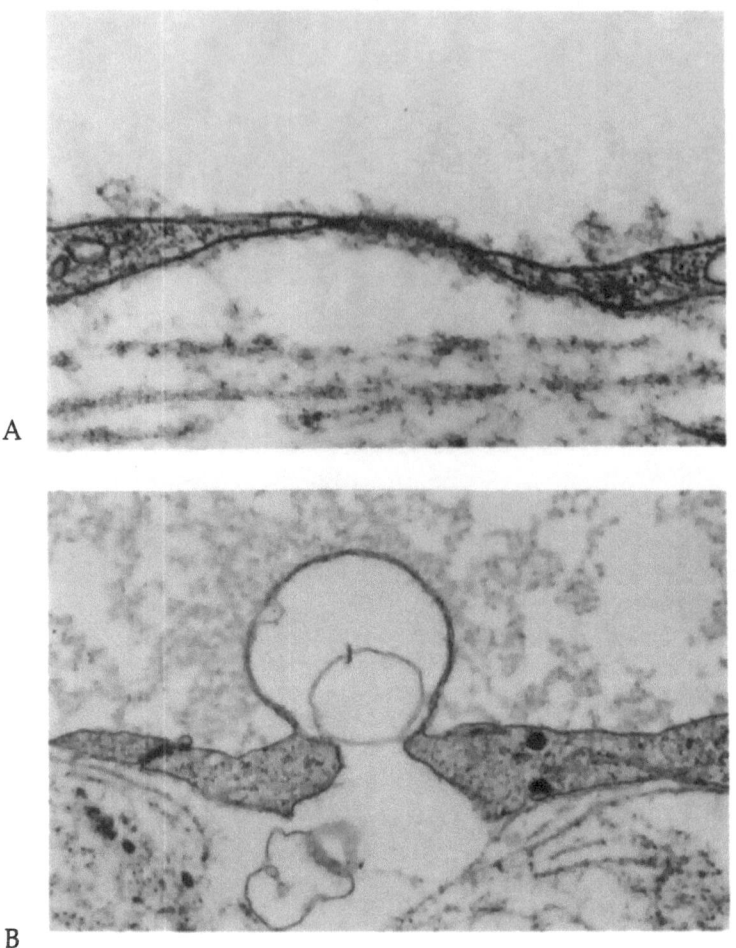

Attenuated tumor endothelium (A) and bizarre endothelial alteration (B) in dog gliomas induced with avian sarcoma virus.

tumors among those pathologic states in which profound alterations could regularly be seen. Once it became apparent that the endothelium is the anatomic location of the barrier to blood-borne protein, studies rapidly focused upon the endothelial cell and the biology of permeability in brain tumors. Although ultrastructural studies of endothelial alterations in human brain tumors are even less quantifiable than those conducted in experimental brain tumors, such as those of my colleagues and I, a spectrum of structural defects including fenestrations have been seen in human specimens: neurilemoma (Hirano et al. 1972); neuroblastoma, glioblastoma, and medulloblastoma (Waggener and Beggs 1976); meningioma (Waggener and Beggs 1976; Long 1973); pituitary adenoma

(Waggener and Beggs 1976; Hirano et al. 1972b; Schechter 1972); heman-gioblastoma (Waggener and Beggs 1976; Tani et al. 1974); choroid plexus papilloma (Waggener and Beggs 1976; Carter et al. 1972); craniopharyn-gioma (Hirano et al. 1973); metastatic renal carcinoma (Hirano and Zimmerman 1972); and lymphoma (Hirano et al. 1974).

The observations in humans, like the parallel ones in experimental brain tumors, have not been linked as yet with any understanding of the genesis of the vascular alterations. Nothing in the structure of capillaries proliferating under the influence of tumor angiogenesis factor, for example, corresponds with the microvascular abnormalities I have considered here (Folkman 1974; Folkman and Cotran 1976). In any event, it seems to me that these abnormalities are not merely a superficial adaptation of normal vascular endothelium, appropriated from host tissue, nor are the endothelial alterations regressive in the degenerative sense. Instead, they appear to be a result of a transformation into a less specialized type of endothelium, a de-differentiation, as if the vasculature were influenced by the neoplastic agency itself or isolated from some regulating factor derived from normal brain tissue.

The most important practical question raised by these observations on the heterotypical vascular endothelium of human brain tumors concerns their implications for the delivery of effective chemotherapy to tumor cells. The presence of open communications between the vascular compartment and the parenchyma indicates that chemotherapeutic agents may have access to tumor tissue through bulk flow and that attributes of such agents that have hitherto been studied most intensively, such as their molecular size, lipid solubility, and degree of ionization, are not the most crucial. It would appear that potentially therapeutic agents should be studied for their uptake and metabolic fate in tumor cells and for their dosage and timing of delivery in relation to the kinetics of tumor cell growth. The sink effect of the extracellular fluid and spinal fluid flow should also be examined. Until these factors are understood and until an experimental brain tumor is destroyed in the light of knowledge derived from such studies, it seems unlikely that any significant progress will be made in the treatment of human brain tumors. Empirical drug trials have yielded very little thus far, and we have no reason to hope that this will be otherwise in the future. Instead, we must look to systematic studies and rigorous biological data in order to move forward.

REFERENCES

Bigner, D. D. et al. Factors influencing the cell type of brain tumors induced in dogs by Schmidt-Ruppin Rous sarcoma virus. *J. Neuropathol. Exp. Neurol.* 31:583–595, 1972a.

Bigner, D. D. et al. Virus-cell relationships in dog brain tumors induced with Schmidt-Ruppin Rous sarcoma virus. *Prog. Exp. Tumor Res.* 17:40–58, 1972b.

Brightman, M. W. Morphology of blood-brain interface. In *The ocular and cerebrospinal fluids*, eds. L. Z. Bito, H. Davson, J. D. Fenstermacher. New York: Academic Press, 1978.

Brightman, M. W., and Reese, T. S. Junctions between intimately apposed cell membranes in the vertebrate brain. *J. Cell Biol.* 40:647–677, 1969.

Brightman, M. W. et al. The blood-brain barrier to proteins under normal and pathological conditions. *J. Neurol. Sci.* 10:215–239, 1970.

Brightman, M. W. et al. A mechanism underlying the lack of a blood-brain barrier to peroxidase in virally induced brain tumors. *J. Neuropathol. Exp. Neurol.* 30:139–140, 1971.

Carter, L. P.; Beggs, J. L.; and Waggener, J. D. Ultrastructure of three choroid plexus papillomas. *Cancer* 30:1130–1136, 1972.

Copeland, D. D.; Talley, F. A.; and Bigner, D. D. The fine structure of intracranial neoplasms induced by the inoculation of avian sarcoma virus in neonatal and adult rats. *Am. J. Pathol.* 83:149–166, 1976.

Cox, D. J.; Pilkington, G. J.; and Lantos, P. L. The fine structure of blood vessels in ethylnitrosourea-induced tumors of the rat nervous system. With special reference to the breakdown of the blood-brain barrier. *Br. J. Exp. Pathol.* 57:419–430, 1976.

Folkman, J. Tumor angiogenesis factor. *Cancer Res.* 34:2109–2113, 1974.

Folkman, J., and Cotran, R. Relation of vascular proliferation to tumor growth. *Int. Rev. Exp. Pathol.* 16:207–248, 1976.

Hashimoto, P. H. On the fenestrated capillary endothelium in the area postrema of the rat and the cat. *Acta Anat. Nippon.* 41:154–155, 1966.

Hashimoto, P. H., and Hama, K. An electron microscope study on protein uptake into brain regions devoid of the blood-brain barrier. *Med. J. Osaka Univ.* 18:331–346, 1968.

Hirano, A., and Zimmerman, H. M. Fenestrated blood vessels in a metastatic renal carcinoma in the brain. *Lab. Invest.* 26:465–468, 1972.

Hirano, A.; Dembitzer, H. M.; and Zimmerman, H. M. Fenestrated blood vessels in neurilemoma. *Lab. Invest.* 27:305–309, 1972a.

Hirano, A.; Tomiyasu, U.; and Zimmerman, H. M. The fine structure of blood vessels in chromophobe adenoma. *Acta Neuropathol.* 22:200–207, 1972b.

Hirano, A.; Ghatek, N. R.; and Zimmerman, H. M. Fenestrated blood vessels in craniopharyngioma. *Acta Neuropathol.* 26:171–177, 1973.

Hirano, A. et al. A comparison of the fine structure of small blood vessels in intracranial and retroperitoneal malignant lymphomas. *Acta Neuropathol.* 27:93–104, 1974.

Hirano, A., and Matsui, T. Vascular structures in brain tumors. *Hum. Pathol.* 6:611–621, 1975.

Klara, P. M., and Brizzee, K. R. The ultrastructural morphology of the squirrel monkey area postrema. *Cell Tissue Res.* 160:315–326, 1975.

Klara, P. M., and Brizzee, K. R. Ultrastructure of the feline area postrema. *J. Comp. Neurol.* 72:409–431, 1977.

Long, D. M. Capillary ultrastructure and the blood-brain barrier in human malignant brain tumors. *J. Neurosurg.* 32:127–144, 1970.

Long, D. M. Vascular ultrastructure in human meningioma and schwannomas. *J. Neurosurg.* 38:409–419, 1973.

Nystrom, S. Pathological changes in blood vessels of human glioblastoma multiforme. *Acta Path. Microbiol. Scand.* 49 (Suppl 137):1–85, 1960.

Peters, A.; Palay, S. L.; and Webster, H. de F. *The fine structure of the nervous system*. Philadelphia: W.B. Saunders Co., 1976.

Rapoport, S. I.; Hori, M.; and Klatzo, I. Testing of a hypothesis for osmotic opening of the blood-brain barrier. *Am. J. Physiol.* 223:323–331, 1972.

Schechter, J. Ultrastructural changes in the capillary bed of human pituitary tumors. *Am. J. Pathol.* 67:109–126, 1972.

Tani, E. et al. Fenestrated vessels in human hemangioblastoma. *J. Neurosurg.* 40:697–705, 1974.

Vick, N. A.; Bigner, D. D.; and Kvedar, J. P. The fine structure of canine gliomas and intracranial sarcomas induced by the Schmidt-Ruppin strain of Rous sarcoma virus. *J. Neuropathol. Exp. Neurol.* 30:354–367, 1971.

Vick, N. A.; and Bigner, D. D. Some structural aspects of dog brain tumors induced with the Schmidt-Ruppin strain of the Rous sarcoma virus. *Prog. Exp. Tumor Res.* 17:59–73, 1972a.

Vick, N. A., and Bigner, D. D. Microvascular abnormalities in virally induced canine brain tumors: structural bases for altered blood-brain barrier function. *J. Neurol. Sci.* 17:29–39, 1972b.

Vick, N. A.; Khandekar, J. D.; and Bigner, D. D. Chemotherapy of brain tumors. The "blood-brain barrier" is not a factor. *Arch. Neurol.* 34:523–526, 1977.

Waggener, J. D., and Beggs, J. L. Vasculature of neural neoplasms. *Adv. Neurol.* 15:27–49, 1976.

Walker, M. D., and The Brain Tumor Study Group. Evaluation of BCNU and/or radiotherapy in the treatment of neoplastic gliomas. *J. Neurosurg.* 49:333–343, 1978.

Westergaard, E. The blood-brain barrier to horseradish peroxidase under normal and experimental conditions. *Acta Neuropathol.* 39:181–187, 1977.

Wilfong, R. F.; Bigner, D. D.; and Self, D. J. Brain tumor types induced by the Schmidt-Ruppin strain of Rous sarcoma virus in inbred Fischer rats. *Acta Neuropathol.* 25:196–206, 1973.

Wilson, C. B. Chemotherapy of brain tumors. *Adv. Neurol.* 15:361–367, 1976.

Yung, W. K.; Blank, N. K.; and Vick, N. A. "Glioblastoma": induction of a reproducible autochthonous tumor in rats with murine sarcoma virus. *Neurology* 26:76–83, 1976.

8

A Model for Brain Metastasis

William R. Shapiro

Numerous animal-brain tumor models have been developed to assist in choosing new chemotherapeutic agents for primary brain tumors (Bigner and Swenberg 1977). None can be used directly to test for hematogenous metastatic disease because each depends on direct tumor (or viral) implantation into the brain, which necessarily traumatizes the brain. In order (1) to circumvent the problem of mechanical disruption of brain tissue so as to examine chemotherapy and its relation to blood-brain barrier function in brain tumors, and (2) to develop a system to test agents specifically for metastatic brain tumors, my colleagues and I developed an animal model of metastatic brain tumor that does not require direct implantation into the brain (Ushio et al. 1977a). We have since used this model to test a series of chemotherapeutic agents, to begin an evaluation of the distribution of chemotherapeutic agents utilizing the marker molecule methotrexate, to examine the effects of radiation therapy, and to define the breakdown of the blood-brain barrier using α-aminoisobutyric acid. These studies are reviewed in this report.

DEVELOPMENT OF THE MODEL

The method for production of the metastatic brain tumor model has been described in detail (Ushio et al. 1977a). Female Wistar rats weighing approximately 150 gm are anesthetized with sodium pentobarbital, and the right common carotid artery is exposed under a dissecting microscope. Using a 32-gauge needle, the right common carotid artery is inoculated with 0.01–0.02 ml of a tumor-cell suspension of Walker 256 carcinoma containing $0.5–1 \times 10^6$ viable cells. The animals are observed, and if nothing further is done, tumor take occurs in about 82% (table 8.1) with a median survival of about 27 days. Approximately 30% of the animals develop intracerebral metastases, and 83% develop extracranial metastases, primarily in the jaw, that prevent eating and eventually kill the animal by inanition. External carotid ligation (table 8.1) increases the take of intracerebral metastatic tumors but does not reduce the extracranial metastases and does not increase survival. Administration of cyclophosphamide (15 mg/kg intravenously) on day 14 reduces the overall take rate to about half,

134

increases the intracerebral metastatic take rate to 100%, and reduces the clinically significant extracranial metastases to 25%, permitting the animals to live twice as long. Cyclophosphamide produces cytopathic effects in the jaw tumor 3–7 days after treatment. In the brain, tumors are distributed in the cerebrum (87%), cerebellum (50%), choroid plexus (62%), pineal body (25%) and pituitary gland (12%). Figure 8.1 shows a coronal section of a rat brain with three metastatic brain tumors in the right cerebral hemisphere. There is also localized hydrocephalus on the right side.

Clinically, the animals develop hemiparesis between days 25 and 35 after inoculation (approximately 2–3 weeks after the initial low-dose cyclophosphamide treatment). They also tend to lose weight beginning at about day 7, but after therapy they gain weight until about day 28 when tumor-bearing animals again begin to lose weight. It is of importance that about half of the animals are cured by the low-dose cyclophosphamide treatment; the other half develop metastatic brain tumors as detailed later.

CHEMOTHERAPY OF THE METASTATIC BRAIN TUMOR MODEL

We have recently completed a set of chemotherapy experiments on the metastatic brain tumor model (Hasegawa et al. 1979a). We also treated subcutaneously implanted tumors to determine the approximate effectiveness of the drug against the tumor when it was implanted entirely outside of the brain where blood-brain barrier phenomena could be excluded. We also treated animals bearing directly implanted intracerebral Walker 256 and compared the results to the intracarotid inoculated metastatic brain tumor model. We tested a variety of drugs based on their use

Table 8.1

SO-CALLED INTRACEREBRAL METASTASES DEVELOPED AFTER CAROTID ARTERY INJECTION OF WALKER 256 CARCINOMA CELLS IN WISTAR RATS

Condition	Percentage of Takes	Median Survival Days	Intracerebral Metastases (percentage)	Extracranial Metastases (percentage)
Control	82	27	30	83
External carotid artery ligation	75	27.5	67	83
Cyclophosphamide*	53	60	100	25

*15 mg/kg intravenously on day 14.

Figure 8.1.

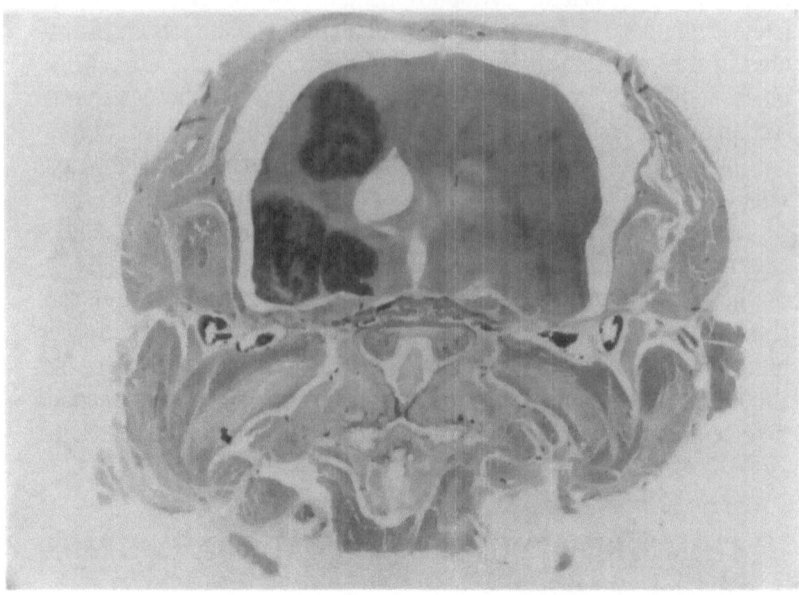

Metastatic rat brain tumor. Coronal section of rat brain 51 days after intracarotid tumor inoculation and 37 days after treatment with intravenous cyclophosphamide (30 mg/kg). Three tumors occupy the right cerebral hemisphere. The rigid lateral ventricle is dilated. (Hematoxylin and eosin.)

against primary brain tumors in patients, choosing doses at or below the animals' LD_{10} (defined as the dose of drug which produces 10% toxic deaths). The drugs included 3 nitrosoureas: 1-(4-amino-2-methyl-5-pyrimidinyl) methyl-3-(-2-chloroethyl)-3-nitrosourea (ACNU), a new water-soluble nitrosourea developed in Japan and found to be effective against primary experimental brain tumors (Hasegawa et al. 1979b); 1-(2-chloroethyl)-3-cyclohexyl-1-nitrosourea (CCNU); and 1-(2-chloroethyl)-3-(4-methyl cyclohexyl)-1-nitrosourea (methyl-CCNU). Other drugs were cyclophosphamide, methotrexate (MTX), procarbazine, and the steroid dexamethasone.

In the subcutaneous tumor studies, the tumor was implanted into the right axilla of Wistar rats and the volume of the tumor was calculated weekly after measuring the tumor's long and short axis. In the intracerebral tumor studies, a 1-mm³ fragment of tumor was inoculated percutaneously with a modified 19-gauge spinal needle into the right cerebral hemisphere of anesthetized Wistar rats. The animals were treated on day 16 after inoculation. Saline or vehicle-treated control animals were used for comparison. The animals with "metastatic" tumors resulting from intra-arterial injections were initially treated with cyclophosphamide on day 14 after inoculation as noted above. They were weighed every other day. As they began losing weight (about day 28) and when they had reached a grade of early weakness, they were divided into control and treated groups of similar weight and grade. The treated animals received the drugs, and the control animals received saline or a vehicle.

The most effective agents against the subcutaneous tumor were the three nitrosoureas and cyclophosphamide. These drugs caused the tumors to shrink with loss of almost all of the tumors within two weeks after treatment. Most of the tumors became palpable again within a week, and all regrew within 3 weeks. Methotrexate produced a definite but transient effect about a week after treatment, but within another week the tumor had increased in size about 10-fold. Procarbazine failed to reduce the size of any of the tumors. The results of chemotherapy of the metastatic and the direct intracerebral inoculated tumor are shown in table 8.2. The maximum increased lifespan for each of the treatments and the maximum longterm survivors are shown; the data represent a distillation of a large

Table 8.2

RESULTS OF CHEMOTHERAPY OF "METASTATIC" RAT BRAIN TUMOR
AND DIRECTLY INOCULATED RAT BRAIN TUMOR

Drug	Dose*	"Metastatic"		Direct Inoculum	
		Increased Lifespan Over Control (percentage)	Longterm Survivors † (60+ days after inoculation)	Increased Lifespan Over Control (percentage)	Longterm Survivors (60+ days after inoculation)
ACNU	30	153	1	224	2 of 4 animals
CCNU	40	169	1	180	1 of 15 animals
	60	186	3		
Methyl-CCNU	40	213	3		
Cyclophosphamide	60	206	1	108	0 of 5 animals
Methotrexate	100	75	1	0	0 of 5 animals
Procarbazine	250	13	0		
Dexamethasone	10‡	0	0		

*Intravenous injection.
†Each drug was assessed in 10 animals with metastatic tumors.
‡Twice daily for 10 days intramuscularly.

series of experiments. The Wilcoxon rank-sum test was used statistically to analyze improvement in lifespan. The median day of death of the treated group was compared to that of the control and the percentage of increased lifespan over control was determined. Longterm survivors were calculated as the number of animals surviving more than 60 days after inoculation.

As can be seen for the metastatic brain tumor model, ACNU, CCNU and methyl-CCNU all significantly increased median survival of treated animals and up to 30% of the animals survived more than 60 days after initial tumor inoculation. Cyclophosphamide was likewise highly effective, but methotrexate was considerably less so and procarbazine and dexamethasone were essentially ineffective. In the directly inoculated tumor model, ACNU and CCNU were both effective, cyclophosphamide somewhat less so, and methotrexate in this model was ineffective. Some intercomparisons between the two models are possible. Cyclophosphamide was more effective in the metastatic tumor model than in the direct intracerebral tumor model, but this result may relate to the fact that the metastatic treated animals had previously been treated with cyclophosphamide. The same may also be true for the methotrexate effect. The nitrosoureas were about equally efficacious although ACNU appeared to be more effective against the directly inoculated tumor than against the metastatic tumor.

These results indicate that the nitrosoureas and cyclophosphamide effectively treated metastatic tumors even after tumors had developed in the brain. Thus, cyclophosphamide, which was used to create the model because it could not cure or prevent brain tumor growth, could be used for therapy once the tumor had grown. None of the treatment protocols cured many of the animals although several rats were longterm survivors. These results, especially in comparison to the directly implanted intracerebral model, have implications for the problems of blood-brain barrier. Some aspects of these are developed in the discussion.

RADIATION THERAPY

Preliminary experiments have now been completed utilizing radiation therapy to treat the metastatic brain tumor model. This work was done in collaboration with Dr. Jae-Ho Kim of Memorial Sloan-Kettering Cancer Center. Both high-energy x-ray and betatron radiation therapy were used (table 8.3). A specific problem was created because the radiation was delivered to the top of the anesthetized animal's heads while the animal was restrained in a special case. Because radiation damaged the animal's mouth by this technique, many died of radiation damage rather than of brain tumor. Nevertheless, there was a marked increase in survival with an increased total dose of radiation therapy. Longterm survivors averaged 50%. Walker 256 carcinoma is sensitive to radiation and this mode of treatment effectively treated a model of epidural spinal cord compression

Table 8.3

RESULTS OF RADIATION THERAPY OF "METASTATIC" RAT BRAIN TUMOR

Total dose (rads)	Schedule (rads × doses)	Maximum Increased Lifespan Over Control (percentage)	Longterm Survivors (60+ days after inoculation)
1,000	1,000 × 1	71	0 of 12 animals
1,500	500 × 3	171	1 of 12 animals
2,000	1,000 × 2	271	4 of 13 animals
2,000	200 × 10	371	5 of 9 animals
3,000	500 × 3 + 300 × 5	329	6 of 11 animals
3,600	(250 × 2) × 3* + (150 × 2) × 3	193	4 of 12 animals

*250 rads twice daily for 3 days followed by 150 rads twice daily for 3 days.

produced in the rat using Walker 256 (Ushio et al. 1977b). Because of the radiation damage to the mouth parts, it was difficult to combine the radiation therapy with chemotherapy although this was attempted. In no case, however, have we been able to achieve longer survival with combined radiation with chemotherapy than was achieved with the radiation alone (see Chapter 24). These experiments continue in an effort to improve therapy of the tumor.

METHOTREXATE CONCENTRATION IN BRAIN TUMOR AND BRAIN AND ITS ALTERATION BY INTRACAROTID MANNITOL

As noted elsewhere, the influence of the blood-brain barrier on chemotherapy remains controversial. Nevertheless, the ability to enhance movement of small water-soluble molecules across such a barrier may improve the results of chemotherapy. Recently, Allen and others (1978) reported a method for enhancing the penetration of methotrexate into the brain and spinal fluid of rats bearing meningeal carcinomatosis. The method is that of Rapoport described in detail elsewhere in this monograph (see Chapter 6). After development of the meningeal carcinomatosis model (Ushio et al. 1977c), we investigated its chemotherapy (Ushio et al. 1977d) and became interested in determining the concentration of methotrexate in the spinal fluid because that drug had been used in treatment protocols. We examined the concentration of methotrexate in the blood, cerebrospinal fluid (CSF), and brain of animals harboring meningeal carcinomatosis and then repeated these studies in other animals after the intracarotic administration of hypertonic mannitol. Methotrexate concentrations were measured by microbiologic assay (Mehta and Hutchison 1977). We found that meningeal carcinomatosis itself increased the concentration of methotrexate in the CSF after intravenous administration (as compared to controls), confirming that meningeal carcinomatosis breaks down the blood-brain barrier or permits neovascularization and thus circumvents the barrier.

Hypertonic mannitol infusion appears to open the barrier by causing loss of fluid from the capillary endothelial cells of the brain in the distribution of the carotid artery infused by mannitol. This loss of fluid causes the endothelial cells to shrink, thus pulling away from their neighboring cells and breaking the tight junctions which characterize capillary blood vessels in brain. Materials up to large protein size (M.W. 70,000 daltons and larger) may then rapidly diffuse through the opened junctions into the surrounding brain. Mannitol appears to perform the same function for methotrexate. Intracarotid mannitol increased the brain concentration of methotrexate on the side of the infused carotid and increased the CSF concentration as well. There was a suggestion that the combination of intracarotid mannitol plus intravenous methotrexate had a therapeutic advantage over intravenous methotrexate alone.

Utilizing similar methodology, we have begun to examine the methotrexate concentration in the brain tumor, the brain adjacent to tumor, and the distant brain in our metastatic brain tumor animals. A typical experiment is shown in figure 8.2, which depicts the concentration of methotrexate in metastatic brain tumor animals for tumor, adjacent brain, and distant brain both without mannitol and with intracarotid mannitol. As can be seen, the methotrexate concentration within the tumor is substantial and is not increased by the addition of mannitol. Similarly, enough methotrexate leaks into the adjacent brain so that intracarotid mannitol produces little further change in concentration of methotrexate in that region. On the other hand, the concentration of methotrexate in the brain distant from the brain tumor is markedly enhanced by mannitol. Whether this increased brain concentration will improve therapy of the disease remains to be seen, and such studies are now underway. These results suggest that within the limitations of our model it may be difficult to demonstrate a sufficiently intact blood-brain barrier in the brain near the tumor to improve therapy by forcibly opening it.

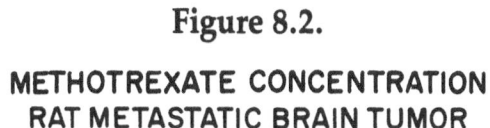

Figure 8.2.

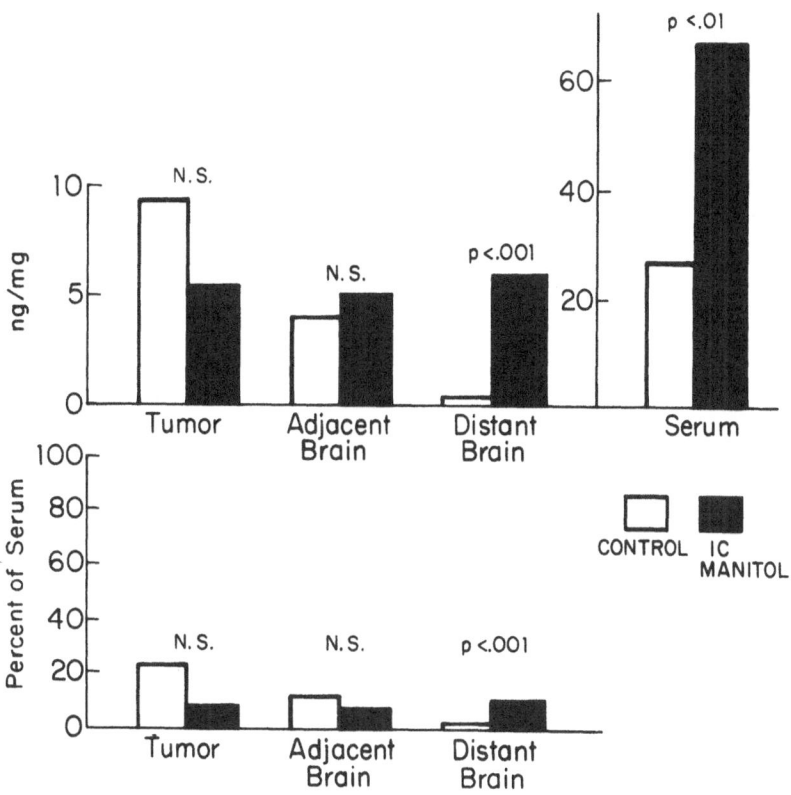

Methotrexate concentration in metastatic rat brain tumor, brain adjacent to tumor, and brain distant from tumor in rats 1 hour after receiving methotrexate 100 mg/kg intravenously without and in conjunction with the intracarotid infusion (ipsilateral to the brain tumor) of hyperosmolar mannitol. In the control rats the methotrexate concentration in the tumor and adjacent brain was high and not significantly changed by the mannitol. Methotrexate failed to enter the distant brain until the hyperosmolar mannitol opened the blood-brain barrier.

TRACER STUDIES OF THE BLOOD-BRAIN BARRIER

Recently Blasberg and others (1978) reported an autoradiographic technique to measure the permeability of normal and abnormal brain capillaries using the synthetic (nonmetabolized) neutral amino acid, α-amino-isobutyric acid (AIB). AIB has slow transport across normal brain capillaries but is concentrated to high levels in brain tissue once the blood-brain barrier is breached. The molecule rapidly gains entrance into cells in the same area by sharing the transport system A-alanine, but because the molecule is not further metabolized, it remains within the cell. By labeling AIB with ^{14}C and using autoradiography, the location of the breakdown in the blood-brain barrier can be depicted.

Blasberg and his colleagues have also used this system to quantify change in the blood-brain barrier secondary to a variety of lesions. In a collaborative effort with our laboratory, rats bearing metastatic brain tumors received intravenous AIB. The brains were sectioned, frozen and autoradiograms developed. One such study demonstrated the presence of the AIB in the immediate area of the metastatic brain tumor (fig. 8.3). This investigation suggests that the barrier is broken down only within the confines of the tumor and not in the surrounding brain. We plan to compare these studies with others using diffusible compounds such as albumin or EDTA, which like methotrexate, would be expected to diffuse into the surrounding brain.

DISCUSSION

Animal models of human cancer must deal with two problems: the pathologic nature of the tumor and its location in the body. If the model is designed to help define and choose effective therapy, it must be possible to predict with reasonable accuracy human tumor response to the therapy under consideration. Although the problem of pathologic similarity between the animal tumor and that of humans must be solved for all cancers, the problem of the location of the tumor is especially important when dealing with brain tumors. Here the question is very specific. Does the location of the tumor within the brain impose unique properties on the tumor that require approaches to chemotherapy differing from those used against tumors situated elsewhere in the body? Animal brain tumor models designed to get at this question have involved direct inoculation of tumor into the brain. Our metastatic brain tumor model was designed to avoid direct trauma to the brain and permit the study of the tumor in situ. In our initial experiments we found that drugs effective against brain tumors in the clinic could also be used to treat metastatic brain tumors. We also found, however, that drugs effective in the treatment of metastatic brain tumor were equally effective against a directly inoculated tumor and against a subcutaneous tumor. One might then reasonably question the need for a metastatic brain tumor model if one can examine chemotherapy in directly implanted intracerebral or subcutaneous tumor models.

We believe that both the intracerebral and the metastatic tumor models are necessary to study brain tumor therapy. Such models measure survival within narrow limits: the minimal increase in growth required to produce cerebral death rather than the larger change required to produce animal death in tumor implanted subcutaneously. Furthermore, previous studies have demonstrated that a drug effect as measured by survival of animals with intracerebrally implanted tumors more closely predicts the

Figure 8.3.

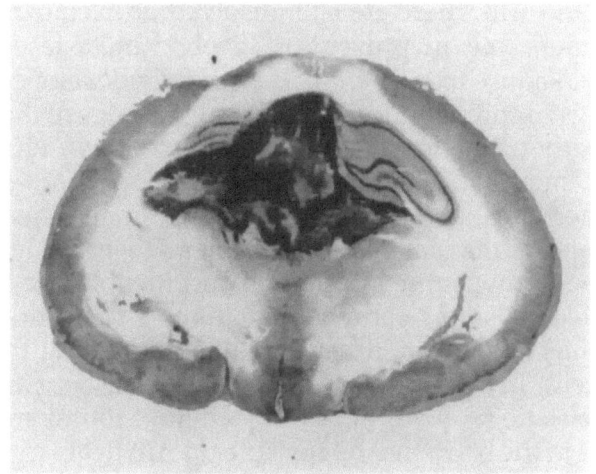

A

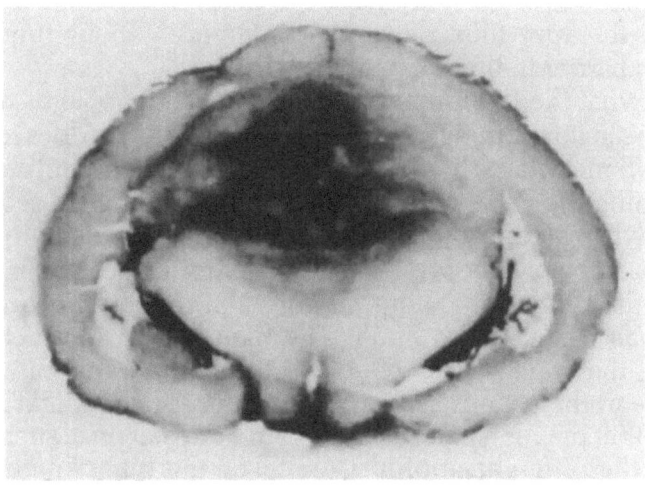

B

Metastatic rat brain tumor after intravenous infusion of amino isobutyric acid (AIB). The AIB occupies the area of the large metastatic brain tumor indicating breakdown of the blood-brain barrier in this region. A. Cresyl-violet section. The brain tumor occupies a central location. B. Autoradiogram. The black areas show the location of the AIB.

results in similarly treated patients where survival is also an endpoint. Finally, the intracerebral tumor model and specifically the metastatic tumor model still represent the only way that one can study blood-brain barrier function in brain tumors, and there is reason to believe that this problem is still important.

Although the blood-brain barrier appears to be broken down in fully grown tumors (Vick et al. 1977) as confirmed by our own studies with methotrexate and AIB, there are still unsolved problems in treating fully developed tumors and in preventing cerebral metastases by systemic chemotherapy. Failure to cure animals with fully developed tumors may mean that drugs simply cannot get at the growing edge of the tumor where blood-brain barrier function may be preserved (Levin et al. 1975). Furthermore, the metastatic brain tumor is developed in animals by intracarotid tumor inoculation and the adding systemic chemotherapy. In this case, it appears that small clusters of hematogenously disseminated cells implant and grow in the intact brain despite systemic chemotherapy because the blood vessels near where the tumors begin their growth still maintain an intact blood-brain barrier, thus preventing the drugs from reaching the cells. In a preliminary observation, Blasberg and coworkers, using our metastatic rat brain tumor model, have found small metastatic tumor nodules in the brain that do not take up AIB near larger tumors that do so avidly (1978). This seems to confirm that the blood-brain barrier breaks down as the tumor grows, presumably as it is supplied with so-called leaky blood vessels. Our model permits us to compare early therapy versus late therapy, thus permitting inferences about function of the blood-brain barrier in these circumstances.

As for what the experiments tell us about the problems of metastatic brain tumors in humans, systemic chemotherapy so far does not appear to prevent CNS metastases in humans or animals. Our model appears to aid in determining the value of such drugs in preventing subsequent tumor take. It may be necessary to develop similar models, using other tumors sensitive to known effective systemic agents. Conceivably, one might utilize a breast tumor, a lung tumor, a trophoblastic tumor, and a melanoma all metastatic to brain. The requirement for such modeling, however, is the availability of effective systemic therapy. Since this is the prerequisite in the patient as well, one can use such animal modeling to test agents that prevent metastasis to brain or treat it once such metastases occur. This then offers an appropriate goal for this type of modeling experiment.

REFERENCES

Allen, J. C. et al. CNS penetration of methotrexate is enhanced by hyperosmolar intracarotid mannitol and meningeal carcinomatosis. *Neurology* 28:351, 1978.

Bigner, D. D., and Swenberg, J. A., eds. *Janish and Schriber's experimental tumors of the central nervous system*, First English Edition. Kalamazoo: Upjohn Co. 1977.

Blasberg, R. G. et al. An autoradiographic technique to measure the permeability of normal and abnormal brain capillaries. *Neurology* 28:363, 1978.

Hasegawa, H.; Shapiro, W. R.; and Posner, J. B. Chemotherapy of experimental metastatic brain tumors. *Cancer Res., in press.*

Hasegawa, H. et al. The effect of 1-(4-amino-2-methyl-5-pyrimidinyl) methyl-3-(2-chloroethyl)-3-nitrosourea hydrochloride (ACNU) on experimental brain tumors. *Cancer Res., in press.*

Levin, V. A., Freeman-Dove, M., and Landahl, H. D. Permeability characteristics of brain adjacent to tumors in rats. *Arch. Neurol.* 32:785–791, 1975.

Mehta, B. M., and Hutchinson, D. J. Microbiological assays of cancer chemotherapeutic agents. *Cancer Treat. Rep.* 61:597–601, 1977.

Ushio, Y. et al. Metastatic tumor of the brain: development of an experimental model. *Ann. Neurol.* 2:20–29, 1977a.

Ushio, Y. et al. Treatment of experimental spinal cord compression caused by extradural neoplasms. *J. Neurosurg.* 47:380–390, 1977b.

Ushio, Y. et al. Meningeal carcinomatosis: development of an experimental model. *J. Neuropath. Exp. Neurol.* 36:224–244, 1977c.

Ushio, Y.; Posner, J. B.; and Shapiro, W. R. Chemotherapy of experimental meningeal carcinomatosis. *Cancer* 37:1232–1237, 1977d.

Vick, N. A.; Khandekar, J. D.; and Bigner, D. D. Chemotherapy of brain tumors: the "blood-brain barrier" is not a factor. *Arch. Neurol.* 34:523–526, 1977.

9
Pharmacokinetics and Metastatic Brain Tumor Chemotherapy

Ronald G. Blasberg

This discussion of pharmacokinetics and metastatic brain tumors covers three topics. First, pharmacokinetics are developed from a physiologic point of view, focusing on the transport steps involved in drug delivery to the tumor cells and the major parameters which affect that delivery. Second, the parameters of drug administration which can be varied by the clinician to achieve optimal drug delivery and an optimal chemotherapeutic effect are discussed and illustrated by a comparison of local and systemic drug administration. Third, current studies using a metastatic brain tumor model and quantitative autoradiography demonstrate considerable variability in the permeability of tumor capillaries and a reduction in blood flow through a metastatic tumor in comparison to normal brain regions.

The distinctive anatomy of the brain has been well described and is generally appreciated to represent the structural basis for comparatively slow exchange of most water-soluble compounds and drugs (with the exception of certain metabolites) between blood and brain or blood and cerebrospinal fluid (CSF) (Brightman 1977). The interfaces for blood-brain-CSF exchange are schematically illustrated in figure 9.1. The tight junctions which circumscribe the endothelial cells of brain capillaries, the specialized ependymal cells of the choroid plexus, and the arachnoidal cells of the external CSF surface are not the only structural components of the so-called blood-brain barrier. In addition, one must consider the permeability characteristics and specific transport systems of the cell membranes as well as the surface area of the endothelial, specialized ependymal, and arachnoidal cells.

PHYSIOLOGY

The movement of most drugs across the capillary endothelium—or any other blood-brain interface—appears to be diffusional or passive. Diffusional or passive transport can be described by first-order transport kinetics: the amount of drug transported across a biologic membrane is directly proportional to its concentration and not to any other factor or series of factors. Drug transport may be measured and expressed quantitatively in various ways (table 9.1). These expressions of permeability may be

146

Figure 9.1.

MODEL OF BLOOD-CSF-BRAIN EXCHANGE

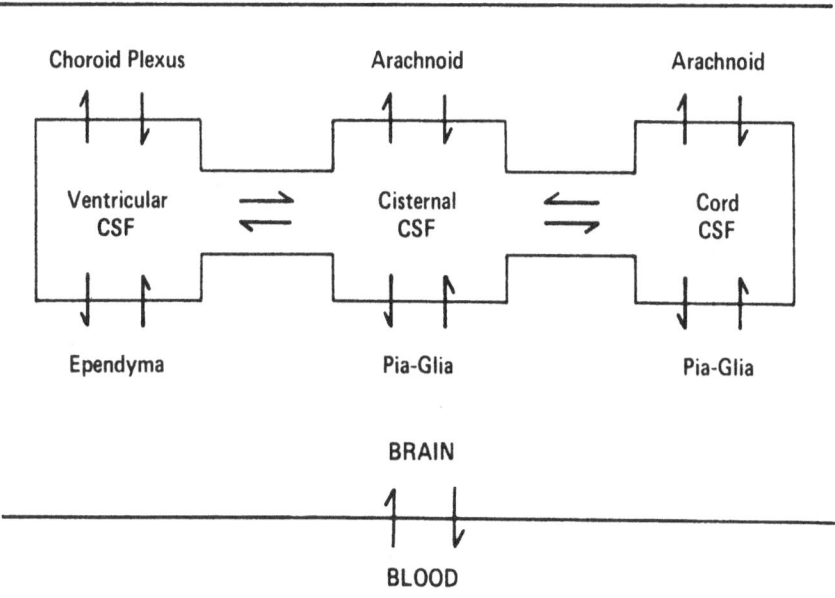

Model of blood–CSF–brain exchange.

Table 9.1

EXPRESSIONS OF PERMEABILITY

Expression	Units	Comment
I Permeability Coefficient (P)	$cm\ sec^{-1}$	physical constant
II Permeability* Surface Area (PS)	$cm^3/g \cdot sec^{-1}$	functional expression; surface area may not be known
III Transfer Constant (K)	$ml/g \cdot min^{-1}$	functional expression; surface area is not known
IV Extraction Fraction (E)	none	single capillary passage
V Brain Uptake Index (BUI)	none	single capillary passage

interrelated under specific conditions such as:

$$PS = -F \ln(1 - \frac{K}{F})$$

$$(1)$$

where F is bloodflow. When K/F is small, less than 0.1, equation (1) reduces to:

$$PS \simeq K$$

$$(2)$$

The relationship between the other expressions of capillary permeability have been described elsewhere (Blasberg 1979).

The permeability coefficient (P) is not the only parameter which determines the amount of drug which crosses a membrane. The size or surface area (S) of the exchanging membrane in a unit mass of tissue will also determine the amount of drug which exchanges in the tissue. Therefore, the permeability–surface area product (PS) or the capillary transfer constant (K) is a more functional index of drug transfer. The PS product and K value reflect the amount of drug transferred across a membrane, such as the capillary endothelium, in a unit mass of tissue over a given period of time. The Ps product and K value were originally expressed in terms of clearance: volume per unit mass of tissue per unit time ($cm^3/gm \cdot min^{-1}$). For simplicity we can assume a tissue density of one; the volume and mass terms will cancel and the units of reciprocal time remain (table 9.1). The units of amount (mg or mMoles) or concentration (mg/ml or mM) do not appear in the P, PS, or K terms. The units of amount or concentration are determined by the units of blood (plasma) activity or concentration and will cancel in the calculation of PS or K.

The amount of drug which moves directly from blood to brain across the capillary endothelium in a gram of brain tissue is determined by the least four parameters: (1) the permeability coefficient (P) of the capillaries with respect to the drug; (2) the luminal surface area (S) of the capillaries in a gram of brain tissue; (3) the activity or concentration of unbound drug in the plasma (C_p); and (4) the length of time (t) the drug circulates through the capillaries. A fifth parameter, blood flow (F) through the capillaries is also important when K/F is large, greater than 0.1 (equation 1). In this case, where the drug permeates the capillaries readily, the amount of drug delivered to the tissue depends in part on the blood concentration and the rate of blood flow. Expressed in another way, if drug transfer across the capillaries is rapid and partly or entirely dependent on the amount of drug brought to the capillary circulation by the arterial system, then the amount of drug which enters the brain is dependent on blood flow. All five of the above considerations are important and are applicable to any organ system or tissue.

There are vast differences in the surface areas of the various interfaces represented in the schematic model of the blood-brain-CSF system in figure 9.1. The capillary endothelium presents a very large surface area; in the human brain it is estimated to be approximately 20 m² or 220 ft².[1]

Significant regional differences are also thought to exist. Gray matter such as cortex is thought to have a 5-fold greater capillary surface area than white matter such as corpus callosum. Therefore, the amount of drug which enters a gram of cortex can be expected to be five times that which enters a gram of corpus callosum after intravascular administration providing the capillary permeability coefficient of the drug is the same in both brain regions. In this case, the difference in the amount of drug which enters the cortex and the corpus callosum is due to the regional differences in capillary surface area and not to any intrinsic difference in the capillaries.

The area of the arachnoidal membrane, which functions as the so-called external CSF surface, can also be estimated.[2] For the human the approximate value is 0.1 m² or 1 ft². The arachnoidal surface area is approximately 1/200 that of the capillary surface area. The pia-glial surface area is not readily determined because of the cortical gyri and sulci; similarily, the surface area of the ependyma and the specialized ependyma over the choroid plexus cannot be accurately measured because of the microvilli on the luminal or CSF surface. Therefore, it is not possible to calculate the permeability (P) of these membranes from the experimental data; the results must be expressed as a permeability–surface area product (PS) or transfer rate constant (K).

PHARMACOKINETICS

This discussion centers on the parameters which affect the vascular delivery and distribution of drug to the brain or to a parenchymal brain metastasis. Pharmacokinetic models are used to illustrate the significant transport steps and to indicate where specific clinical control or intervention is possible. The pharmacokinetics of intrathecal chemotherapy for meningeal metastases is not discussed; this topic has been reviewed elsewhere (Blasberg et al. 1977; Blasberg 1977).

The first simplified model of drug transport—blood-to-brain— illustrates the parameters which are important during the initial phase of drug administration (fig. 9.2). A two-compartment model with a unidirectional transfer constant (K_i) is presented. Plasma drug levels are assumed

---

[1]The value for the capillary surface area of the human brain was calculated by assuming (a) the gray-to-white matter volume ratio is approximately 0.6/0.4 and (b) the capillary surface area of gray and white matter in the human is similar to that which has been determined in the Rhesus monkey: 192 and 38 cm²/cm³, respectively (Levin et al. 1976). The capillary surface area for rat cortex has been calculated to be 240 cm²/gm tissue (Crone 1963); the higher value for rat cortex is consistent with the higher rates of cortical blood flow and glucose utilization measured in the rat in comparison to the cat and monkey (Sokoloff et al. 1977; Sakurada et al. 1978; Kennedy et al. 1978).

[2]The arachnoidal surface area was estimated by assuming that the geometry of the outer CSF surface is represented by a sphere 14 cm in diameter and a cylinder 2 cm in diameter and 60 cm long.

to be high in comparison to brain levels during the initial phase of drug administration, and insignificant amounts of drug move back across the capillaries—brain-to-blood—during this period. The amount of drug which enters the brain (A_{br}) during the initial phase following drug administration is the product of the capillary transfer constant (K_i) and the plasma arterial integral of free or unbound drug ($\int C_p dt$). These relationships clearly indicate what can be done to increase A_{br}: an increase in either K_i or $\int C_p dt$ or an increase in both parameters will increase the amount of drug which enters the brain.

The capillary transfer constant—blood to brain—(K_i) reflects the permeability coefficient (P) and the surface area (S) of the capillaries in a unit mass of tissue with respect to a particular drug (equation 1). An obvious way for the chemotherapist to increase K_i is to choose a drug which permeates the capillaries more rapidly. Drugs such as epipodophyllotoxin, 5-fluorouracil, and dianhydrogalactitol have low permeability coefficients (P) and, therefore, low capillary transfer constants (K) in normal brain, whereas the P values of BCNU and CCNU are high (table 9.2). The close correlation between the permeability coefficient (P) and partition coefficient (log octanol/water solubility) illustrates the association between

Figure 9.2.

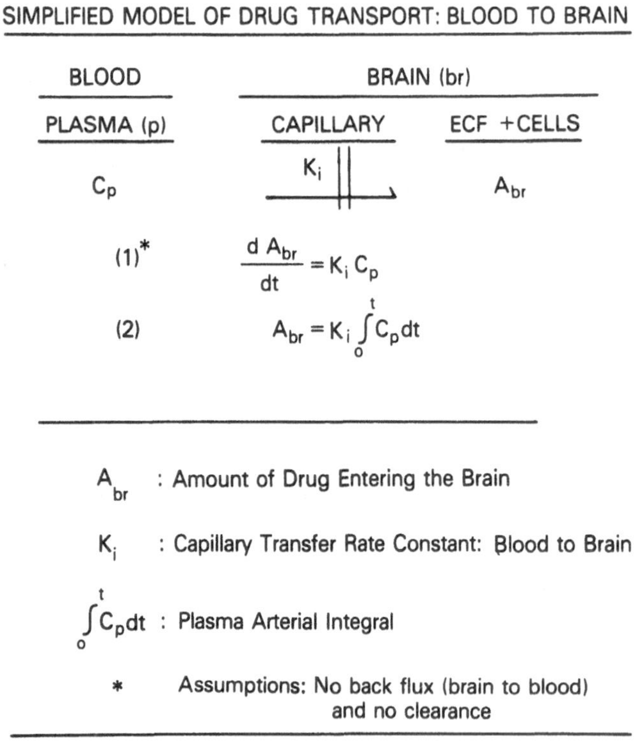

SIMPLIFIED MODEL OF DRUG TRANSPORT: BLOOD TO BRAIN

BLOOD	BRAIN (br)	
PLASMA (p)	CAPILLARY	ECF +CELLS
C_p	K_i	A_{br}

$(1)^*$ 　　$\dfrac{d\,A_{br}}{dt} = K_i\,C_p$

(2) 　　$A_{br} = K_i \displaystyle\int_{0}^{t} C_p\,dt$

A_{br}　: Amount of Drug Entering the Brain

K_i　: Capillary Transfer Rate Constant: Blood to Brain

$\displaystyle\int_{0}^{t} C_p\,dt$　: Plasma Arterial Integral

*　　Assumptions: No back flux (brain to blood) and no clearance

Simplified model of initial drug transport: blood to brain.

Table 9.2

CAPILLARY PERMEABILITY COEFFICIENTS: RAT BRAIN

	Drug	Permeability (P) (cm/sec × 10⁷)	Molecular Weight	Partition Coefficient*
Impermeable	Sucrose	1.2	342	−3.7
	Epipodophyllotoxin	1.2	657	−2.8
Slightly Permeable	Sodium	7.4	24	−3.0
	5-Fluorouricil	17	130	−1.0
	Dianhydrogalactitol	25	150	−1.3
Moderately Permeable	Procarbazine	190	221	0.1
Very Permeable	BCNU	1,500	214	1.5
	CCNU	1,000	234	2.8
	Tritiated Water	1,600	20	—

*Log octanol/water.
SOURCE: Levin et al. 1976.

permeability and lipophillicity. Presumably those drugs which are able to dissolve readily in the lipid portion of the endothelial membrane also pass more rapidly across the entire endothelial cell and enter the brain parenchyma.

It is also possible to design and synthesize drugs with specific characteristics, such as a high octanol/water partition coefficient, in order to achieve a higher P or K value. This has recently been achieved with an alkylating agent, spirohydantoin mustard (NSC-172112) (Peng et al. 1975). The log partition coefficient of spirohydantoin mustard is 2.6 (John Driscoll, personal communication), and its blood-to-brain transport appears to be limited by the rate of blood flow (Kobayashi and Blasberg, unpublished observations, 1978).

An alternative to choosing or synthesizing a drug with a high P or K value is to alter the capillaries such that the P or K value of a particular drug increases. Rapoport and coworkers (1978) demonstrated that it is possible to transiently and reversibly open the blood-brain barrier by an intracarotid infusion of a hyperosmolal solution. Using this technique, they obtained up to a 20-fold increase in the P value for sucrose. It is not clear, however, whether increasing the permeability of normal brain capillaries by hyperosmolal therapy will significantly increase the amount of drug delivered to the cells of a metastatic brain tumor.

Clinical and experimental studies have demonstrated that the capillaries in most regions of a metastatic brain tumor are considerably more permeable than the surrounding brain tissue (Vick et al. 1977). Whether the magnitude of higher permeability of tumor capillaries is sufficient for adequate drug deliver to the tumor cells has not been determined quantitatively. One particular region in question is the brain adjacent to tumor. It has been suggested that the leading edge of tumor growth is protected from effective systemic chemotherapy with water soluble drugs by tight capillaries and a reduced extracellular space (Levin et al. 1975). There are new quantitative autoradiographic methods to measure focal capillary permeability in and around a brain tumor which will help resolve some of these conflicting studies. Preliminary results with this technique are presented in the last section of this chapter.

The plasma arterial integral, $\int C_p dt$, has been used as an index of drug exposure. If the arterial plasma level (C_p) is maintained constant, the $\int C_p dt$ is simply the $C_p \times T$ product. If the plasma level is not maintained constant, the plasma arterial integral can be obtained graphically or mathematically from the drug concentration time course in the arterial blood (plasma) during and after drug administration. There are several ways by which the chemotherapist can influence and control the plasma arterial integral. They include such obvious parameters as the dose or amount of drug administered and the site of administration (table 9.3). These parameters primarily affect the concentration of drug in the plasma (C_p).

Until recently, the clinician had little influence over the time the drug circulated throughout the body. Drug clearance from the plasma and body tissues is not readily controlled. With the advent of so-called rescue techniques as an adjunct to antimetabolite chemotherapy, it is possible to more precisely control the time (T) parameter. Citrovorum factor rescue after high-dose methotrexate therapy has been well described; other methotrexate rescue agents include L-asparaginase, carboxypeptidase, and

Table 9.3

PARAMETERS OF CLINICAL INFLUENCE

I. Choice of Drug

II. Administration

    A. site (local vs. systemic)
    B. amount (dose)
    C. rate (bolus vs. infusion)
    D. multiple-dose scheduling

III. Adjuvants
    A. inhibitors of drug metabolism and excretion
    B. rescue technique

thymidine (Chabner and Johns 1977). Another rescue possibility includes uridine after N-(phosphonacetyl)-L-aspartate (NSC-224131) or PALA therapy (Johnson 1977). Without rescue techniques, the time parameter conceptually extends to infinity, but there is a lower limit or base plasma concentration below which the drug no longer has a biologic effect. The plasma arterial integral should be corrected for the minimally effective plasma concentration (C_{mp}) if it is used as an index of drug exposure (IDE):

$$IDE = \int (C_p - C_{mp})\, dt \qquad (3)$$

providing $C_p > C_{mp}$ during the time of exposure (0 to T).

There are inherent limitations associated with correlating the index of drug exposure with chemotherapeutic effect and drug toxicity. The complex interrelationships between plasma concentration and in vivo biologic effect, such as enzyme inhibition or cell death, are not likely to be described accurately by simple first order kinetics. Furthermore, the time or duration of drug exposure at effective drug levels may be critical, particularly for antimetabolites and cell-cycle–specific drugs. The time parameter is not specifically indicated by the index of drug exposure. One could have a comparatively high IDE due to very high plasma levels ($C_p - C_{mp}$). If the plasma halflife of the drug is short, however, plasma drug levels (C_p) will rapidly fall to the minimally effective concentration (C_{mp}) and the time or duration of effective drug exposure will be short. The biologic effect of a cell-cycle–specific drug is likely to be small, irrespective of the initial value of C_p, if the duration of drug exposure is short.

The clinical experience with cytosine arabinoside illustrates this point. Cytosine arabinoside is rapidly inactivated by deamination and the plasma halflife of the active drug is short (Ho and Frei 1971). The therapeutic response to an intravenous bolus of cytosine arabinoside has been shown to be small. To achieve an optimal response with this cell-cycle–specific drug, it is necessary to infuse cytosine arabinoside in order to maintain effective plasma concentrations over an extended period of time (Frei et al. 1969).

After the initial phase of drug administration and passage across the capillary endothelium, several other parameters affect the amount of drug in the brain and metastatic brain tumor. A simplified model of drug transport and clearance illustrates some of these parameters (fig. 9.3). This model represents a later phase, following drug administration, in which the amount of drug in the brain is not solely determined by the capillary transfer rate constant (K_i) and the plasma arterial integral ($\int C_p dt$). At least two other parameters must be considered: (1) back diffusion or reverse transport of drug from brain to blood and (2) the clearance of drug from the brain and/or tumor by metabolism and/or movement into the CSF. The effect of these parameters is to reduce the amount of drug in the brain exchangeable pool (A^*_{br}) as indicated by the equations in figure 9.3. The magnitude of the reduction depends on the magnitude of the rate constants for brain-to-blood back transport (k_o) and drug clearance (k_c).

The transfer constant for brain-to-blood efflux, k_o, is more conveniently expressed in terms of an amount per gram of tissue because the

Figure 9.3.

SIMPLIFIED MODEL OF DRUG TRANSPORT AND CLEARANCE

BLOOD	BRAIN (br)	
PLASMA (p)	CAPILLARY	ECF + CELLS

C_p K_i → ← k_o A_{br}^* k_c →

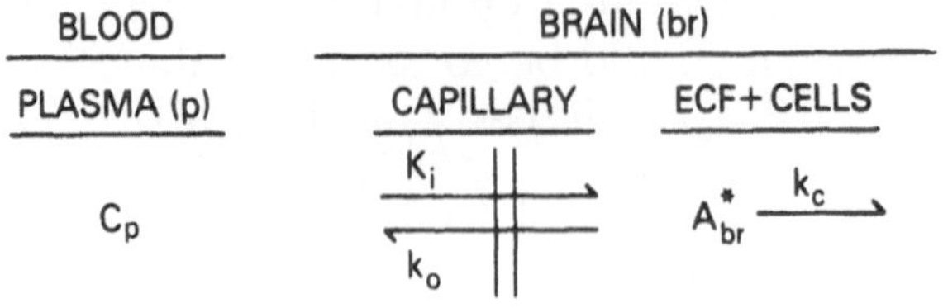

(1)
$$\frac{d A_{br}}{dt} = K_i C_p - k_o A_{br} - k_c A_{br}$$

(2)
$$A_{br} = K_i e^{-(k_o + k_c)t} \int_0^t C_p e^{(k_o + k_c)\tau} d\tau$$

A_{br}^* : Amount of Drug in the Exchangeable Pool

k_o : Capillary Transfer Rate Constant: Brain to Blood

k_c : Brain Clearance and Inactivation Rate Constant

Simplified model of drug transport and clearance.

concentration of drug in the extracellular fluid (ECF) is not readily measurable. Therefore, the transfer constant is expressed as a lower case k_o in contrast to an upper case K_i where the plasma levels can be readily measured and expressed as a concentration. The expressions K and k are not interchangeable, nor would the values K_i and k_o be expected to be equal for passively exchanging solutes. Although the ECF concentration of drug is not readily measured, it is the ECF concentration of drug which determines the amount which is transported back across the capillaries (brain to blood). The ECF concentration of drug can be influenced by at least three factors: (1) cellular uptake and binding will remove drug from the ECF and lower its concentration in this compartment although the total amount of drug in the tissue as a whole (amount per gram tissue) will remain the same; (2) movement through the ECF to another brain region by diffusion or bulk flow could reduce or increase the concentration of drug in the ECF of a particular region; and (3) ECF biotransformation or metabolism.

Cellular uptake from the ECF is probably the most important factor in addition to the permeability coefficient–surface area product of the capillaries, which determines the magnitude of k_o and regulates the ECF concentrations of drug. In contrast to drug inactivation, cellular uptake and binding effectively traps drug within the cells by removing it from the ECF but not from the tissue as a whole. Operationally, k_0 is a lumped constant which reflects several different processes that affect the clearance of drug from the ECF and is expressed as the transfer constant for brain-to-blood efflux.

The rate constant for brain clearance, k_c, is also expressed in terms of an amount per gram of tissue. Operationally, k_c is also a lumped constant which represents all the drug clearance processes of the tissue including: (1) metabolism and inactivation in both cellular and extracellular compartments and (2) diffusion and bulk flow to distant sites such as CSF.

The simplified model of drug transport and clearance states that the amount of drug in the brain exchangeable pool (A_{br}^*) at time (T) after administration is due to the interaction of several parameters (fig. 9.3). A_{br}^* will always be equal to or less than the amount of drug which enters the brain (fig. 9.2, equation 2), and the amount less will depend on the magnitude of the lumped constants k_0 and k_c (fig. 9.3, equation 2). The equilibrium or steady state amount of drug in the brain or metastatic tumor could be relatively low compared to plasma levels irrespective of K_i and T, providing k_0 or k_c are large in comparison to K_i. If the rate of net drug loss from the brain ($k_0 + k_c$) is high relative to the rate of drug entry into the brain (K_i), the amount of exchangeable drug in the tissue will remain low in comparison to plasma concentrations; that is, the brain-to-blood partition coefficient will be low. Therefore, drug loss from the brain or tumor could be a limiting factor in achieving adequate brain (tumor) concentrations of drug, particularly for those drugs which cross the capillaries slowly and are rapidly metabolized or transformed to inactive compounds in the tissue.

This exercise in pharmacokinetic modeling attempts to illustrate some of the interrelated parameters which determine the activity of a drug in an organ after intravascular administration; however, by necessity, the model is much simpler than the system actually is. The parameters, k_0 and k_c, are summated or lumped constants because the concentration of drug in the ECF and various cellular compartments and the individual rate constants for cell uptake, cell metabolism, and ECF diffusion and bulk flow cannot be readily measured. Furthermore, the regional heterogeneity of the brain, including different cell types, capillary surface area, and ECF volume complicate the interpretation of pharmacokinetic data obtained from the experimental animal as well as its extrapolation to the human situation.

CLINICAL INFLUENCE

The chemotherapist can influence drug delivery to the brain and to a metastatic brain tumor. The parameters which the chemotherapist can control are discussed briefly in the preceding section and are outlined in table 9.3. In this section I review in more detail the parameters of drug administration and indicate several important interrelationships that may be useful in the clinic.

The site of drug administration may be conveniently described as *local* for intra-arterial infusion or *systemic* for oral, intramuscular, or intravenous administration. Although intracarotid (local) infusion is technically more complex and involves an increased risk of complications for the patient, a significant advantage may be gained with specific drugs. Several important criteria for optimal drug delivery have emerged from a pharmacokinetic model of drug distribution and a comparison of intracarotid and intravenous drug administration (Fenstermacher and Cowles 1977). The major difference between local and systemic intravascular drug administration is primarily observed during the initial or first capillary passage. It is only during the initial passage of drug through brain and tumor capillaries that intracarotid administration offers any significant advantage over intravenous administration. The magnitude of that advantage is proportional to the ratio of cardiac output and blood flow in the arterial vessel being infused. After the initial capillary passage, the concentration of drug in the arterial blood during the second and subsequent passages through the brain and tumor capillaries will be similar for both local and systemic intravascular administration and no significant intraarterial versus intravenous advantage will be observed.

A second important consideration is the rate of drug inactiviation, metabolism, and excretion. Rapid degradation and excretion during the first passage of drug through the brain (tumor) and lungs will reduce the amount of drug which enters the systemic circulation and will reduce the systemic toxicity for a given amount of administered drug. Stated in another way, for the same degree of systemic toxicity, considerably larger amounts of drug can be delivered to the brain (tumor) by the intraarterial route (in comparison to the intravenous route) if the rates of biotransformation, metabolism, and excretion during the first passage are high.

Other considerations, which may be important with respect to the amount of drug which enters the brain (tumor) but do not increase the advantage of intraarterial versus intravenous infusion, include the drug extraction fraction (E) and blood flow (F). The extraction fraction (E) is the fraction of drug in the blood that equilibrates between the plasma and tissue compartments during a single capillary passage (Crone 1963). For an E of 1.0, equilibration is complete: virtually all the drug is extracted from the blood by the brain (tumor) during the initial capillary passage. In this case, the amount of drug which enters the brain (tumor) is dependent on the total amount of drug which reaches the capillary network by way of the circulation, namely, blood flow (F) and blood concentration (C_p). For E values less than 1.0, equilibration between plasma and tissue compartments is not complete during a single capillary passage and the amount of

---

[3] The advantage of intra-arterial over intravenous administration may be expressed in terms of the ratio of their peak concentrations or in terms of the ratio of their indices of drug exposure (IDE) or their $C_p \times t$ products.

drug which enters the brain (tumor) during the initial passage is not totally determined by blood flow. The permeability–surface area product (PS) of the capillary network assumes increasing importance for drugs with decreasing E values. Below an extraction fraction of 0.1, blood flow has little effect on the amount of drug which enters the tissue; drug entry is primarily determined by the PS product or K_i value. The relationship between E and F and PS or K_i is given by:

$$PS = -F \ln (1 - E) \tag{4}$$

$$K = E^*F \tag{5}$$

The amount of drug which crosses the capillaries and enters the brain (tumor) depends on the parameters already discussed: the arterial plasma concentration (C_p), the PS product or K_i values, and blood flow (F) where K_i/F or the extraction fraction (E) is greater than 0.1. The amount of exchangeable drug in the brain (tumor) was also shown to depend on the efflux and clearance rate constants, k_o and k_c, respectively. The increased amount of drug which enters the brain (tumor) during intraarterial infusion is primarily due to the higher value of C_p which is achieved during intraarterial administration in comparison to that achieved by intravenous infusion. On completion of the infusion, the difference in the magnitude of C_p after local versus systemic administration will be small and little or no further advantage from the intraarterial infusion can be expected.

The drug must exert its principal effect during the time course of intraarterial infusion if an intraarterial infusion of drug is to have a significant chemotherapeutic advantage over the simpler and less hazardous systemic routes of administration. Therefore, the cell kinetics of the tumor and the organ tissue manifesting drug toxicity, the mechanism of drug action, and the optimal concentration and time course over which that concentration of drug is maintained to achieve an optimal chemotherapeutic effect should be known before a specific drug is chosen for intraarterial infusion. All too often we have limited information on the cell kinetics or the time course for optimal drug activity, and pharmacokinetic modeling is used to explain the clinical manifestations of chemotherapy rather than to aid in establishing chemotherapeutic protocols.

Therefore, an ideal drug for local intraarterial infusion should have the following characteristics: (1) the time course of drug action should be short, certainly no longer than that of the intraarterial infusion; (2) the physical characteristics of the drug should be such that it rapidly equilibrates across brain (tumor) capillaries and cell membranes—a specific affinity, binding, or trapping within tumor cells could provide an additional advantage; (3) a significant fraction of the drug should be taken up by the brain (tumor) or be biotransformed or metabolized during the first passage through the brain (tumor) capillaries or be excreted by the lungs. These processes will reduce the amount of drug delivered to the systemic circulation and correspondingly reduce systemic toxicity.

Neither the pharmaceutical industry nor most drug-screening programs are looking specifically for an ideal intraarterial drug, particularly with respect to uptake by the brain (tumor). Indeed, most of the drugs that have been injected or infused intraarterially were chosen because they demonstrated a significant effect after systemic administration. If we wish to use the intraarterial route for local chemotherapy, we should seek a new class of drugs. Several highly labile drugs have demonstrated a selective advantage for intraarterial infusion (Seligman 1962; Davis and Ross 1965; Meyza and Cobb 1971). A new drug, spirohydantoin mustard (NSC-172112), has certain characteristics ideal for intraarterial CNS chemotherapy; it has a short biologic halflife and permeates brain capillaries readily (Plowman et al. 1977). The rapidly acting and degraded alkylating agents and the nitrosoureas are probably closest to the ideal intraarterial drug at the present time.

The last three parameters in table 9.3, dose, rate and schedule of drug administration, affect the concentration and time course of drug activity in the blood and subsequently in the tissue. The effect of dose on drug plasma levels (C_p) is straightforward. The rate of drug administration and the schedule of repetitive courses of chemotherapy introduces a time factor (t) which may have a significant bearing on the total dose of drug which can be administered. This has been convincingly demonstrated for methotrexate: a single dose of 350 mg/kg is required to produce a lethal effect (LD_{50}) in rats, whereas less than 2.4 mg/kg total dose or amount of drug infused over 96 hours produces a similar effect (Zaharko 1974). The duration or time of drug exposure at adequate concentrations has been shown to be critical for several antimetabolites and cell-cycle–specific drugs (Skipper et al. 1970).

The duration of adequate drug levels in the plasma (C_p) will also determine the amount of drug which crosses the capillaries and enters the brain (tumor) when the values for E, PS, and K_i are low. This is readily appreciated if one considers drug recirculation through the capillary network of the brain (tumor). Recirculation will occur several times after administration until the drug is cleared from the vascular compartment. During this time drug molecules will exchange across the capillary endothelium according to the influx (K_i) and efflux plus clearance ($k_o + k_c$) constants. If the drug exchanges passively across the capillaries and the values of K_i and ($k_o + k_c$) are low, equilibration between plasma and tissue compartments will require several circulation times. The number of circulation times or duration of drug exposure is directly proportional to ($k_o + k_c$) providing the plasma level (C_p) is maintained constant:

$$t_{1/2} = \frac{\text{in } 2}{k_o + k_c} \qquad (6)$$

where $t_{1/2}$ is the equilibration half-time. The equilibrium partition coefficient (λ) of drug distribution between brain (tumor) and blood (plasma) is related to the transfer and clearance constants by:

$$\lambda = \frac{K_i}{k_o + k_i} \qquad (7)$$

If the brain (tumor) to blood partition coefficient or exchangeable space is known, the number of circulation times or duration of drug exposure to achieve half equilibration between blood and tissue compartments is inversely proportional to the influx constant (K_i) (table 9.4). If the capillaries of the brain (tumor) are highly permeable to the drug ($K_i > 10^{-1} \, min^{-1}$), the half-time of equilibration with blood will be seconds. If the capillaries are moderately permeable with respect to the drug ($10^{-1} > K_i > 10^{-3} \, min^{-1}$), the half-time of equilibration between tissue and blood will be minutes to several hours. If the capillaries are relatively impermeable ($K_i < 10^{-3} \, min^{-1}$), the half-time of equilibration could require days to weeks. The time parameter, expressed as an equilibration half-time, assumes increasing importance as the value of K_i decreases. Therefore, an adequate concentration of drug in the blood may have to be maintained for an extended period of time—by continuous infusion or multiple dose scheduling—in order to achieve adequate brain (tumor) concentrations of the drug. If the drug is cell-cycle–specific or an antimetabolite, additional time during which adequate drug levels are maintained in the tissue may be required to achieve optimal drug activity.

In summary, the time parameter or duration of exposure may have considerable importance with respect to both drug equilibration between blood and brain (tumor) and the period necessary for optimal drug activity

Table 9.4

RELATIONSHIP OF BLOOD-BRAIN EQUILIBRATION HALFTIME* TO THE
BLOOD-TO-BRAIN TRANSFER RATE CONSTANT (K_i)

K_i	Equilibration Halftime Exchangeable Space †	
min^{-1}	0.15	0.80
10^{-1}	1.0 min	5.5 min
10^{-2}	10 min	55 min
10^{-3}	1.7 hr	9.2 hr
10^{-4}	17 hr	3.9 days
10^{-5}	7.2 days	39 days
10^{-6}	72 days	385 days

*Equilibration half-time = exchangeable space in $2/K_i$ when the plasma concentration (C_p) is kept constant.

†Exchangeable space is the fraction of brain (tumor) volume which equilibrates with the blood −0.15 and 0.80 are equivalent to the extracellular space and total tissue water, respectively, assuming a brain (tumor)-to-plasma partition coefficient of 1.0.

once the drug has achieved an adequate concentration in the target tissue. Control of the time parameter may be achieved through various means: (1) variation in the rate and duration of drug infusion or multiple dose scheduling; (2) inhibition of drug clearance by the use of inhibitors of drug metabolism and excretion; and (3) the use of rescue techniques.

PRELIMINARY OBSERVATIONS

The relationship of capillary permeability and blood flow to drug equilibration within brain (tumor) tissue has been discussed. Questions raised at this workshop focused on the relative importance of these parameters with respect to drug delivery and distribution in different regions of the tumor and surrounding brain tissue. With the advent of quantitative autoradiographic techniques, it is possible to measure local cerebral blood flow and capillary permeability in brain regions as small as 100–200 microns in diameter (Sakurada et al. 1978; Blasberg et al. 1978a,b). Measurements of local blood flow and capillary permeability were made using these techniques within and around a Walker 256 metastatic brain tumor developed by Shapiro and coworkers (Ushio et al. 1977).

The blood flow studies demonstrated a significant reduction in capillary flow through large tumor regions (fig. 9.4). Differences in capillary flow within large tumor masses were observed, but a sharp demarcation was not seen between low and high flow regions within the tumor mass to correspond to necrotic central cells and viable peripheral cells within the tumor mass. The decrease in capillary blood flow appeared to extend beyond the tumor margins into neighboring cortex and may in part reflect the effects of cerebral edema. Two small foci of tumor in the right lateral margin of cortex also show small decreases in flow. In other brain regions where the tumor mass was less than 1 mm in diameter, no decrease in flow could be observed on the autoradiograph.

The measurement of local capillary permeability expressed as a blood-to-brain transfer constant (K_i) demonstrated a significant increase in the permeability of the capillaries in large tumor regions (fig. 9.5). There was considerable variability in capillary permeability within the tumor mass, but a clear difference in capillary permeability corresponding to necrotic central tissue and viable tissue at the periphery of the tumor was not consistently seen. The tumor margins exhibited both abrupt and gradual permeability gradients between tumor and brain tissue; in some regions the brain adjacent to tumor had tight capillaries whereas in other regions brain tissue capillaries demonstrated increased permeability. A small tumor focus is visible in the right superior lateral cortex in the hematoxylin and eosin stained section of fig. 9.5B. The capillaries of this tumor focus and other tumor foci less than 1 mm in diameter did not demonstrate increased permeability (fig. 9.5A).

These preliminary observations suggest that the Walker 256 metastatic brain tumor has diminished capillary blood flow and increased capillary permeability in the larger tumor foci and in some surrounding brain tissue

Figure 9.4.

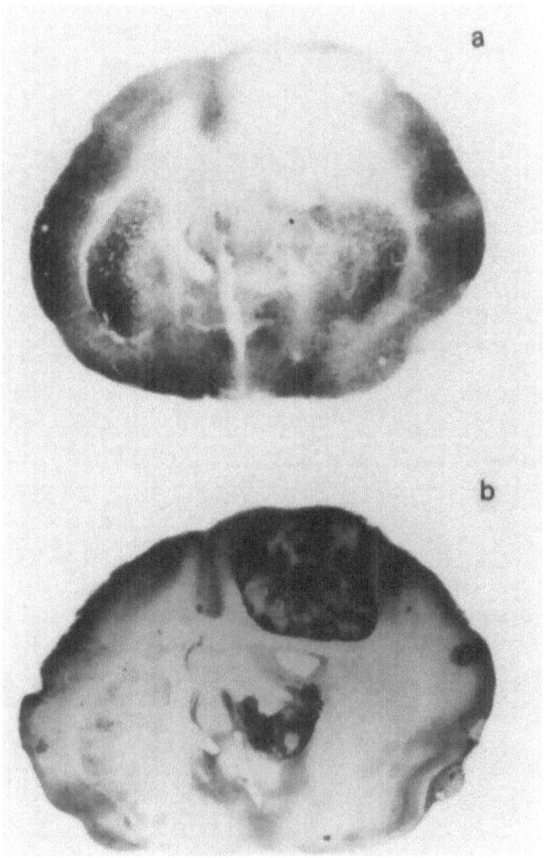

Iodo-[^{14}C] antipyrine blood flow study and histopathology of a Walker 256 metastatic brain tumor in the rat. An anesthetized rat was administered tracer iodo-[^{14}C] antipyrine (30 μCi) by constant intravenous infusion, arterial blood was sampled, and the animal was decapitated after 60 seconds. A. An autoradiographic image after a 7-day exposure on x-ray film of a brain section cut 20 microns thick in a cryostat was obtained. Optical density measurements of the autoradiographic image can be quantitatively correlated to ^{14}C activity and to capillary blood flow; a region of low optical density corresponds to a region of low blood flow. The autoradiogram demonstrates a greater reduction in blood flow through the larger tumor masses (0.1–0.2 ml/gm/min) in comparison to the smaller lesions (0.5–0.8 ml/gm/min), and the reduction in flow extended beyond the larger tumor margins into neighboring cortex (0.4–0.9 ml/gm/min); cortical blood flow contralateral to the tumors was 1.3 ml/gm/min. B. The tumor margins are sharp, and regions of central necrosis are evident in the brain section neighboring the section used for autoradiography (A). (Cresyl violet.)

Figure 9.5.

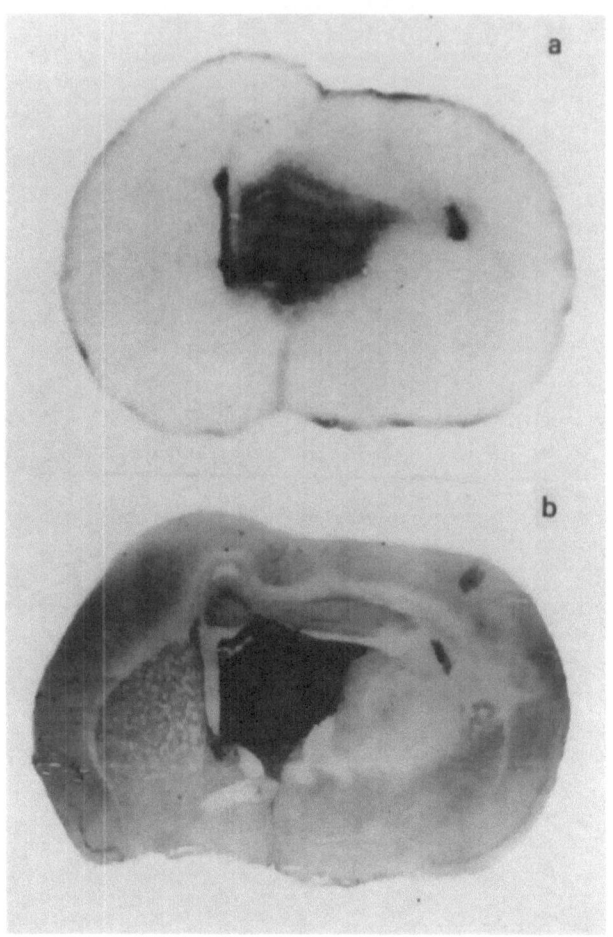

^{14}C-α-aminoisobutyric acid (AIB) capillary permeability study and histopathology of a Walker 256 metastatic brain tumor in the rat. An anesthetized rat was administered a bolus intravenous injection of tracer ^{14}C-AIB (50 μCi), arterial blood was sampled, and the animal was decapitated after 10 minutes. A. An autoradiographic image after a 14-day exposure on x-ray film of a brain section cut 20 microns thick in a cryostat was obtained. Optical density measurements of the autoradiographic image can be quantitatively correlated to ^{14}C activity and to a blood-to-brain transfer rate constant (K_i); a region of high optical density corresponds to a region of high capillary permeability. The autoradiogram demonstrates a variable increase in the permeability of tumor capillaries to AIB ranging 2–100 times higher than that of normal rat cortex ($K_i = 2 \times 10^{-3}$ min^{-1}). B. The tumor margins are sharp, and there is some evidence of central necrosis of the brain in the section neighboring the section used for autoradiography (A). (Hematoxylin and eosin.)

free of tumor cells. A critical tumor size, greater than 1 mm in diameter, appears to be necessary before these changes are demonstrable. It is also apparent from these preliminary studies that quantitative autoradiographic techniques can be expanded to the study of drug delivery to a brain tumor and to the distribution within and around the tumor.

REFERENCES

Blasberg, R. G.; Patlak, C. S.; and Shapiro, W. R. Distribution of methotrexate in the CSF and brain after intraventricular administration. *Cancer Treat. Rep.* 61:633–641, 1977.

Blasberg, R. G. Pharmacodynamics and the blood-brain barrier. In *Modern concepts in brain tumor therapy: laboratory and clinical investigations.* N.C.I. Monograph 46, D.H.E.W. Publication No. (NIH) 77-1236, 1977.

Blasberg, R. G. An outline of problems associated with quantifying the effects of microwave irradiation on blood-brain barrier function. *Radio. Sci.* (Suppl.):

Blasberg, R. G. et al. An autoradiographic technique to measure the permeability of normal and abnormal brain capillaries. *Neurology* 28:363, 1978a.

Blasberg, R. G.; Patlak, C. S.; and Fenstermacher, J. D. Experimental basis for an autoradiographic technique to measure the permeability of normal and abnormal brain capillaries. *Soc. Neurosc. Abstr.* 4:243, 1978b.

Brightman, M. W. Morphology of blood-brain interfaces. In *Ocular and cerebrospinal fluids,* eds. L. Z. Bito, H. Dawson, J. D. Fenstermacher. New York: Academic Press, 1977.

Chabner, B. A., and Johns, D. G. Folate antagonists. In *Cancer—A Comprehensive Treatise,* vol. 5, ed. F. F. Becker. New York: Plenum Press, 1977.

Crone, C. The permeability of capillaries in various organs as determined by use of the "indictor diffusion" method. *Acta Physiol. Scand.* 58:292–305, 1963.

Davis, W., and Ross, W. C. A highly reactive sulphur mustard gas derivative for localized infusion studies. *J. Med. Chem.* 8:757–759, 1965.

Fenstermacher, J. D., and Cowles, A. L. Theoretical limitations of intracarotid infusions in brain tumor chemotherapy. *Cancer Treat. Rep.* 61:519–526, 1977.

Frei, E. et al. Dose schedule and antitumor studies on arabinosyl cytosine (NSC 63878). *Cancer Res.* 29:1325, 1969.

Ho, D. H., and Frei, E. III. Clinical pharmacology of 1-β-D arabinofuranosyl cytosine. *Clin. Pharmacol. Ther.* 12:944–954, 1971.

Johnson, R. K. Reversal of toxicity and antitumor activity of N-(phosphonacetyl)-L-aspartate by uridine or carbonyl-DL-aspartate *in vivo. iochem. Pharmacol.* 26:81–84, 1977.

Kennedy, C. et al. Local cerebral glucose utilization in the normal conscious macaque monkey. *Ann. Neurol.* 4:293–301, 1978.

Levin, V. A.; Freeman-Dove, M.; and Landahl, H. D. Permeability characteristics of brain adjacent to tumor in rats. *Arch. Neurol.* 32:785–791, 1975.

Levin, V. A.; Landahl, H. D.; and Freeman-Dove, M. A. The application of brain capillary permeability coefficient measurements to pathological conditions and the selection of agents which cross the blood-brain barrier. *J. Pharmacokin. Biopharm.* 4:499–519, 1976.

Meyza, J., and Cobb, L. M. The clinical trial of an alkylating agent with a short half-life designed for intra-arterial chemotherapy. *Cancer* 27:369–373, 1971.

Peng, G. W.; Marquez, V. E.; and Driscoll, J. S. Potential central nervous system antitumor agents. Hydantoin derivatives. *J. Med. Chem.* 18:846–849, 1975.

Plowman, J. et al. Initial studies on the penetration of spirohydantoin mustard into the cerebrospinal fluid of dogs. *Pharmacology* 15:359–366, 1977.

Rapoport, S. I. et al. Regional cerebrovascular permeability to [^{14}C] sucrose after osmotic opening of the blood-brain barrier. *Brain Res.* 150:653–657, 1978.

Sakurada, O. et al. Measurement of local cerebral blood flow with iodo [^{14}C] antipyrine. *Am. J. Physiol.* 234:H59–H66, 1978.

Seligman, A. M. Enzyme alterable alkylating agents: a new approach to regional chemotherapy by intra-arterial infusion of new short-lived alkylating agents. *Ann. Surg.* 156:429–441, 1962.

Skipper, H. E. et al. Implications of biochemical, cytokinetic, pharmacologic, and toxicologic relationships in the design of optimal therapeutic schedules. *Cancer Chemother. Rep.* 54:431–450, 1970.

Sokoloff, L. et al. The [^{14}C]deoxyglucose method for the measurement of local cerebral glucose utilization: theory, procedure, and normal values in the conscious and anesthetized albino rat. *J. Neurochem.* 28:897–916, 1977.

Ushio, Y. et al. Metastatic tumor of the brain: development of an experimental model. *Ann. Neurol.* 2:20–29, 1977.

Vick, N.; Khandekar, J. D.; and Bigner, D. D. Chemotherapy of brain tumors; the blood-brain barrier is not a factor. *Arch. Neurol.* 34:523–526, 1977.

Zaharko, D. S. Pharmacokinetics and drug effect. *Biochem. Pharmacol.* 23(suppl. 2):1–8, 1974.

10
Human Cancer Immunology

Herbert F. Oettgen
Hiroshi Shiku
Toshitada Takahashi
Thomas Carey
Lois Resnick
Ryuzo Ueda
Michael Pfreundschuh
and Lloyd J. Old

Much work in cancer immunology is based on the assumption that cancer cells can be distinguished from normal cells by the presence of distinctive antigens on their surface. The evidence supporting this assumption comes primarily from transplantation experiments in inbred mice and rats with tumors induced by chemical carcinogens or viruses. The demonstration that these tumors are immunogenic in syngeneic hosts, or even in the host in which the tumor originated, represents the cornerstone of the field of cancer immunology. Not all transplanted tumors in experimental animals are immunogenic, however. In the view of some, nonimmunogenic tumors raise serious questions about the general validity of the immunosurveillance concept and thus the whole field of cancer immunology. Others contend that lack of immunogenicity in transplantation experiments may be related to any aspect of the recognition-rejection complex and need not indicate the absence of tumor-specific antigens. This view is supported by the surprising array of escape routes by which tumors of known antigenicity escape immunologic destruction.

Rather than argue the merits or deficiencies of the immunosurveillance concept, it seems far more reasonable and important at this point to test the central hypothesis of the field: a change in cell surface antigenicity is an invariable consequence of transition to the malignant state regardless of whether it leads to rejection. Because transplantation techniques may give us misleading information about the existence of tumor-specific antigens in experimental tumors and are not admissible in the study of human cancer, the emphasis must be on in vitro methods. Of these, serologic techniques are the most sensitive and precise, but certain antigens may not elicit the production of antibody and their detection may thus depend on measurements of cellular immunity.

TUMOR-SPECIFIC CELL SURFACE COMPONENTS

Tumor-specific cell surface components comprise a number of distinct categories (Old and Boyse 1973). Antigens that are recognized primarily by their capacity to cause rejection of tumors are known as tumor-specific transplantation antigens (TSTA). It appeared at first that a distinction could be made between chemically induced tumors, each of which possesses a unique TSTA, and virus-induced tumors, which share a TSTA common to all tumors induced by the same virus. It now seems likely that this distinction is relative rather than absolute: individually distinct TSTA may be characteristic of tumors generally, but this will often be over-shadowed by the presence of cross-reacting antigens in virus-induced tumors.

The antigens demonstrable primarily by serologic techniques are a diverse group. There are antigens that belong to the envelope of oncogenic viruses that bind from the cell surface. Other cell surface antigens, while not structural components of the virus, are either coded by the viral genome or under control by the viral genome. The TL (thymus leukemia) antigens fall into a class of their own. In normal mice their inheritance is Mendelian, like other alloantigens, and their expression is confined to thymocytes. Some mouse strains, however, do not carry the antigens on their thymocytes. When leukemias occur in such TL-negative strains, the leukemia cells frequently do express TL antigens. This anomalous appearance of TL antigens on malignant cells, arising from a progenitor cell on which they were not expressed, indicates that derepression of TL-coding genes accompanies malignant transformation.

Despite the enormous volume of literature addressing the question of tumor-specific surface antigens of human cancers, the existence of such antigens must still be considered speculative. The general impression by many tumor immunologists as well as others that tumor-specific antigens have been demonstrated in many types of human cancer is simply not justified. The critical issue is specificity, and defining the specificity of a serologic or cell-mediated immune reaction is much easier in the mouse than in man. In laboratory animals, the availability of inbred strains permitted the transplantation studies that established the existence of distinctive cell surface antigens in tumors. The serologic definition of these antigens in the mouse and rat has also depended on inbred populations to provide the necessary reagents.

In the absence of these advantages, the human cancer serologist is still attempting to evolve approaches that can cope with the issue of specificity. Antisera prepared against human cancer cells in foreign species, while at first appearing tumor-specific, have in every instance turned out to be directed against normal cellular products, which are either present in higher concentration in tumor cells or are found in restricted normal cell populations. Surveys of human sera for reactivity with cell surface antigens of allogeneic tumor cells, usually cell lines considered representative of one type of cancer, form the basis for many reports in the literature. They are rarely, if ever, interpretable as tumor-specific reactions, however, because unknown participation of alloantibodies in the reactions observed is extremely difficult to exclude.

To develop as unambiguous a serologic typing system as possible, we turned several years ago to analyzing autologous serum reactivity to cell surface antigens of human cancer. Because we considered continued availability of target cells for repeated testing important, our studies have been restricted to tumor types that can be grown in culture with some degree of regularity, namely malignant melanoma, renal cancer and astrocytoma. Another essential feature has been the extensive use of absorption tests to establish specificity by determining the occurrence of antigen on a wide range of normal and malignant tissues.

STUDIES WITH MALIGNANT MELANOMA

The serologic assays we chose initially were mixed hemadsorption (MHA) (Metzgar and Olenick 1968) and immune adherence (IA) (Tachibana and Klein 1970). More recently, we have included C3 mixed hemadsorption (C3-MHA) (Irie et al. 1975) and the protein A assay (PA). The initial step, incubation of the patient's serum with his own cultured tumor cells, is the same in all assays. They differ in how the final indicator, a sheep or human red blood cell, is attached to the antibody-coated target cell. Between them, the assays detect both IgM and IgG classes of antibodies and both complement-fixing and noncomplement-fixing antibodies (fig. 10.1).

Figure 10.1.

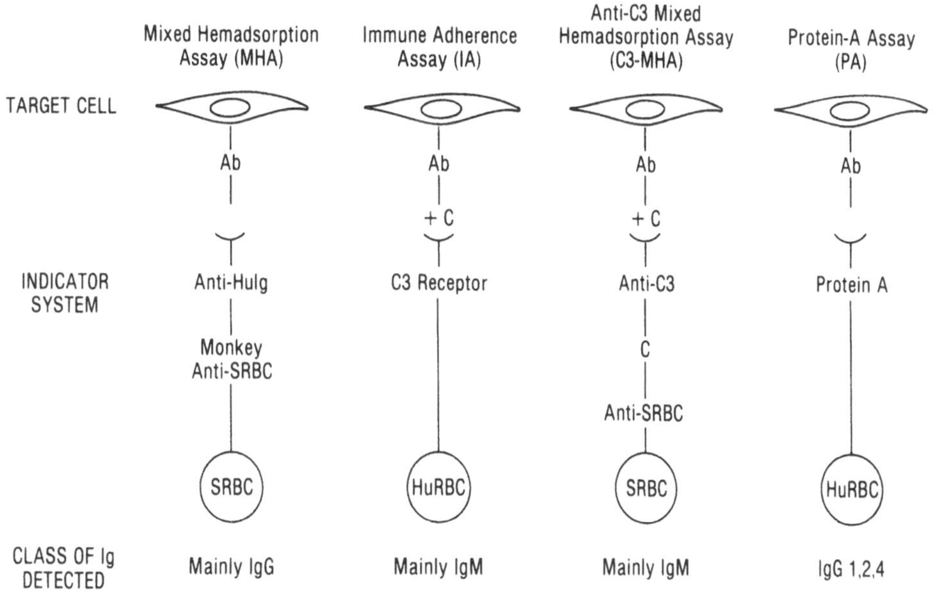

Serologic assays.

Results obtained in IA and MHA assays of sera from the first 30 patients are summarized in table 10.1. Several sequential serum samples were tested from almost all patients. In more than two-thirds of the patients, the period of observation was 6 months or longer, and the number of sequential serum samples was 6 or more. Antibody to surface antigens of cultured autologous target cells was detected in the serum of 18 patients, 17 by IA and 9 by MHA. As might be expected, MHA and IA assays do not always give concordant results since a substantial difference in titers in the two assays is not uncommon. Of more significance, some antibody-antigen systems are detected only by one of the techniques, not by both. Application of several serologic techniques is therefore an important aspect of comprehensive serologic analysis.

Table 10.1

RESULTS OF IA AND MHA ASSAYS OF SERA TAKEN FROM PATIENTS WITH MALIGNANT MELANOMA AND TESTED ON AUTOLOGOUS CULTURED MELANOMA CELLS

Patient	Antibody Titer		Patient	Antibody Titer	
	IA	MHA		IA	MHA
AA	—	—	AW	—	—
AD	—	—	AX	1/16	1/4
AG	—	—	AY	—	—
AH	1/160	1/4	AZ	1/32	—
AI	—	—	BC	1/4	1/64
AL	1/4	—	BD	1/96	1/64
AN	1/320	1/16	BG	1/128	—
AO	1/4	1/4	BH	—	—
AP	1/4	—	BI	—	1/128
AQ	—	—	BO	—	—
AR	1/4	—	BR	—	—
AS	—	—	BS	1/64	—
AT	1/32	1/64	BT	—	—
AU	1/32	1/512	BV	1/160	—
AV	1/16	—	BW	1/64	—

A few individual cases show how these reactions were analyzed. Simultaneous titrations in IA assays of individual serum specimens collected from patients AH and BD over periods of 24 or 10 months, respectively, are shown in figures 10.2 and 10.3. Antibody titers remained essentially unchanged in the case of patient AH. By contrast, sera from patient BD showed a progressive fall in antibody titers.

Figure 10.2.

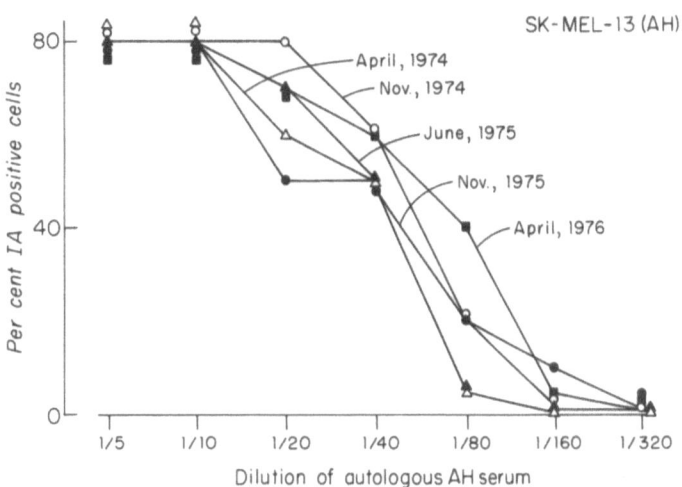

Constant reactivity of sequential serum samples tested on autologous melanoma cells. (Shiku et al. 1976.)

Figure 10.3.

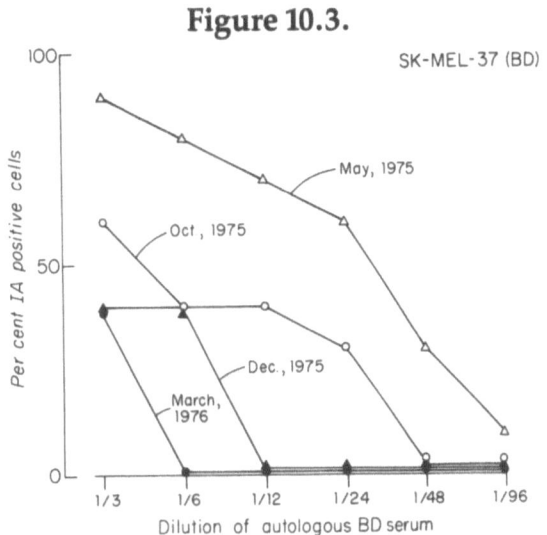

Changing reactivity of sequential serum samples tested on autologous melanoma cells. (Shiku et al. 1976.)

The specificity of the autologous reaction was determined by absorption tests (figs. 10.4, 10.5 and 10.6). Autologous reactivity was removed from BD serum only by absorption with autologous melanoma cells—not by absorption with autologous normal blood cells or allogeneic melanoma cells (fig. 10.4). By contrast, autologous reactivity was removed from AH serum by absorption not only with autologous melanoma cells but also with two allogeneic melanoma cell lines. Absorption with a third melanoma line and a renal cancer line was negative (fig. 10.5). In the case of AN, the antigen that reacted with autologous antibody was not restricted to melanoma but was also found on allogeneic lymphocytes, monkey kidney cells, and allogeneic fibroblasts (fig. 10.6).

The results of absorption tests performed in these three cases are summarized in tables 10.2, 10.3 and 10.4. Patient BD (table 10.2) is an example of autologous antibody against an individually specific melanoma antigen. Absorption tests with a wide array of autologous and allogeneic normal tissues, allogeneic melanoma cells and non-melanoma cancer cells, and xenogeneic tissues were negative. In contrast, patient AH's antibody reacted not only with the patient's own melanoma cells but also with some but not all allogeneic melanoma cells. Absorption tests with

Figure 10.4.

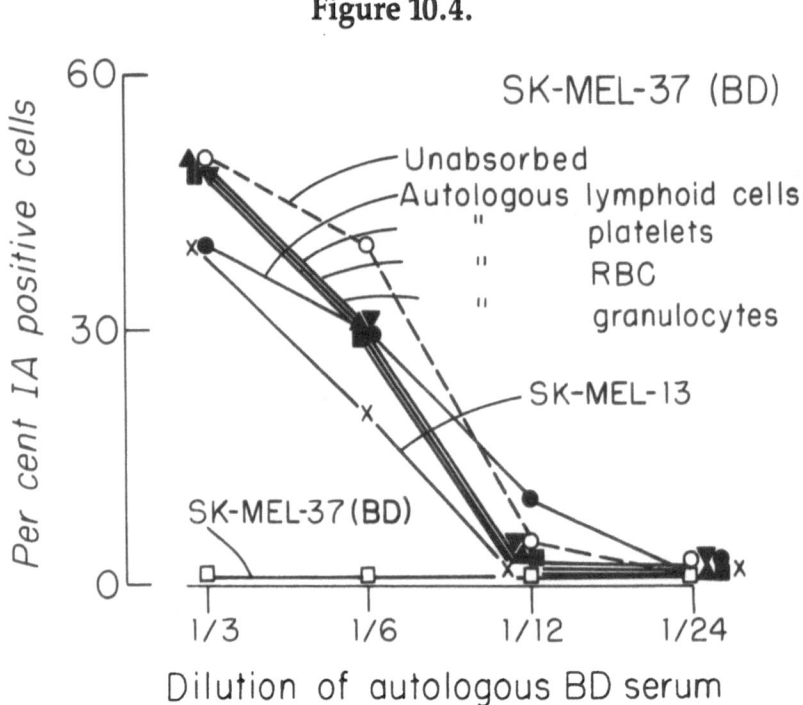

Qualitative absorption analysis: an individually specific melanoma cell surface antigen. (Shiku et al. 1976.)

Figure 10.5.

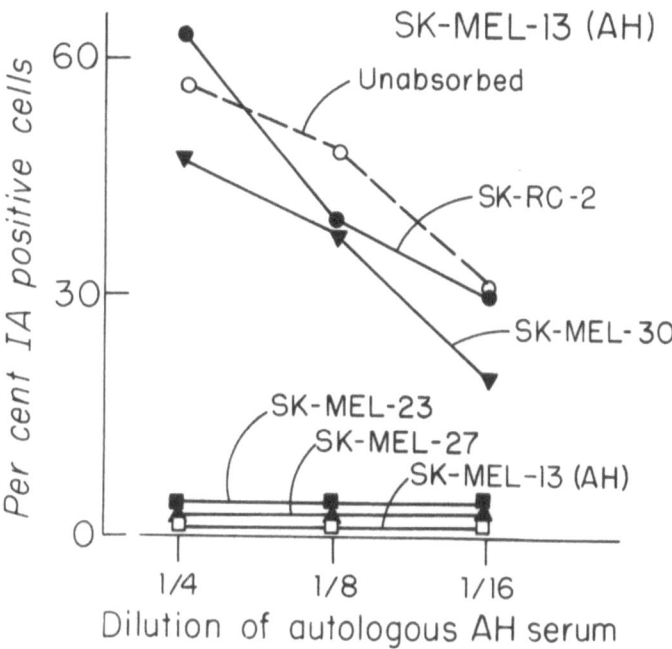

Qualitative absorption analysis: a shared melanoma-specific cell surface anti-gen. (Shiku et al. 1976.)

Figure 10.6.

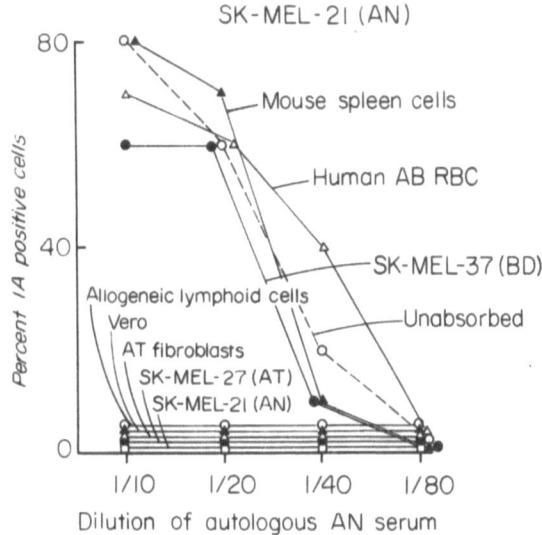

Qualitative absorption analysis: a melanoma cell surface antigen of wide distri-bution. (Shiku et al. 1977.)

autologous and allogeneic normal cells, non-melanoma cancer cells and xenogeneic tissues were again negative. Thus the antigen detected by AH's antibody on autologous melanoma cells represents a shared melanoma antigen (table 10.3). In the case of patient AN (table 10.4), the specificity of the reaction is no longer restricted to melanoma cells. The

Table 10.2

ABSORPTION OF IA REACTIVITY FROM SERUM OF PATIENT BD
TESTED AGAINST AUTOLOGOUS MELANOMA CELLS (SK-MEL-37)

Positive Absorption	Negative Absorption

Autologous cultured melanoma cells:
  SK-MEL-37 (BD)
	Autologous normal cells:
	  Lymphoid cells
	  Platelets
	  Granulocytes
	  Red blood cells
	
	Autologous cultured normal cells:
	  BD Fibroblasts
	
	Allogeneic normal cells:
	  Pooled buffy coat leukocytes
	  A red blood cells
	  B red blood cells
	  AB red blood cells
	  O red blood cells
	
	Xenogeneic cells or serum:
	  Sheep red blood cells
	  Guinea pig kidney
	  Fetal bovine serum
	
	Oncornaviruses:
	  SSV-1
	  RD-114
	  MuLV (AKR)
	
	Microorganisms:
	  BCG

SOURCE: Shiku et al. 1976.

antigen detected in AN's melanoma cells by antibodies in his own serum shows a very wide distribution which includes allogeneic normal and malignant tissues and even tissues from monkey, mouse and chicken.

On the basis of extensive absorption analysis (table 10.5), three general classes of cell surface antigens detected by autologous sera on melanoma cells can be distinguished: (1) individually distinct or unique antigens confined to autologous melanoma cells: AU, BD and BI; (2) shared melanoma antigens: AH; and (3) antigens not restricted to melanoma and recognized by widely reactive autoantibodies: AV, AN,

Negative Absorption
Allogeneic cultured melanoma cells:
SK-MEL-8   (AD)
SK-MEL-13   (AH)
SK-MEL-15   (BO)
SK-MEL-19   (AL)
SK-MEL-22   (AO)
SK-MEL-23   (AP)
SK-MEL-27   (AT)
SK-MEL-28   (AU)
SK-MEL-29   (AV)
SK-MEL-30   (AW)
SK-MEL-36   (BC)
MeWo   (BI)
Allogeneic cultured nonmelanoma cells:
SK-RC-2   (Renal cell cancer)
SK-RC-4   (Renal cell cancer)
T-24   (Bladder cancer)
J-82   (Bladder cancer)
ME-180   (Cervical cancer)
SK-LC-LL   (Lung cancer)
SK-L7   (Leukemia)
Sal III   (Breast cancer)
Allogeneic cultured normal cells:
AT Fibroblasts
Allogeneic cultured fetal cells:
WI-38   (Fetal lung fibroblasts)
PHEL-6   (Fetal lung fibroblasts)

Table 10.3

ABSORPTION OF AI REACTIVITY FROM SERUM OF PATIENT AH
TESTED AGAINST AUTOLOGOUS MELANOMA CELLS (SK-MEL-13)

Positive Absorption	Negative Absorption

Autologous cultured melanoma cells:
  SK-MEL-13   (AH)
 	
Allogeneic cultured melanoma cells:
  SK-MEL-23   (AP)
  SK-MEL-27   (AT)
  SK-MEL-29   (AV)
  MeWo   (BI)
	Autologous normal cells:
	  Lymphoid cells
	  Platelets
	  Granulocytes
	  Red blood cells
	
	Autologous cultured normal cells:
	  AH Fibroblasts
	
	(Allogeneic normal cells:
	(from patients whose cultured melanoma cells absorb reactivity from AH serum)
	  AT and AV:
	    Lymphoid cells
	    Platelets
	    Granulocytes
	    Red blood cells
	  AP:
	    Lymphoid cells
	
	Allogeneic cultured normal cells:
	(from patients whose cultured melanoma cells absorb reactivity from AH serum)
	  AT Fibroblasts
	  AV Fibroblasts
	  BI Fibroblasts
	
	Allogeneic normal cells:
	  Pooled buffy coat leukocytes
	  A red blood cells
	  B red blood cells
	  AB red blood cells
	  O red blood cells
	
	Zenogeneic cells or serum:
	  Sheep red blood cells
	  Guinea pig kidney
	  Fetal bovine serum

SOURCE: Shiku et al. 1976.

Negative Absorption

Oncornaviruses:
  SSV-1
  RD-114
  MuLV (AKR)

Microorganisms:
  BCG
  Corynebacterium parvum

Allogeneic cultured melanoma cells:
  SK-MEL-8   (AD)
  SK-MEL-15   (BO)
  SK-MEL-19   (AL)
  SK-MEL-22   (AO)
  SK-MEL-28   (AU)
  SK-MEL-30   (AW)
  SK-MEL-37   (BD)

Allogeneic cultured nonmelanoma cells:
  SK-RC-2   (Renal cell cancer)
  SK-RC-4   (Renal cell cancer)
  T-24   (Bladder cancer)
  J-82   (Bladder cancer)
  SK-LC-LL   (Lung cancer)
  SK-LU1   (Lung cancer)
  Sal III   (Breast cancer)
  A1Ab   (Breast cancer)
  ME 180   (Cervical cancer)
  HeLa   (Cervical cancer)
  SK-OV-3   (Ovarian cancer)
  HT-29   (Colon cancer)

Allogeneic cultured normal cells:
  AU Fibroblasts
  FB Fibroblasts
  FB Normal kidney cells

Allogeneic cultured fetal cells:
  WI-38   (Fetal lung fibroblasts)
  PHEL-8   (Fetal lung fibroblasts)

Table 10.4

ABSORPTION OF IA REACTIVITY OF AN SERUM FOR
AUTOLOGOUS MELANOMA SK-MEL-21

Positive Absorption	

Autologous
  cultured melanoma cells:
    SK-MEL-21   (AN)
 	
Allogeneic
  cultured melanoma cells:
    SK-MEL-13   (AH)
    SK-MEL-19   (AL)
    SK-MEL-27   (AT)
    SK-MEL-28   (AU)
    MeWo   (BI)
  cultured normal cells:
    AH fibroblasts
    AT fibroblasts
	Allogeneic
	  cultured nonmelanoma cells:
	    SK-LMS-1 (leiomyosarcoma)
	    Sal III (breast cancer)
	    HEp-2 (larynx cancer)
	    SK-LC-LL (lung cancer)
	    WI-38 (fetal lung fibroblasts)
	    PHEL-6 (fetal lung fibroblasts)
	  normal cells:
	    Lymphoid cells (including BD)
	    Granulocytes (including BD)
	
	Xenogeneic
	  cultured monkey kidney cells

SOURCE: Shiku et al. 1977.

and AT. If not recognized, this latter class of antibodies can introduce considerable confusion into the serologic analysis. For instance, several older studies have claimed tumor specificity on the basis of serologic reactions with malignant cells but not with normal fibroblasts from the same individuals. We now see that this sort of control is inadequate. AV and AT fibroblasts did not react with autologous serum in direct tests but could remove reactivity for autologous melanoma cells in absorption tests. Nor can absorption with peripheral lymphocytes, a convenient source of normal cells, be depended upon to prove tumor specificity even in autologous systems. AV's reactivity for autologous melanoma was not removed by autologous lymphocytes but was absorbed by fibroblasts. As these autoantibodies may arise unexpectedly, it cannot be assumed that sequential serum specimens drawn from the same patient will be detecting the same specificities. The possible presence of these broadly reactive antibodies to cell surface components will have to be taken into account when monitoring and interpreting changes in serologic activity of patients to autologous cancer cells (Carey et al. 1976; Shiku et al. 1976; Shiku et al. 1977).

STUDIES WITH RENAL CANCER AND ASTROCYTOMA

Our serologic analysis of renal cancer and astrocytoma is not as far advanced as our melanoma studies. It seems, however, that the three

Negative Absorption	

Allogeneic
  cultured melanoma cells:
    SK-MEL-37   (BD)
  cultured normal cells:
    BD fibroblasts
  cultured nonmelanoma cells:
    ME 180 (cervical cancer)
  normal cells and serum:
    Platelets
    Erythrocytes
    Serums
	Xenogeneic cells and serum:
	  Sheep erythrocytes
	  Fetal bovine serum
	  Mouse spleen cells
	  Mouse erythrocytes
	  Cultured mouse fibroblasts
	  Cultured chicken fibroblasts

classes of antigens detected in our investigation of malignant melanoma—individually specific, shared tumor-specific and widely distributed—are also found in these two cancers. A summary of absorption tests on sera from 5 patients with renal cancer is shown in table 10.6. Patient AX represents the first class of individually specific antigens. The antibodies in the serum of patients AB, AQ, and BM detected class II antigens, shared by each patient's own as well as other patients' renal cancer cells but not found in tissues other than renal cancer. Class III antigens found not only in autologous renal cancer cells but also in other types of cancer and monkey kidney were detected by the serum of patient AR. An advantage in the serologic analysis of renal cancer has been that normal kidney cells from our patients can be cultured with relative ease (Ueda et al. 1978).

In our investigation of astrocytoma the findings have been similar. As shown in table 10.7, sera from patients BC and AC contained antibodies specific for antigens which were found only on the patients' own astrocytoma cells and on no other cell tested. The antigen detected by AJ's serum on his own astrocytoma cells was shared not only by the cells of other astrocytomas but also by melanomas, neuroblastomas and sarcomas. The antigen is not found in cancers of other types or in normal tissues. The antibodies in AK's serum again represent autoantibodies of the widely reactive type, reacting with antigens found in a wide range of neoplastic and normal tissues, including tissues of foreign species (Pfreundschuh et al. 1978).

Table 10.5

CELL SURFACE ANTIGENS OF HUMAN MALIGNANT MELANOMAS
DEFINED BY ABSORPTION TESTS WITH AUTOLOGOUS SERUM

Antigen System Serologic Test	AU* MHA	BI† MHA	BD‡ IA
Absorbed with:			
Autologous cells:			
Cultured melanoma cells	+	+	+
Cultured skin fibroblasts	−	−	−
Lymphoid cells	−		−
Erythrocytes	−		−
Allogeneic cells and serum:			
Cultured melanoma cells	−	−	−
Cultured skin fibroblasts	−	−	−
Cultured nonmelanoma cells	−	−	−
Lymphoid cells	−	−	−
Erythrocytes	−	−	−
Serum	−		−
Xenogeneic cells and serum:			
Cultured monkey kidney cells	−		−
Cultured chicken fibroblasts	−		−
Cultured mouse fibroblasts	−		−
Mouse spleen cells	−		−
Mouse erythrocytes	−		−
Sheep erythrocytes	−	−	−
Fetal bovine serum	−	−	−
Classification of antigen:	Melanoma specific individual	Melanoma specific individual	Melanoma specific individual

*See Carey et al. 1976.
†Takahashi et al., unpublished results.
‡See Shiku et al. 1976.
SOURCE: Shiku et al. 1977.

To summarize our findings in malignant melanoma, renal cancer and astrocytoma: By typing with autologous sera, three classes of cancer cell surface antigens have been defined. Class I antigens are specific for each patient's individual tumor. Class II antigens are shared by tumors of the

	AH‡ IA	AV IA	AN IA	AT MHA
	+	+	+	+
	−	+		+
	−	−		+
	−	−		−
	+ or −	+ or −	+ or −	+
	−	+ or −	+ or −	+
	−	+	+ or −	+
	−	−	+	+
	−	−	−	
	−	−	−	−
	−	+	+	+
	−	+	−	+
	−	+	−	+
	−	+	−	+
	−	−	−	−
	−	−	−	−
	−	−	−	−
	Melanoma specific shared	Not melanoma specific	Not melanoma specific	Not melanoma specific

same type (malignant melanoma or renal cancer) or, in the case of astrocytoma, by tumors of some types but are not found on tumors of other types or normal tissues. Class III antigens are found on a wide range of neoplastic and normal tissues, including tissues of foreign species.

Table 10.6

CELL SURFACE ANTIGENS OF HUMAN RENAL CANCER DEFINED BY
ABSORPTION TESTS WITH AUTOLOGOUS SERUM (C3-MHA)

Absorbed With	Antigen System				
	AX	AB	AQ	BM	AR
Autologous cells:					
Cultured renal cancer cells	+	+	+	+	+
Cultured skin fibroblasts	−	−	−	−	
Cultured normal kidney cells	−				
Allogeneic cells:					
Cultured renal cancer cells	−	+	+	+	+
Cultured skin fibroblasts	−	−	−	−	
Cultured nonrenal cancer cells	−	−	−	−	+
Erythrocytes	−	−	−	−	−
Xenogeneic cells:					
Cultured monkey kidney cells	−	−	−	−	+
Sheep erythrocytes	−	−	−	−	−

STUDIES WITH OTHER HUMAN CANCERS

As for the definition of surface antigens in other human cancers, the challenge is to learn how to establish these cancers in tissue culture. Our present rate of success (particularly with the common human cancers of colon, lung, breast, ovary and pancreas) is too low to permit applications of the approach outlined here. One way we are exploring is to see if passage through athymic (nude) or asplenic-athymic mice facilitates growth in vitro. Other approaches involve using feeder layers, changing the source of the serum supplement, or adding growth factors that are being found to be required for the propagation of a number of differentiated cell populations. Until the problem of cell culture is solved, progress in the serology of many types of human cancer will be greatly limited.

In cancers that are amenable to autologous serologic typing, important new areas of investigation have become accessible. Undoubtedly, biochemical characterization of the cell surface antigens of melanoma, renal cancer and astrocytoma which is now feasible with available serologic reagents will define in more precise terms the individually unique versus common antigens, just as comparable studies of histocompatibility antigens have clarified these issues. Equally important, such studies may give insight into the genetic origin of these specific surface components of melanoma cells and their relation to other cell surface com-

Table 10.7

CELL SURFACE ANTIGENS OF HUMAN ASTROCYTOMA DEFINED BY
ABSORPTION TESTS WITH AUTOLOGOUS SERUM

Absorbed With	Antigen System BC Serologic Assay PA	AC C3-MHA	AJ C3-MHA	AK C3-MHA
Autologous cells:				
Cultured astrocytoma cells	+	+	+	+
Cultured skin fibroblasts	−	−		+
Allogeneic cells:				
Cultured astrocytoma cells	−	−	+	+
Cultured neuroblastoma cells	−	−	+	+
Cultured melanoma cells	−	−	+	+
Cultured sarcoma cells	−	−	+	
Cultured nonastrocytoma cancer cells	−	−	−	+
Cultured meningioma cells	−	−	−	
Cultured normal glial cells	−	−	−	
Cultured fetal brain cells	−	−	−	+
Cultured skin fibroblasts			−	+
Ery., Ly., Gran., Plat.	−	−	−	−
Xenogeneic cells or serum:				
Cultured monkey brain	−		−	
Cultured monkey kidney		−	−	
Cultured rat glioblastoma	−	−	−	+
Sheep erythrocytes	−	−		−
Fetal bovine serum	−	−	−	−

ponents, particularly antigens coded by the major histocompatibility complex. Genetic analysis of individually distinct antigens is obviously not possible by conventional Mendelian genetics, but somatic cell genetics with interspecies hybrids segregating mouse or human chromosomes provide the techniques to do so.

It is also possible now to determine if any of the various mechanisms by which antigenic tumors in experimental animals escape immunologic control play a role in the progression of human cancer. Examples of known escape routes are (1) immunoselection, selection of the least antigenic clones among variants arising in a tumor; (2) antigenic modulation, temporary cessation of antigen synthesis in the presence of antibody; (3) fluctuation of antigen expression in short-term cycles independent of the presence of antibody, a phenomenon quite prominent in some melanoma cell lines; and (4) shedding of antigen into the circulation, creating a smoke screen which deflects the immunologic attack away from the tumor.

IMMUNOTHERAPY

The detection and characterization of tumor-specific cell surface antigens provides the basis for new approaches to immunotherapy. For most practical purposes, what we euphemistically call immunotherapy of cancer today is limited to the use of so-called nonspecific immunopotentiators, biologic or synthetic products which enhance the immune response to unrelated antigens. The expectation has been that immunopotentiators will also augment the immune response to the putative tumor antigens. The role that these materials may play in therapy is still being defined in clinical trials, and I do not evaluate the current status of that field in this chapter. It is clear, however, that specific immunization must be explored if the full potential of immunologic therapy is to be realized.

Attempts have been made to immunize cancer patients with cancer cells or cancer cell extracts, derived from their own or, more often, other patients' cancers. Interpretation of these studies has been difficult, however, because there was no acceptable way of estimating whether the preparations used for immunization in fact contained tumor-specific antigens or whether the patient responded to them. The serologic reagents which we are now developing on the basis of initial autologous typing permit us to accomplish both: to develop vaccines of defined antigenicity, and to monitor the serologic response to immunization and correlate it with the therapeutic effect. Let me illustrate this with a few examples but caution you that our experience is too limited to interpret the meaning of changes in serologic reactivity and the causal relation between them and vaccination.

Patient BD, 66 years old, developed malignant melanoma and was treated by surgery. One year later the tumor recurred, and this is when our study began. By IA assays, serum reactivity against autologous melanoma cells was highest at the time when recurrent melanoma was resected; it then fell and remained at a low level. At the time of maximal IA reactivity, titers in MHA assays were low, but they rose during vaccination with irradiated autologous melanoma cells and BCG and then fell despite continued vaccination (fig. 10.7). This patient shows the importance of using more than one serologic assay for the detection of autologous serum reactivity. In addition, we found that serum taken at the peak of IA reactivity and serum taken at the peak of MHA reactivity showed different specificity by absorption tests. The antigenic system detected at the peak of IA reactivity was individually distinct and was absorbed by autologous melanoma only. The antigenic system detected at the peak of MHA reactivity was of the shared melanoma-specific class, cross-reactive with three allogeneic melanomas but not other tissues.

In another patient, BG, vaccination with autologous tumor cells and BCG led to increased production of widely reactive autoantibodies to class III antigens (fig. 10.8).

Figure 10.7.

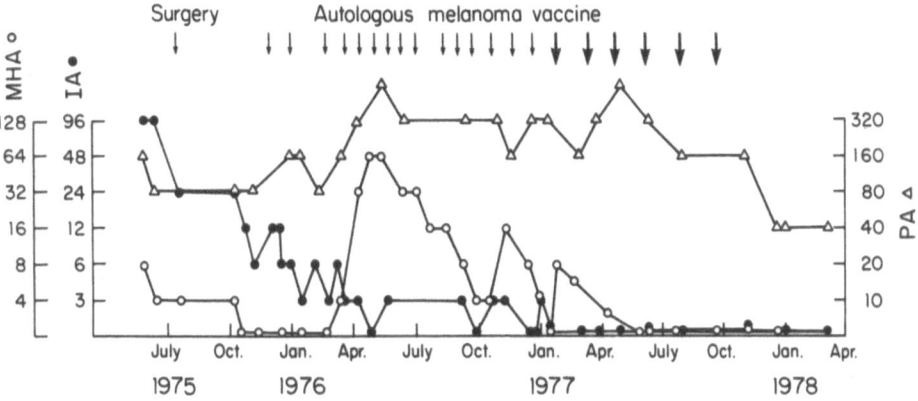

Changes in titers of antibodies to class I and II antigens associated with the administration of autologous melanoma cell vaccine. (Shiku et al. 1978.)

Figure 10.8.

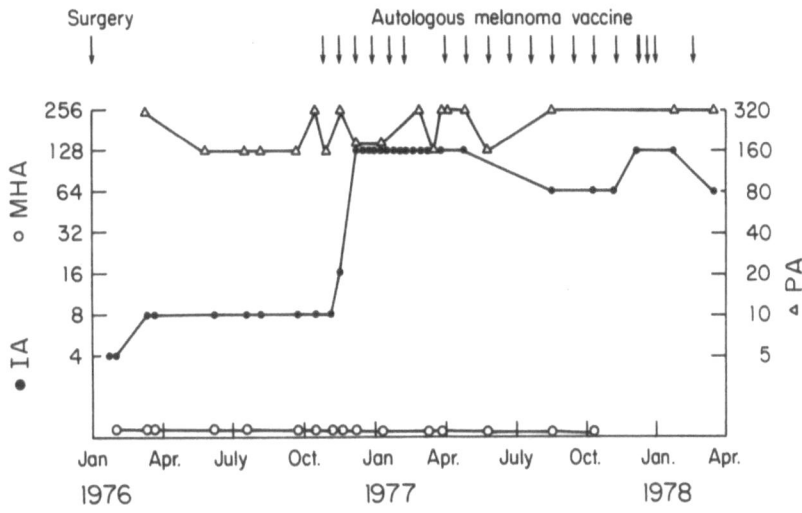

Changes in titers of antibodies to class III antigens associated with the administration of autologous melanoma cell vaccine. (Shiku et al. 1978.)

CONCLUSIONS

We are only just beginning to learn how cancer patients respond to immunization with their own cancer cells. We realize, of course, that unaltered autologous cancer cells may not be an effective stimulus for the immune system, and so we are beginning to explore modifications aimed at increasing the immunogenicity of cancer-specific antigens. In cases where shared antigens exist, immunization with allogeneic tumor cells which carry the relevant antigen may be more effective (Mitchison 1970). The immunogenicity of individually specific antigens on autologous cancer cells may be enhanced by chemical modifications (Lachmann and Sikora 1978), infection of the cells with nonpathogenic viruses (Boone et al. 1978; Wallack et al. 1977), or by fusing the cells with normal allogeneic cells, a procedure referred to as somatic cell hybridization (Pontecorvu 1975). Purified antigens, suitably modified, may turn out to be a more effective immunogen than whole cells. There are precedents for successful application of each of these approaches in experimental animals. The serology that has now been developed makes it possible to monitor the preparation of these various vaccines and the changes they induce in the patients' immune response to their own cancer cells.

REFERENCES

Boone, C. W. et al. Melanoma skin test antigens of improved sensitivity prepared from vesicular stomatitis virus-infected tumor cells. *Cancer* 41:1781–1787, 1978.

Carey, T. E. et al. Cell surface antigens of human malignant melanoma: mixed hemadsorption assays for humoral immunity to cultured autologous melanoma cells. *Proc. Natl. Acad. Sci. USA* 73:3278–3282, 1976.

Irie, K.; Irie, R.; and Morton, D. L. Detection of antibody and complement complexed *in vivo* on membranes of human cancer cells by mixed hemadsorption techniques. *Cancer Res.* 35:1244, 1975.

Lachmann, P. J., and Sikora, K. Coupling PPD to tumor cells enhances their antigenicity in BCG-primed mice. *Nature* 271:463–464, 1978.

Metzgar, R. S., and Olenick, S. R. The study of normal and malignant cell antigens by mixed agglutination. *Cancer Res.* 28:1366–1371, 1968.

Mitchison, N. A. Immunologic approaches to cancer. *Transplant Proc.* 2:92–103, 1970.

Old, L. J., and Boyse, E. A. Current enigmas in cancer research. *The Harvey Lectures*, Series 67:273–315, 1973.

Pfreundschuh, M. et al. Serological analysis of cell surface antigens of human malignant brain tumors. *Proc. Am. Assoc. Cancer Res.* 19:198, 1978.

Pontecorvu, G. Production of mammalian somatic cell hybrids by means of polyethylene glycol treatment. *Som. Cell Genet.* 1:397–400, 1975.

Shiku, H. et al. Cell surface antigens of human malignant melanoma. II. Serological typing with immune adherence assays and definition of two new surface antigens. *J. Exp. Med.* 144:873–881, 1976.

Shiku, H. et al. Cell surface antigens of human malignant melanoma. III. Recognition of autoantibodies with unusual characteristics. *J. Exp. Med.* 145:784–789, 1977.

Shiku, H. et al. Cell surface antigens of human cancer. In *Biological markers of neoplasia: basic and applied aspects*, ed. R. W. Ruddon. Amsterdam: North-Holland Publishing Co., 1978.

Tachibana, T., and Klein, E. Detection of cell surface antigens on mononuclear cells. I. The application of immune adherence on a microscale. *Immunology* 19:771–782, 1970.

Ueda, R. et al. Serological analysis of cell surface antigens of human renal cancer. *Proc. Am. Assoc. Cancer Res.* 19:198, 1978.

Wallack, M. K.; Steplewski, Z.; and Koprowski, H. A new approach to specific active immunotherapy. *Cancer* 39:560–564, 1977.

Part 2
The Diagnosis
of
Brain Metastases

11

Clinical Manifestations of Brain Metastasis

Jerome B. Posner

The neurologic signs and symptoms caused by a brain metastasis can be divided into two categories: focal and generalized (table 11.1). Focal symptoms include hemiparesis or hemiplegia, visual field deficits, aphasia, focal seizures and ataxia; they usually identify the site of the metastasis but at times may falsely localize the lesion. A brain metastasis can cause focal symptoms or signs in one (or more) of several ways (table 11.1; fig. 11.1):

Table 11.1

BRAIN METASTASIS: PATHOGENESIS OF SIGNS AND SYMPTOMS

I. Focal Symptoms (Signs)
  A. Examples
      Hemiparesis (hemiplegia)
      Visual field defects
      Aphasia
      Focal seizures
      Ataxia

  B. Causes
      Direct effect of metastasis (plus hemorrhage or cyst)
      Secondary effect of edema
      Remote effect of cerebral herniation (false localizing signs)

II. Generalized Symptoms (Signs)
  A. Examples
      Headache
      Confusion—memory loss
      Lethargy
      Vomiting
      Ataxia

  B. Causes
      Increased intracranial pressure
      Hydrocephalus

Figure 11.1.

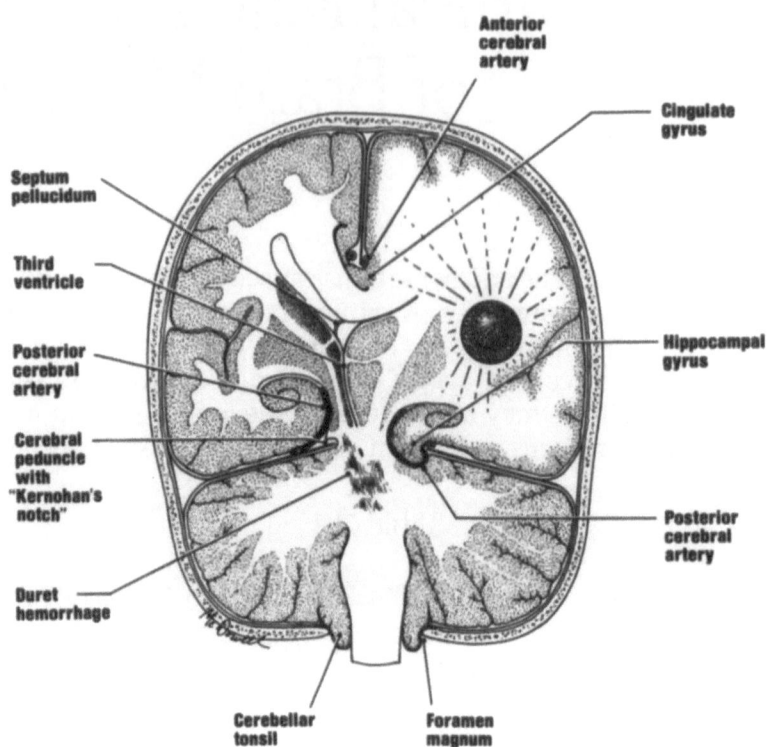

Septum pellucidum

Third ventricle

Posterior cerebral artery

Cerebral peduncle with "Kernohan's notch"

Duret hemorrhage

Anterior cerebral artery

Cingulate gyrus

Hippocampal gyrus

Posterior cerebral artery

Cerebellar tonsil

Foramen magnum

Mechanism(s) of symptom production by a brain metastasis. This schematic coronal section of the brain enclosed in the skull illustrates the changes caused by a frontal brain metastasis. The lesion itself underlies the arm area of the motor strip and causes weakness of the contralateral arm. The edema surrounding the metastasis involves most of the motor area and would be likely to cause a contralateral hemiplegia. Because of the size of the brain metastasis and the surrounding edema, several areas of normal brain have herniated into other compartments, producing compression both of themselves and of the brain in the compartments into which they have herniated: (1) Herniation of the cingulate gyrus under the falx, compressing not only the contralateral frontal lobe and the anterior cerebral arteries. Such herniation could cause bilateral frontal ischemia with weakness of the legs, urinary incontinence and mental changes. (2) Herniation of the uncus of the temporal lobe into the tentorial notch. Temporal herniation compresses the posterior cerebral artery leading to infarction in the ipsilateral occipital lobe. Uncal herniation also stretches the ipsilateral oculomotor nerve and compresses the brainstem and diencephalon, causing changes in state of consciousness. (3) Compression of the opposite cerebral peduncle against the tentorium causes a hemiparesis which is ipsilateral to the side of the lesion (a false localizing sign). (4) Downward displacement of the brainstem alters consciousness. (5) Hydrocephalus. The lateral ventricle which is enlarged as a result of obstruction of the Sylvian aqueduct by compression. Any combination of the mechanisms illustrated in this figure may play a role in producing the symptoms caused by a brain metastasis.

(1) The tumor itself can destroy nervous system tissue and lead to a clinical state in which the neurological signs and symptoms identify the site of the tumor (for example, homonymous hemianopsia due to an occipital tumor). In addition, hemorrhage, cyst formation or necrosis within the tumor can compress or destroy normal brain tissue.

(2) A brain metastasis engenders cerebral edema. The edema often affects function of the brain at a distance from the metastasis, leading to focal signs and symptoms more widespread than those caused by the metastasis alone but still pointing to the general area of the tumor (for example, hemiparesis due to an anterior frontal tumor).

(3) The brain metastasis and its surrounding cerebral edema increase local tissue pressure (Reulen 1976), which in turn shifts cerebral structures and causes cerebral herniations (Zulch and colleagues, 1974). Cerebral herniations may produce false localizing signs. False localizing symptoms and signs are focal neurologic abnormalities caused by shifts of intracranial structures which suggest the presence of a tumor in an area where it does not in fact exist (Collier 1904; Gassel 1961; Talalla and McKissock 1971). An example is hemiparesis ipsilateral to a brain metastasis caused by massive swelling of the hemisphere, shifting of the midbrain, and compression of the opposite cerebral peduncle against the tentorium cerebelli, Kernohan's notch (Kernohan and Wollman 1929).

Generalized symptoms include headache, confusion, lethargy and papilledema. Two mechanisms are usually responsible for generalized symptoms: increased intracranial pressure from the metastasis and its surrounding edema, and hydrocephalus caused by obstruction of CSF. (See fig. 1.6B, Chapter 1.)

Some signs may be either focal or generalized. For example, ataxia may result from a cerebellar lesion or may be a sign of hydrocephalus. In a given patient, there is likely to be more than one symptom, and the causes of the symptoms are likely to be multiple (fig. 11.1). For example, brain metastases may lead to seizures which are usually focal in onset but which may spread from the initial focus and produce generalized convulsions with no localizing value.

SIGNS AND SYMPTOMS

Presenting Symptoms

The presenting symptoms of brain metastases are summarized in table 11.2. This table includes the results from four recent series of patients with diagnosed and treated brain metastases. The series by Young (see Posner 1974) and by Gamache and colleagues (1979) are from Memorial Sloan-Kettering Cancer Center. The first series includes 162 patients with single or multiple metastases who were treated with radiation therapy. In the second group 94 patients with presumably single metastases were treated by surgical extirpation. There are no striking differences in symptoms between these two groups except for the higher incidence of visual field deficits in the surgical group. The four series summarized here are similar to other reports (Van Eck et al. 1965; Stortebecker 1954). Headache, focal weakness (hemiparesis or monoparesis), mental disturbances and seizures are the most common presenting symptoms. Other less frequent symptoms include gait ataxia (a common presenting sign with cerebellar metastases), aphasia, visual field abnormalities, and sensory changes. The figures in table 11.2 add up to more than 100% in each list because many patients presented with more than one symptom.

HEADACHE is a presenting complaint in about half of patients with brain metastases. The headache may be focal or generalized. When the headache is focal, it has localizing value. Simionescu (1960) reported that the headache in 72% of his patients was localized at the site of the metastasis. The headache is often diffuse or located bilaterally in frontal or occipital regions, however, and then has no localizing value. The typical brain metastasis headache is mild at first, usually occurring upon awakening and disappearing shortly after arising. Untreated, the headaches generally increase in frequency, duration, and severity until they become constant, and other signs of increased intracranial pressure develop (drowsiness, nausea and vomiting).

Table 11.2

PRESENTING SYMPTOMS OF BRAIN METASTASES

Symptom	Series (Number of Patients)			
	Paillas and Pellet (178)	Hildebrand (50)	Young (162) (Posner 1974)	Gamache et al. (94)
Headache	44%	26%	53%	43%
Focal Weakness	18	30	40	34
Mental and Behavior Disturbances	22	30	31	34
Seizures	19	6	15	21
Ataxia	—	—	20	—
Aphasia	1	4	10	—
Visual Field Defect	1	6	—	13
Sensory Change	10	2	—	—

In the series of Paillas and Pellet (1976), 44% of patients had headaches as a presenting symptom, and this number increased to 62% by the time the diagnosis was established.

Headaches as an isolated symptom are more common in patients with multiple metastases than in those with single lesions and are also more common in patients with cerebellar metastases than in those with cerebral metastases. Occasionally large frontal lesions may be accompanied by severe and recurrent headache without other evidence of neurologic dysfunction. In a series of 37 patients with cerebellar tumor (Levy and Posner, unpublished data), headache was a presenting complaint in 70% whereas it is less than 50% in patients with cerebral tumors. The headaches were often occipital, thus suggesting the site of the lesion, but at times they were bifrontal or diffuse and had no localizing value.

The pathogenesis of brain tumor headache was carefully studied by Wolff and his colleagues (Dalessio 1972), who concluded that the headache results from traction on pain-sensitive intracranial structures. These pain-sensitive structures include the dura at the base of the brain, cranial nerves, and the large venous sinuses. The presence of headache thus implies a focal or diffuse increase in intracranial pressure. Occasionally, particularly in cerebellar tumors with markedly increased intracranial pressure, headaches may be paroxysmal (often precipitated by cough or postural change) and sometimes accompanied by other neurologic symptoms such as visual obscurations, changes in consciousness, drop attacks, nausea and vomiting, and syncope (Ekbom et al. 1974; Kremer 1958; Symonds 1956). Paroxysmal headaches are thought to be related to sudden transient increases in intracranial pressure called plateau waves (Lundberg 1960).

Because headaches caused by a metastasis are usually accompanied by increased intracranial pressure, one might expect a high incidence of papilledema in such patients. In fact, the contrary is true. In Young's series, headaches were present in 53% of patients but papilledema was present in only 26% (Posner 1974). In Levy and Posner's patients with cerebellar tumors, headaches were present in 70% of patients and papilledema in only 25% (unpublished data). Paillas and Pellet (1976) reported a 62.3% incidence of headaches after confirmation of the diagnosis, but only 43% of those patients had papilledema.

FOCAL WEAKNESS is the second ranking complaint in most series. The weakness may range from gradually developing mild mono- or hemiparesis to acute hemiplegia. Focal weakness was a presenting complaint in 18% of the Paillas and Pellet series (1976) but was present in 67% of patients by the time the diagnosis was confirmed. The presence of focal weakness accurately locates the tumor in the contralateral cerebral hemisphere, but since the effects of the tumor and its surrounding edema are so widespread, it does not accurately localize the lesion to the motor area of that hemisphere. If only one extremity is weak, the tumor is more likely to be located in the white matter directly below the cortical area subserving that function.

Focal weakness may also be caused by a brain metastasis in the frontal lobe anterior to the motor cortex or in the parietal lobe posterior to the motor cortex. Paillas and Pellet (1976) noted that although metastatic tumors are more frequently found in the parietal lobe than in the frontal lobe, motor disturbances are more common than sensory disturbances. Our own experience is similar: motor deficits are much more common than sensory deficits even when tumors are located posterior to the Rolandic fissure.

MENTAL DISTURBANCES are the initial complaint in about a third of patients. Mental and behavioral changes may be a result of either focal disturbances of brain function or generalized cerebral abnormalities. Focal abnormalities of mental function, when present in pure form, have localizing value. Such disorders include aphasia, agnosia, apraxia, amnesia (Brown 1972; Horenstein 1971) and occasionally affective changes such as mania or depression (Malamud 1967). The patient often complains of being perplexed at his inability to carry out certain simple acts. Examples include patients who are otherwise intellectually intact but who cannot read (alexia) or calculate (acalculia) because of a left parietal metastasis. Dressing apraxia resulting from a right parietal lesion is a common presenting complaint. Unilateral or bilateral lesions of the limbic system may produce loss of recent memory with preservation of other cognitive functions. Occasionally limbic lesions cause behavioral changes which resemble functional psychoses rather than organic brain disease (Malamud 1967).

Much more commonly, however, mental and behavioral changes are nonspecific and result from multiple cerebral metastases or from lesions which increase intracranial pressure. Typically in the early stage, patients are awake and alert although they may sleep more than usual. Patients may complain of difficulty with memory and concentration or the families note that the patients are more irritable and forgetful. Occasionally the presenting complaint is issued by business colleagues who complain that the patient's judgment has become poor.

The most common neurologic symptom associated with nonspecific mental changes is headache since both are generally related to intracranial pressure, but mental changes may occur in the absence of any other neurologic symptoms. If a diagnosis is not made and the patient is not treated, symptoms usually progress to loss of alertness, increasing drowsiness, increasing forgetfulness, and finally loss of orientation, first for time and later for place and person.

SEIZURES, either focal or generalized, are the fourth commonest presenting complaint in most series. Seizures are more common in patients with multiple metastases, particularly malignant melanoma (since these lesions frequently reside in the cortex rather than the subcortical white matter), than they are in patients with a single lesion. The seizures are usually focal in onset and have localizing value. Characteristically a focal motor seizure begins with a clonic jerking of the face or one extremity. The seizure may progress to involve the other extremity on the same side (Jacksonian march) or may generalize. Frequently the patient suffers paralysis of the extremities after the seizure (Todd's paralysis). The paralysis is usually transient with recovery occurring in several hours to days. On occasion a single seizure or repetitive seizures lead to permanent paralysis of the involved extremities.

In the Paillas and Pellet series (1976) seizures were a presenting complaint in 19% of patients, but by the time the diagnosis was confirmed, 39% suffered from seizures. Simionescu (1960) reports a rate of 29% for seizures.

Such a high incidence raises the question of whether patients with brain metastases, particularly if located near the motor center, should be treated prophylactically with anticonvulsant drugs. We have chosen not to do so in most instances, in part because our incidence of seizures is lower than that reported in other series and in part because we have had difficulty maintaining stable blood levels of anticonvulsant drugs in these patients, who are usually taking other drugs as well. The inability to maintain stable blood levels leads to anticonvulsant toxicity alternating with ineffective therapy. Adrenal steroid (especially dexamethasone) metabolism is also altered by phenytoin, the most widely used anticonvulsant (Haque et al. 1972). Seizures can be a difficult problem, however, not only because they may cause increased weakness but because they increase cerebral blood flow and thereby raise intracranial pressure. These changes may tip an otherwise stable patient into an episode of cerebral herniation.

OTHER PRESENTING SYMPTOMS. In Young's series, gait ataxia was a prominent presenting complaint (Posner 1974). Ataxia suggests a cerebellar or brainstem tumor but occasionally is the result of a large frontal lobe metastasis. Gait ataxia may also result from hydrocephalus caused by obstruction of CSF pathways (Maurice-Williams 1975). Ataxia due to hydrocephalus can be relieved by shunting. Rarely parietal lesions cause unilateral ataxia as an isolated sign (Appenzeller and Hanson 1966).

Aphasia was a prominent presenting complaint in about 10% of Young's series (Posner 1974). It was an isolated complaint in only 1% of patients reported by Paillas and Pellet (1976) and 4% by Hildebrand (1978). Aphasia is an excellent localizing symptom when occurring in the absence of other cognitive changes but nonaphasic naming difficulties, which are a result of more generalized brain dysfunction, often can be confused with aphasia (Strub and Black 1977). Sensory changes were an uncommon complaint in all of the series despite the fact that the parietal lobe, site of the sensory cortex, was involved in many patients.

Visual abnormalities, usually a hemianopia, were a prominent presenting complaint only in the series of Gamache and others (1979). Patients with hemianopia are often aware that they are having some visual difficulty although they are unable to specify its nature.

PRESENTING SIGNS. In most series, signs and symptoms are lumped together. Young, however, described the presenting signs and symptoms of brain metastases separately in 162 consecutive cases treated by radiation therapy at Memorial Sloan-Kettering Cancer Center (Posner 1974). These signs and symptoms are listed in table 11.3. The major finding from this series is that careful neurologic examination often reveals neurologic signs never mentioned by the patient. Thus, although only 40% of patients complained of focal weakness, careful neurologic examination revealed some evidence of mono- or hemiparesis in two-thirds of patients. Often the findings were only subtle facial weakness, drift of an outstretched extremity, or spasticity or reflex hyperactivity on one side.

More striking was the high incidence of impaired cognitive or behavioral function in patients at the time of diagnosis. Three-quarters of patients were unable to perform normally in the standard tests of mental status (Strub and Black 1977). This figure is higher than most reported elsewhere in the literature, but it does suggest, nevertheless, that careful testing of patients suspected of having brain metastasis will often reveal subtle and unexpected changes in cognitive function. Paillas and Pellet (1976) report mental disturbances at the time of diagnosis in 24% of patients, but Elkington (1935) reported them in 75% of patients, and Garde and others (1958) in 50%. Part of the discrepancies among these reports may have to do with the definition of mental disturbances since these are not clearly defined in most series. In the Paillas and Pellet series mental disturbances at time of diagnosis or after confirmation of diagnosis are listed as 24%. They list generalized asthenia, including clouding of consciousness and torpor, in an additional 24%. We consider both these symptoms to be mental disturbances. Thus their combined incidence of 48% approaches closely our somewhat higher incidence.

One exception to the rule that neurologic findings are more prominent than symptoms occurs with cerebellar tumors. These patients often complain of difficulty walking at a time when neurologic findings are absent or minimal.

Table 11.3

PRESENTING SYMPTOMS AND SIGNS OF CEREBRAL METASTASES (162 PATIENTS)

Symptoms	Percentage of Patients	Signs	Percentage of Patients
Headache	53	Hemiparesis	66
Focal weakness	40	Impaired cognitive function	77
Behavioral and mental change	31	Unilateral sensory loss	27
Seizures	15	Papilledema	26
Ataxia	20	Ataxia	24
Aphasia	10	Aphasia	19

MODE OF ONSET OF NEUROLOGIC DYSFUNCTION

The signs and symptoms of a brain metastasis usually begin insidiously and evolve subacutely (over days or a few weeks) or rarely chronically (over weeks or months) as presented in table 11.4. Sometimes the onset of neurologic symptoms is sudden (as in hemorrhage into a tumor). Paillas and Pellet (1976) report an acute onset of symptoms in 83 of 178 patients (47%). There were two types of acute onset, seizures (19%) and a stroke-like syndrome with hemiplegia (18%). Other acutely developing neurologic signs (such as sensory loss, aphasia, dementia) were less common. Van Eck and colleagues (1965) indicate that 30 of their 104 patients with brain metastases had a "more or less acute onset of symptoms" but do not further specify. Our own experience has been that if seizures are excluded (15%, Posner 1974), then acute or apoplectic onset of neurologic symptoms occurs in less than 10% of patients.

The pathogenesis of gradually developing symptoms is a slowly increasing space-occupying mass with surrounding edema. The pathogenesis of the acutely developing symptoms other than seizures is more perplexing. In some instances the acute onset heralds hemorrhage into previously silent metastatic tumor. This mode of onset is particularly common in patients with choriocarcinoma (either uterine or testicular in origin) and malignant melanoma, but hemorrhage into a brain metastasis can occur with any primary tumor (Mandybur 1977). Hemorrhage is confirmed by finding blood in the CSF or by CT scan (see Chapter 12). In many instances patients with brain metastasis suffer the apoplectic onset of hemiplegia or other neurologic signs without evidence of hemorrhage. In these patients the pathogenesis is not clear. Perhaps the tumor compromised arterial circulation and caused a cerebral infarct (Mori et al. 1978). Sometimes no explanation for the acute onset can be found even at autopsy.

Table 11.4

BRAIN METASTASIS: ONSET OF SYMPTOMS AND SIGNS

Gradual
    subacute (days to weeks)
    insidious (weeks to months)

Abrupt
    seizures
    "stroke"-like

Episodic

The most unusual presentation of a brain metastasis is episodic loss of neurologic function suggesting transient ischemic attacks. The pathogenesis of the episodic loss of neurologic function is not certain but symptoms probably result from local seizures unrecognized by the patient (Fisher 1978).

COURSE OF NEUROLOGIC DYSFUNCTION

Patients with a gradual onset of neurologic signs and symptoms generally run a subacute course (table 11.5). Once neurologic signs and symptoms have appeared, progression is generally inexorable with a median survival of about one month if the patient receives no treatment (Lang and Slater 1964). In rarer instances, symptoms of brain metastasis slowly progress over months to occasionally as long as a year. At any time during the gradual progression of clinical symptoms, there can be a sudden worsening of the patient's condition.

A patient with an initially acute onset of symptoms may follow one of several courses. Commonly there is a period of stability after the acute onset, followed by rapid deterioration over days to weeks. Less commonly, a patient with an acute onset of symptoms will experience improvement, probably due to resolution of the hemorrhage in the metastasis. The initial improvement may mislead the physician to believe that the patient has suffered a stroke. The situation becomes clear only after several days to weeks when neurologic signs again worsen, reflecting the typical natural history of a brain metastasis.

Paillas and Pellet (1976) have reported a three-stage course in which there is an acute onset of neurologic symptoms which they believe represents a tumor embolus occluding a blood vessel. There is then a phase of improvement which may last weeks to years, followed by progressive

Table 11.5

BRAIN METASTASIS: COURSE OF SYMPTOMS AND SIGNS

Progressive
     subacute
     chronic

Abrupt Worsening Followed by
     progression
     stability
     improvement

"Three-stage course"

neurologic symptoms. The phase of improvement represents return of function to an ischemic area, and the secondary increase in neurologic symptoms represents the growth of tumor from the embolus. We have only rarely encountered this series of events in our patients.

The importance of these unusual modes of onset and course is that they suggest cerebral vascular disease rather than tumor and can be mistaken for such. The apoplectic onset, three-stage course, and transient attacks have all been grouped together by Michel (1976) under the term *pseudovascular forms*. He observed 31 such cases in a series of 200 patients. This is more frequent than in our experience.

UNUSUAL INTRACRANIAL METASTATIC PROBLEMS (Table 11.6)

Sagittal Sinus Occlusion

Sagittal sinus occlusion from an epidural metastasis (fig. 11.2) causes increased intracranial pressure due to interference with venous drainage. Because the occlusion is gradual in onset, however, it does not usually produce severe or acute neurologic damage. Characteristically the patient either is asymptomatic or has a mild generalized headache. On examination, florid papilledema is found and severe hemorrhages over the optic disc are common. The presence of florid papilledema in the absence of significant neurologic signs or symptoms, and particularly in the absence of mental changes, indicates that the brain is uninvolved and suggests sagittal sinus occlusion. A Towne view of the skull revealing a bony metastasis overlying the posterior portion of the sagittal sinus strongly suggests the diagnosis, which can be confirmed by arteriography.

Table 11.6

BRAIN METASTASES: UNUSUAL CLINICAL SYNDROMES

Sagittal sinus occlusion (pseudotumor)
Subdural effusion
Multiple small metastases
Silent occipital lesions
Cerebellar lesions

Figure 11.2.

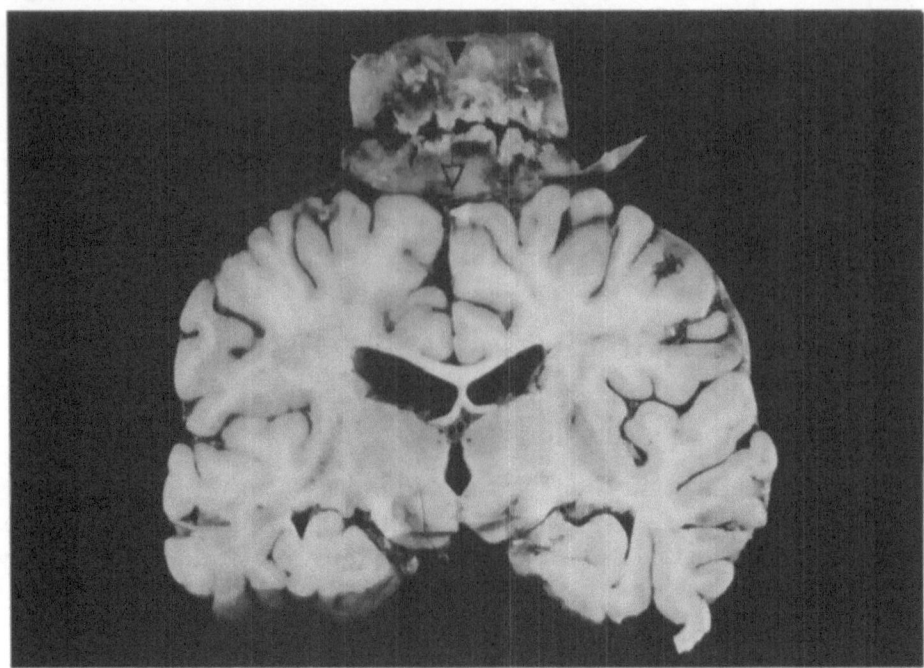

Sagittal sinus occlusion. This patient had carcinoma of the breast. The tumor involved the skull (black arrow) and dura (open arrow) and occluded the sagittal sinus (white arrow). The patient was asymptomatic except for papilledema and mild headache.

Subdural Effusions

Many tumors, particularly those of the breast and prostate, metastasize to the subdural space and produce effusion or hemorrhage (fig. 11.3). The clinical history is progressive, usually unilateral, headache associated with increasing drowsiness and hemiparesis. The clinical symptoms cannot be separated from those of brain metastasis, but diagnostic tests often reveal a subdural collection rather than a metastatic brain tumor. The importance of recognizing subdural effusions is that surgical evacuation relieves the neurologic signs promptly. When evacuating a subdural effusion or hematoma in any patient with a history of cancer, material should be sent to the laboratory for cytologic examination. If malignant cells are present, postoperative radiation therapy is advisable.

Multiple Metastases Presenting as Confusional States

In some patients, particularly those with malignant melanoma, less frequently with oat-cell carcinoma, breast carcinoma, and reticulum-cell

Figure 11.3.

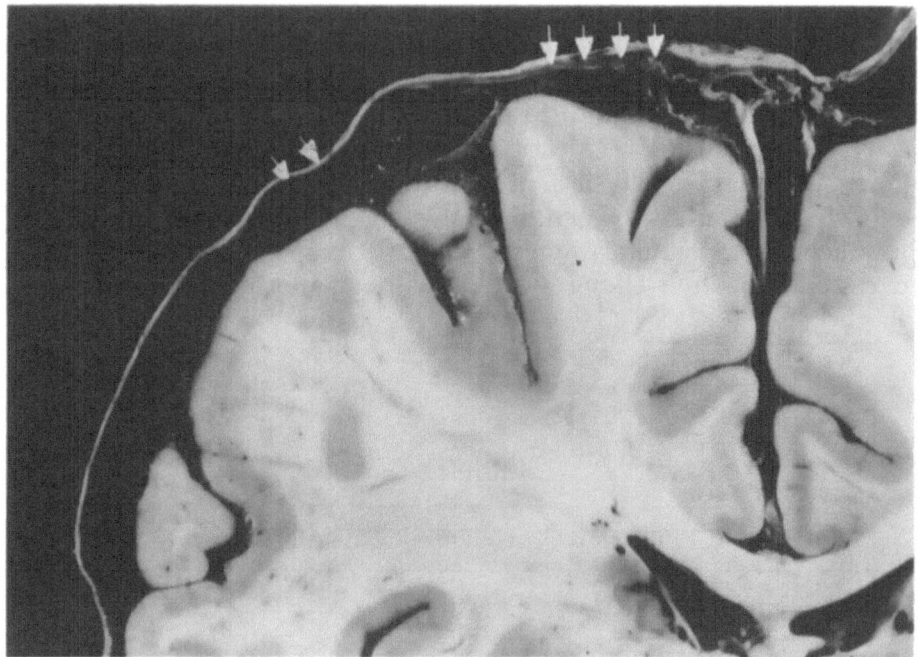

Subdural metastasis with hematoma formation. This patient had carcinoma of the lung widely seeding to the subdural space (arrows). There was no skull or epidural tumor. Bleeding from the metastatic tumor produced a subdural hematoma.

sarcoma, the brain is studded with multiple small metastases which may not be visible on gross inspection. This form of metastatic brain tumor, called *encephalitic* (Madow and Alpers 1951), is characterized pathologically by diffuse invasion of the cortex by tumor. The meninges may or may not be involved. These patients present with subacute mental changes including abnormalities of alertness, orientation and other cognitive functions. Because there may be no focal neurologic signs and no history of headache, the patient is often thought to be suffering from a toxic or metabolic encephalopathy rather than widespread brain metastases.

Automobile Accident Syndrome

Patients with posterior parietal or occipital metastases may develop a homonymous hemianopsia of which they are unaware. The characteristic presenting complaint is multiple, usually minor, automobile accidents in which the same side of the car is involved. Careful examination usually reveals a visual field defect of which the patient is unaware.

Cerebellar Metastases with Gait Ataxia

Early in the course of a cerebellar metastasis, the patient frequently complains of unsteadiness of gait with or without other neurologic symptoms. The most common associated symptom is early morning headache. There are usually few findings on physical examination; specifically there is no nystagmus, and point-to-point tests in the upper and lower extremities are normal. The gait appears normal except for minor difficulty in tandem walking. The physician may attribute the minimal gait difficulty to generalized weakness or cachexia rather than to cerebellar metastasis. If the patient's complaints are ignored, other signs and symptoms, including increasing difficulty walking, develop within a short period of time.

Table 11.7

APPROACH TO THE DIAGNOSIS OF BRAIN METASTASIS

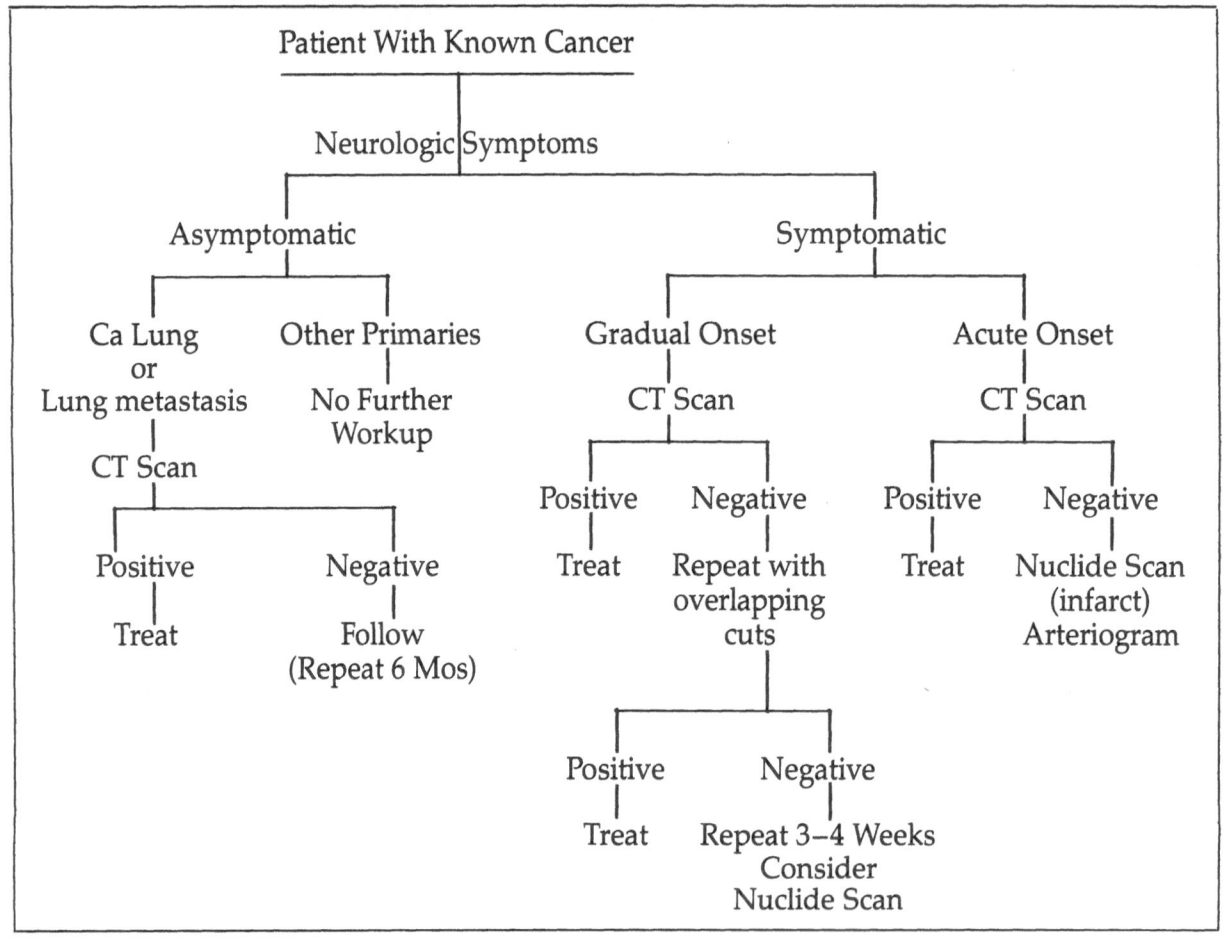

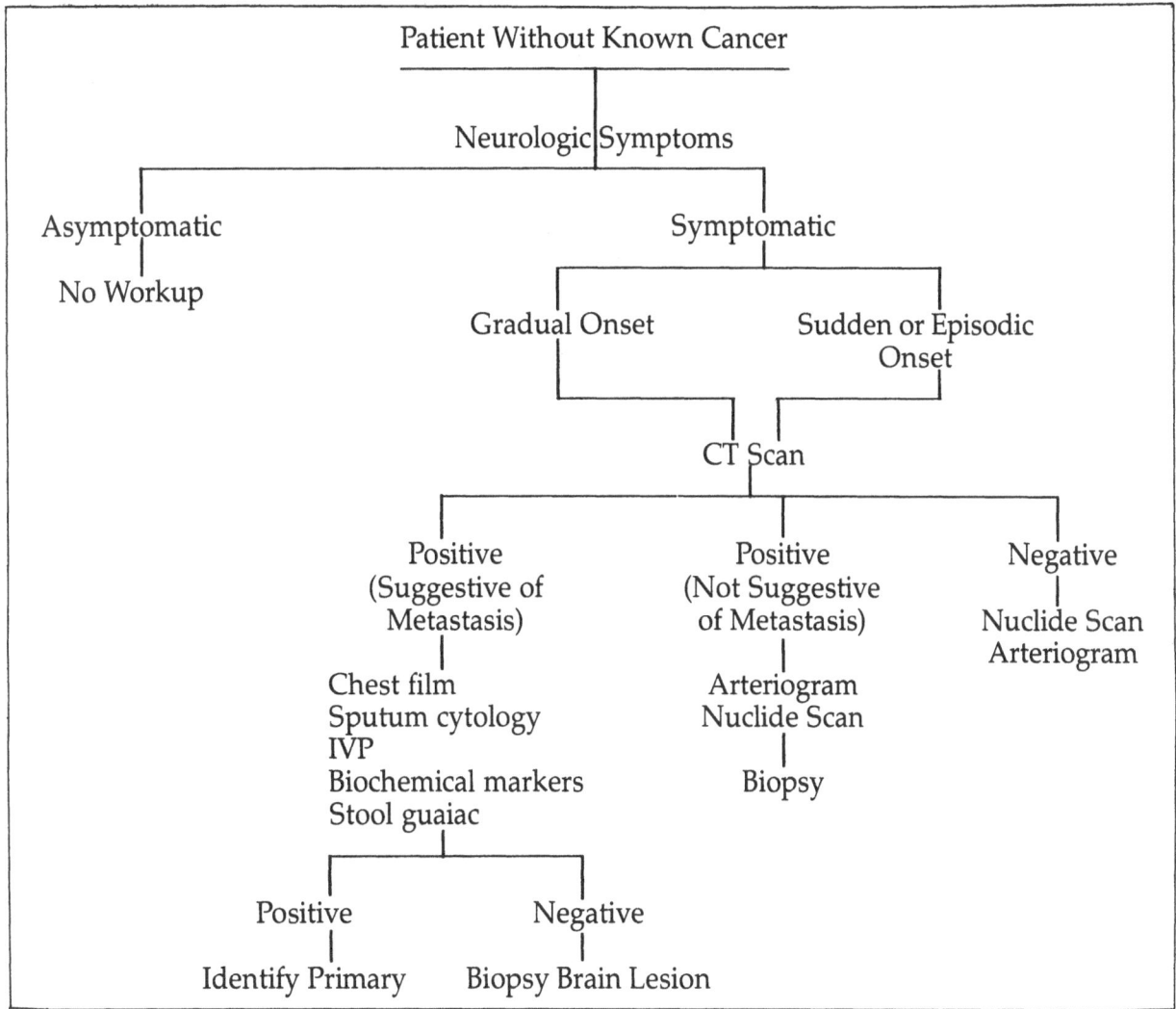

DIAGNOSIS

The physician should suspect a brain metastasis whenever a patient with present or previous cancer develops neurologic symptoms (table 11.7) or when diagnostic tests suggest a brain tumor (see Chapter 12).

The best diagnostic test when a brain metastasis is suspected is computed tomography (CT). This diagnostic test, including its pitfalls, is discussed in detail in Chapter 12. It is sufficient to say here that the test is exceedingly sensitive. It is positive in over 90% of patients with symptomatic brain metastases and sometimes detects asymptomatic brain metastases (Jacobs et al. 1977). In the absence of a CT scan, the best test is a radionuclide brain scan. This test is described in Chapter 13. In my opinion the CT scan is far superior to the radionuclide scan, not only because it is more sensitive but because it gives additional information, including the

Table 11.8

BRAIN METASTASIS: DIFFERENTIAL DIAGNOSIS

I. Primary Brain Tumors
    Meningioma
    Glioma
    Others

II. Vascular Disease

    A. Central Hemorrhage
        into metastasis
        secondary to thrombocytopenia
        hypertensive
        vascular anomaly

    B. Cerebral Embolus
        Nonbacterial thrombotic endocarditis
        Tumor embolus
        Not related to cancer

    C. Cerebral Thrombosis
        Compression of artery or vein by tumor
        Thrombosis
            arterial
                arteriosclerotic
                DIC
            venous
                sinus thrombosis
                DIC

III. Infections

    A. Cerebral Abscesses
        Especially Hodgkin's disease and lymphoma.

    B. Viral Infection—Progressive multifocal
        leukoencephalopathy.

IV. Degenerative Disease
    Related to cancer—"remote effect"
    Not related to cancer (e.g., multiple sclerosis)

size of the ventricles and shifts of cerebral structures. If a CT scan is negative, it is highly unlikely that the radionuclide brain scan will be positive.

When a patient suspected of harboring a brain metastasis has a normal CT scan, it is our policy to repeat the CT scan with overlapping cuts directed at the area of concern. The scan should probably be repeated 2–3 weeks later if the symptoms persist. In my experience, neither radionuclide brain scanning, arteriography nor pneumoencephalography will demonstrate a brain metastasis if the CT scan is negative. EEG, arteriography, pneumoencephalography and CSF examination are far inferior to CT and are not discussed in this monograph, but there is ample literature describing their indications and contraindications. Positron emission tomography, described elsewhere in this monograph (Chapter 14), is at present a research procedure and is unlikely to play a major role in clinical diagnosis because the CT scan will probably remain a more sensitive test.

Differential Diagnosis

Some considerations in the differential diagnosis of brain metastases are listed in table 11.8. The physician's most important task is to correctly identify benign brain tumors and other nonneoplastic masses which masquerade as brain metastases. The CT scan plays an important role in raising the initial suggestion that a brain tumor may be a meningioma (see Chapter 12) rather than a metastasis. The CT scan does not help distinguish brain abscesses from brain metastases, however, and clinical suspicion of a brain abscess (for example, in an immunosuppressed patient such as one with Hodgkin's disease) may require biopsy to establish the diagnosis.

Since a small but significant percentage of brain metastases may have a stroke-like onset, the physician must distinguish true cerebrovascular disease from brain metastasis, and here not only the CT scan but the radionuclide brain scan and the cerebral arteriogram may help. Although the differential diagnosis may be difficult, the physician's role is always to consider the possibility that the patient's neurologic symptoms may be due to disease other than brain metastasis, even if the patient is suffering from widespread cancer, and to carry out the appropriate diagnostic workup before therapy is undertaken.

REFERENCES

Appenzeller, O., and Hanson, J. C. Parietal ataxia. *Arch. Neurol.* 15:264–269, 1966.

Brown, J. W. *Aphasia, apraxia and agnosia. Clinical and theoretical aspects.* Springfield, Ill.: Charles C Thomas, 1972.

Collier, J. The false localising signs of intracranial tumour. *Brain* 27:490–508, 1904.

Dalessio, D. J. *Wolff's headache and other pain*. New York: Oxford University Press, 1972.

Ekbom, K.; Hornsten, G.; and Johansson, T. Posterior cranial fossa tumors. Headaches, oculostatic disorders and scintillation camera findings. *Headache* 14:119–132, 1974.

Elkington, J. S. C. Metastatic tumors of the brain. *Proc. R. Soc. Med.* 28:1080–1096, 1935.

Fisher, C. M. Transient paralytic attacks of obscure nature: the question of non-convulsive seizure paralysis. *Canad. J. Neurol. Sci.* 5:267–273, 1978.

Gamache, F. W.; Posner, J. B.; and Patterson, R. H., Jr. Involvement of the central nervous system by metastatic tumor. In *Neurological Surgery*, 2nd Ed., ed. J. R. Youmans, Philadelphia: W. B. Saunders Company, 1979.

Garde, A.; Tommasi, M.; and Aimard, G. Les complication neurologiques des neoplasmes visceraux. In *Congres de Psychiatrie et de Neurologie de Langue Francais, LVIe Session*. Paris: Masson et Cie, 1958.

Gassel, M. M. False localizing signs. A review of the concept and analysis of the occurrence in 250 cases of intracranial meningioma. *Arch. Neurol.* 4:70–98, 1961.

Haque, N. et al. Studies on dexamethasone metabolism in man: effect of diphenylhydantoin. *J. Clin. Endocrinol. Metab.* 34:44–50, 1972.

Hildebrand, J. *Lesions of the nervous system in cancer patients*. New York: Raven Press, 1978.

Horenstein, S. Amnestic, agnosic, apractic, and aphasic features in dementing illness. In *Dementia*, ed. C. W. Wells. Philadelphia: F. A. Davis, 1971.

Jacobs, L.; Kinkel, W. R.; and Vincent, R. G. "Silent" brain metastasis from lung carcinoma determined by computerized tomography. *Arch. Neurol.* 34:690–693, 1977.

Kernohan, J. W., and Wollman, H. W. Incisura of the crus due to contralateral brain tumor. *Arch. Neurol. Psychiatry* 21:274–287, 1929.

Kremer, M. Sitting, standing, and walking. *Br. Med. J.* 2:121–126, 1958.

Lang, E. F., and Slater, J. Metastatic brain tumors. Results of surgical and nonsurgical treatment. *Surg. Clin. North Am.* 44:865–872, 1964.

Lundberg, N. Continuous recording and control of ventricular fluid pressure in neurosurgical practice. *Acta Psychiat. Neurol. Scand.* [*Suppl.*] 149:1–193, 1960.

Madow, L., and Alpers, B. J. Encephalitic form of metastatic carcinoma. *Arch. Neurol. Psychiatry* 65:161–173, 1951.

Malamud, N. Psychiatric disorder with intracranial tumors of limbic system. *Arch. Neurol.* 17:113–123, 1967.

Mandybur, T. I. Intracranial hemorrhage caused by metastatic tumors. *Neurology* 27:650–655, 1977.

Maurice-Williams, R. S. Mechanism of production of gait unsteadiness by tumors in the posterior fossa. *J. Neurol., Neurosurg. Psychiatry* 38:143–148, 1975.

Michel, D. Diagnostic, prognostic et traitement des metastases intracraniennes. A propos de 200 observations. Cited by Paillas and Pellet, 1976.

Mori, K. et al. Occlusive arteriopathy and brian tumor. *J. Neurosurg.* 49:22–35, 1978.

Paillas, J. E., and Pellet, W. Brain metastasis. In *Handbook of Clinical Neurology*, eds. P. J. Vinken and G. W. Bryn. New York: American Elsevier Publishing Co., 1976.

Posner, J. B. Diagnosis and treatment of metastases to the brain. *Clin. Bull.* 4:47–57, 1974.

Reulen, H. J. Vasogenic brain oedema. *Br. J. Anaesth.* 48:741–752, 1976.

Simionescu, M. D. Metastatic tumors of the brain. A follow-up study of 195 patients with neurosurgical considerations. *J. Neurosurg.* 17:361–373, 1960.

Stortebecker, T. P. Metastatic tumors of the brain from a neurosurgical point of view. A follow-up study of 158 cases. *J. Neurosurg.* 11:84–111, 1954.

Strub, R. L., and Black, T. W. *The mental status examination in neurology.* Philadelphia: F. A. Davis, 1977.

Symonds, C. Cough headache. *Brain* 79:557–568, 1956.

Talalla, A., and McKissock, W. Acute "spontaneous" subdural hemorrhage. An unusual form of cerebrovascular accident. *Neurology* 21:19–32, 1971.

Van Eck, J. H. M.; Go, K. G., and Ebels, E. J. Metastatic tumors of the brain. *Psychiatr. Neurol. Neurochir.* 68:443–462, 1965.

Zulch, K. J.; Mennel, H. D.; and Zimmerman, V. Intracranial hypertension. In *Handbook of Clinical Neurology*, eds. P. J. Viken and G. W. Bruyn. New York: American Elsevier Publishing Co., 1974.

12

Computed Tomography of Metastatic Disease of the Brain

Michael D. F. Deck

Development of the new method of radiologic diagnosis known as computed tomography (CT), computer-assisted tomography or computerized axial tomography (CAT) by Hounsfield (1973) has revolutionized the diagnosis and management of cranial and intracranial metastatic disease. Since installation of a CT scanner at Memorial Sloan-Kettering Cancer Center in December 1975, approximately 9,500 patient examinations have been performed, 60% of which were examinations of the skull and brain. During the period of December 1, 1975 to August 15, 1978, 460 patients were found to have CT appearances consistent with intracerebral or calvarial metastases. Computed tomography is, without question, the technique of choice for the diagnosis of metastatic disease of the brain and skull vault, and this dominant role is reflected by a significant decrease in other diagnostic procedures such as plain skull radiography, radionuclide brain scanning, electroencephalography, and cerebral arteriography (table 12.1). The decrease in these diagnostic modalities has occurred despite an increase in the number of patients seen and treated by the Department of Neurology and the Division of Neurosurgery.

The effect of CT scanning on the use of plain skull radiography is most dramatically shown by the number of neuroskulls. Although many centers require plain skull films before scheduling a CT examination, this has not been the policy at my institution. In fact, plain films are usually obtained only after the CT scan at the request of the radiologist in order to demonstrate areas such as the sella turcica, orbits or base of the skull (Weinstein et al. 1977). The cost effectiveness of using CT as the primary diagnostic modality and only using plain skull films and radionuclide scanning when required is easily demonstrated.

The use of cerebral angiography has decreased less than may be expected because most patients being considered for surgical excision of a solitary metastasis undergo the procedure in order to map the cerebral arteries and veins and plan the surgical approach to the tumor. Cerebral angiograms performed for diagnostic purposes represent approximately 50% of the total. A similar decrease in cerebral angiography has been widely reported (Larson et al. 1977). Pneumoencephalography is per-

208

Table 12.1

FREQUENCY OF DIAGNOSTIC BRAIN STUDIES AT
MEMORIAL SLOAN-KETTERING CANCER CENTER

Examination	1975	1978	Change (%)
Skull radiography	1245	826	↓34
"Neuro-skulls" (6 views)	(663)	(214)	↓68
Radionuclide brain scanning	1087	280	↓74
Cerebral angiography	170	115	↓32
Pneumoencephalography	73	71	↓ 3
Electroencephalography	1320	584	↓56
Echoencephalography	13	0	
Neurologic CT	—	2052	
Total examinations	3908	3926	

formed only occasionally for diagnostic purposes, usually prior to insertion of Ommaya reservoirs for intrathecal chemotherapy. The air in the cerebral ventricles permits accurate positioning of the intraventricular catheter under fluoroscopic control in the operating room.

TECHNICAL CONSIDERATIONS

CT Equipment

The first CT scanners to be introduced were designed specifically for the cranial cavity (dedicated head scanner). Soon thereafter whole-body scanners were developed, and it became rapidly apparent that their resolution of intracranial structures equalled that of the dedicated head scanners. Whole-body scanners now available can scan in 1–2 seconds and produce images that are significantly superior to those of the earlier head scanners. This sophisticated technology is now becoming available to the majority of patients in the United States.

Whole-body scanners permit considerable flexibility in patient positioning, rapid examinations, and variation in resolution by adjusting the radiation dosage (tissue density resolution is approximately proportional to the radiation dose to the part of the body being studied). Although the radiation dose from CT is generally at acceptable levels, there is considerable variation among different types of CT scanners and certain special techniques (thin collimators, overlapping sections, multiple studies) may result in doses of 50 R or more.

Contrast Enhancement

During the introductory period of CT scanning, intravenous iodinated contrast agents such as those used for intravenous pyelography or arteriography were seldom employed, but with greater experience most authorities consider their use essential in order to demonstrate small metastases and differentiate the metastasis from surrounding edema (Bardfeld et al. 1977). The importance of a nonenhanced CT examination may be argued (Butler and Kricheff 1978), particularly if the demand for CT examinations far exceeds the capacity of the facility. At Memorial Hospital, contrast enhancement is used on all patients with suspected or previously defined metastasis unless contraindicated by a history of allergy to the contrast medium, or by incipient renal failure. Nonenhanced scans are performed prior to contrast enhancement on all patients with melanoma or choriocarcinoma, patients suspected of harboring an intracerebral hemorrhage, and patients who have undergone a surgical procedure within the previous four weeks. In fact, the nonenhanced scan is only omitted when the demand for CT scans reaches dramatic levels (Latchaw et al. 1978).

At Memorial Hospital contrast enhancement is achieved with an intravenous bolus injection of 100 ml methylglucamine iothalamate (Conray) 60% given over 2–3 minutes. (Children receive 1.5 ml/kg body weight.) Other workers have advocated different techniques such as 50 ml of methylglucamine diatrizoate 60% (Hypaque or Renografin) (New et al. 1975) or 300 ml of 30% methylglucamine diatrizoate (Renografin) with rapid infusion of the first 200 ml and slow infusion of the last 100 ml during the scan (Butler and Kricheff 1978; Huckman 1975; Kramer et al. 1975). Even larger amounts of contrast are used by Hilal and Chang (1978), who inject 125 ml of methylglucamine diatrizoate 76% as a 5-minute bolus. With the advent of ultra-fast scanners (less than 5 seconds), contrast enhancement may be used for dynamic studies of cerebral bloodflow similar to radionuclide flow studies and the volume and rate of injection may then have to be modified.

Subarachnoid contrast enhancement during CT may be achieved with metrizamide (Amipaque), a recently approved contrast agent developed for myelography. The efficacy of this technique has yet to be fully evaluated, but it has already proven to be useful in studying the posterior fossa cisterns and the suprasellar area, permitting accurate demonstration of the optic nerves, cerebellopontine angle and brainstem (fig. 12.1). Metrizamide has also proven effective in studying cerebrospinal fluid dynamics and differentiating atrophy from communicating hydrocephalus (normal-pressure hydrocephalus).

Figure 12.1.

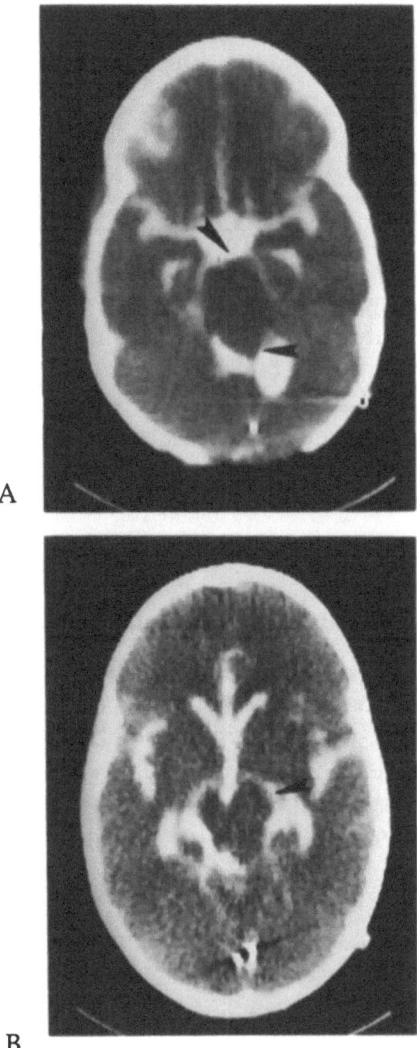

A

B

Metrizamide cisternogram in a child with a brainstem glioma. A. Section through the fourth ventricle demonstrates the enlarged pons and deformity of the ventricular floor (arrows). B. Section through the cerebral peduncles indicates tumor extension (arrow) into the right cerebral peduncle.

INTERPRETATION OF CT SCANS

Metastases of the Skull Vault and Base

Dedicated head or whole-body CT scanners are capable of exquisite resolution of bony structures when appropriate window settings are utilized. Kido and others (1978) found CT scanning to be more sensitive than plain skull films but less sensitive than radionuclide bone scanning in the detection of calvarial lesions and our experience is similar. CT not only demonstrates the precise location of lytic metastases (inner table, outer table, diploic, or through-and-through destruction) (fig. 12.2) but also demonstrates the extent of accompanying soft tissue mass intracranially or beneath the scalp. Contrast enhancement is usually essential to delineate the intracranial extent of such tumors (fig. 12.3.) In addition, many patients with calvarial metastases also have intraparenchymal deposits requiring contrast enhancement for accurate demonstration. Destructive lesions near the vertex escape detection unless the supreme CT section encompasses the skull cap and careful bone window images are available.

Small osseous metastases may escape detection by CT and yet be seen on plain skull films. Becker and others (1978), using a phantom, found that 4 mm in diameter was the critical size for CT detection because of the effect of volume averaging, but resolution could be improved by the use of lower kVp and thinner sections. Metastatic lesions in the skull base are frequently seen better on CT than on plain films, provided the CT images are of high quality without movement artefacts. In suspicious cases, however, complex motion tomography is necessary for confirmation of lesions around the sella turcica, sphenoid sinus, petrous bones and clivus.

Intracerebral Metastases

The Nonenhanced Scan The presence of intracerebral metastatic deposits may be established by CT with an accuracy that exceeds all other radiographic modalities, and generally the appearance of the metastatic lesions is sufficiently specific to render additional studies, such as cerebral angiography, unnecessary. Metastatic deposits are delineated by the surrounding edema, the change in tissue density, contrast enhancement, displacement of adjacent visible structures such as the cerebral ventricles or cortical gray matter, or rarely, calcification within the deposit.

Brain edema, due to a change in the tumor vasculature with breakdown of the blood-brain barrier, is almost always present but the extent of the edema varies and often exceeds the tumor volume considerably. CT demonstrates edema as an area of diminished density involving the white matter with finger-like extensions into the gyri (fig. 12.4). The edema sometimes extends from the frontal pole to the occipital pole and frequently is visible on several CT sections above and below the level of the contrast-enhanced tumor. If multiple metastatic deposits are present, the edema of adjacent lesions may coalesce.

The metastatic deposit itself may have a lesser or greater density than normal brain, depending on its cellular density, vascularity and degree of necrosis. The majority of metastatic nodules have a density similar to normal brain but appear to be more dense or "hyperdense" because of surrounding edema (New et al. 1975). Small metastases may not be detected on the precontrast study because of absence of surrounding edema and similar density to the surrounding brain.

Figure 12.2.

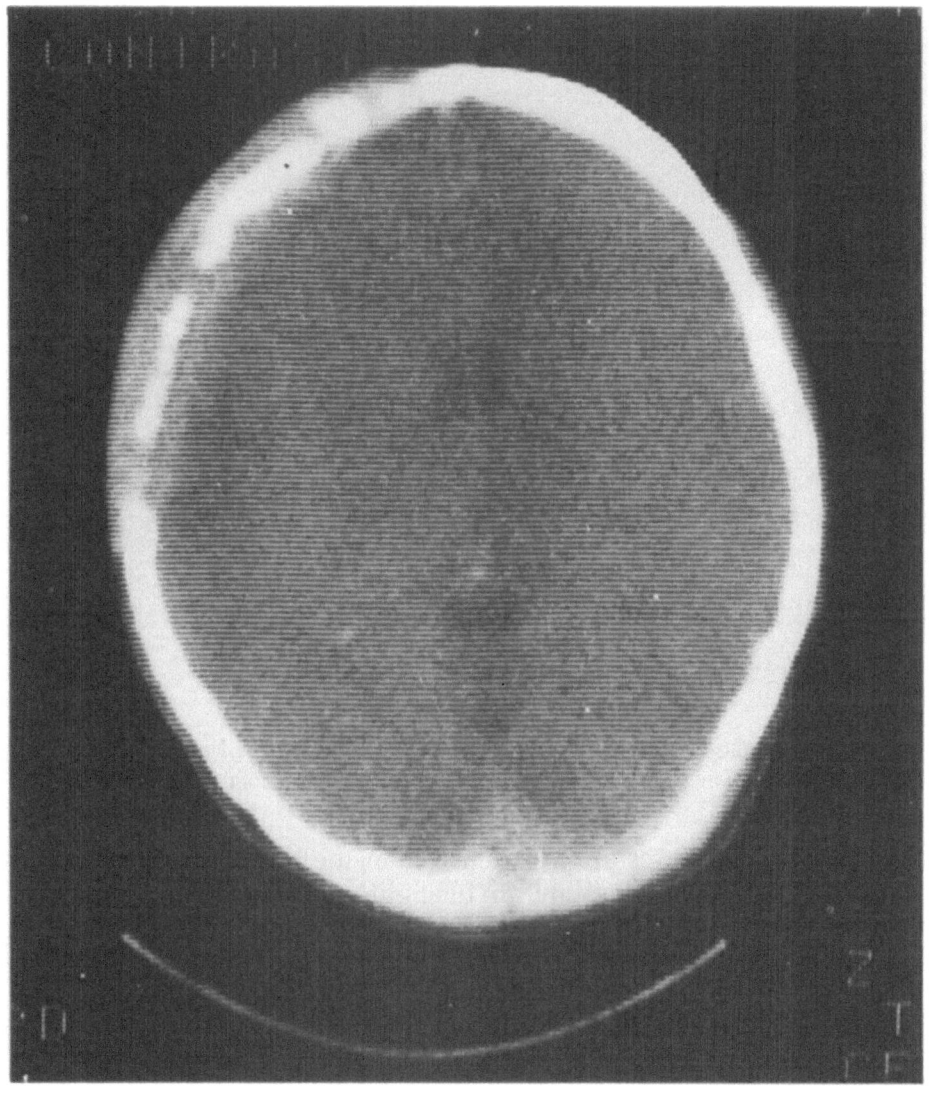

Diffuse calvarial metastases from carcinoma of the breast. Note the contrast enhancement of the epidural tumor over the cerebral convexity and near the sagittal sinus.

Figure 12.3.

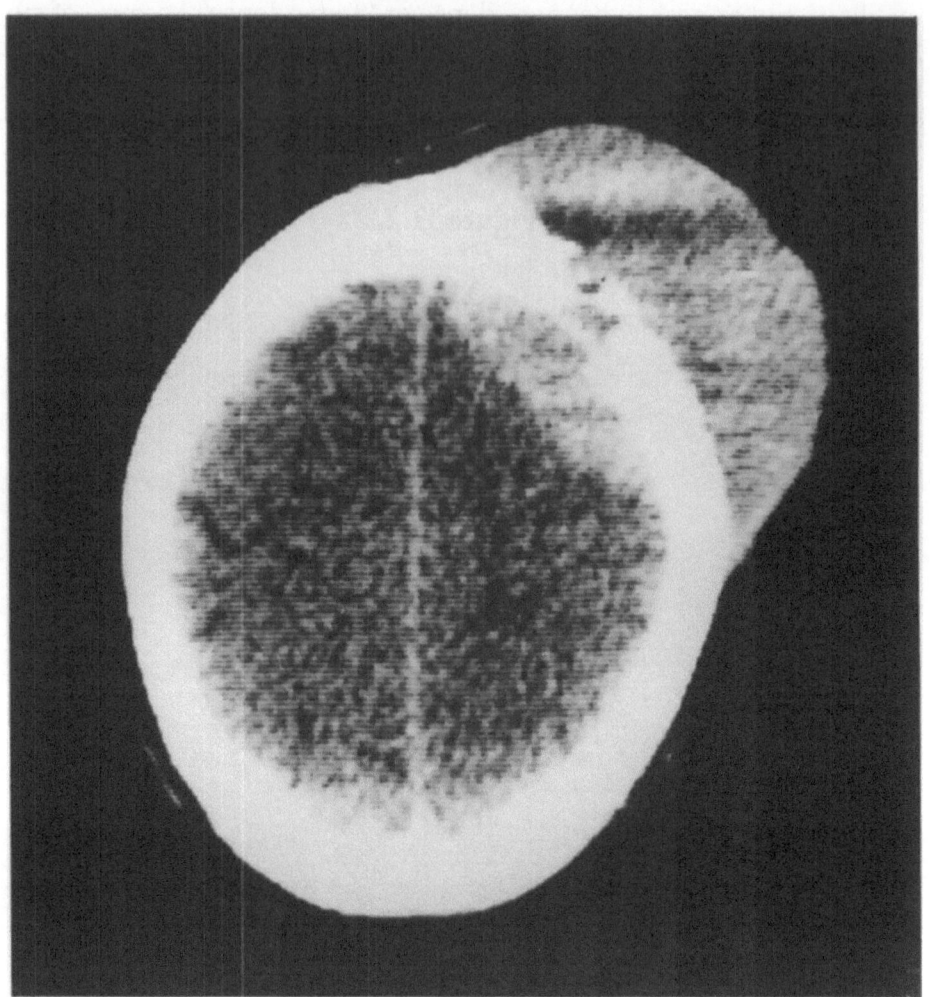

Hodgkin's disease with a calvarial deposit. Note the contrast enhancement, bone destruction, and large intracranial and extracranial components.

Certain metastases are less dense than the brain, or "hypodense," sometimes with a surrounding rim of slightly increased density presumably due to necrosis in the center, to marked vascularity in the central area, or occasionally due to a fluid-containing cyst (fig. 12.5). Classification of metastases according to their precontrast density (Deck et al. 1976) is unfortunately subject to many exceptions, but metastases from lung, breast, kidney, colon and lymphoma tend to be hypodense or isodense (fig. 12.6).

Metastatic lesions may be hyperdense because of dense cellular structure, fresh hemorrhage within or adjacent to the deposit, or rarely calcification within the neoplastic deposit. Adenocarcinoma deposits from

Figure 12.4.

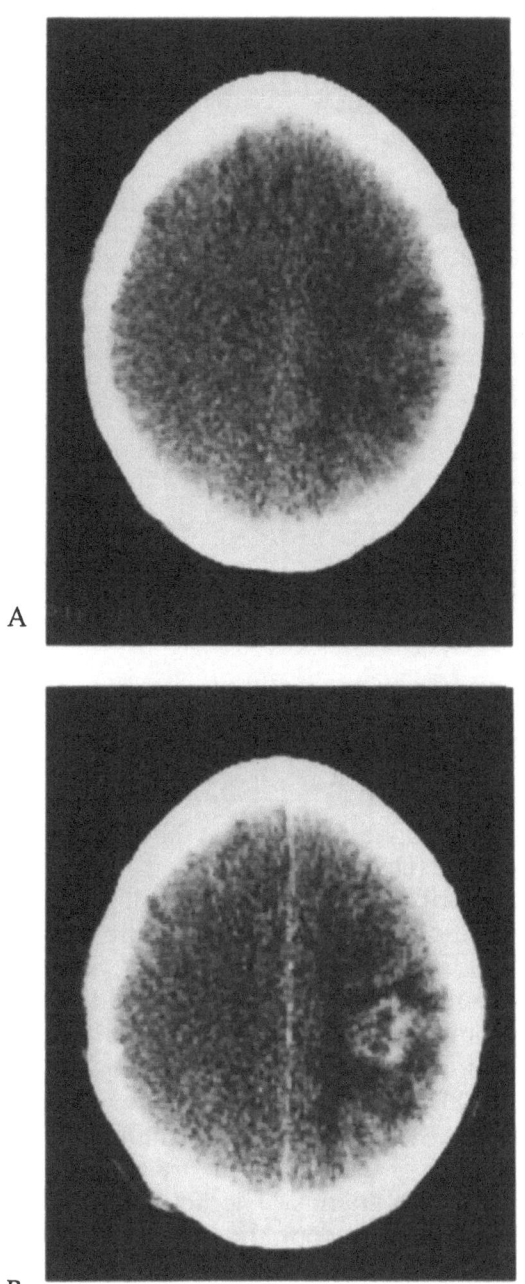

A

B

Hypodense metastatic epidermoid carcinoma of the lung. A. Precontrast scan demonstrates edema in the right frontoparietal convexity. B. Contrast-enhanced CT scan demonstrates the heterogeneous ring-like enhancement of the metastatic deposit.

Figure 12.5.

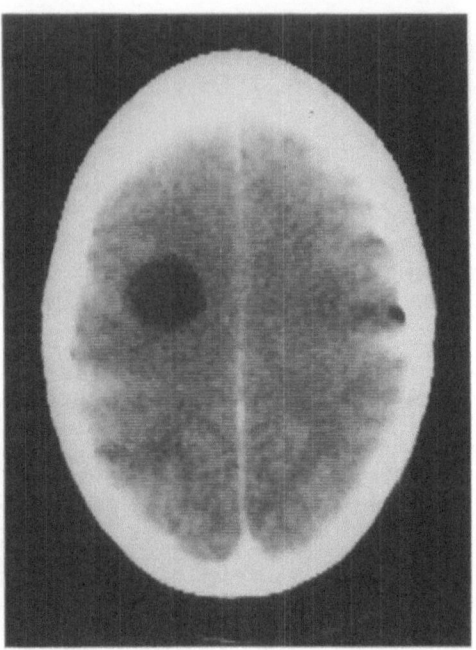

Cystic metastasis from carcinoma of the breast. This lesion has a density of water on the CT scan. There is no contrast enhancement of its margin.

colon, lung and occasionally breast may be slightly denser than the surrounding brain tissue (Deck et al. 1976).

Melanoma, chorionic carcinoma deposits, and rarely, hypernephroma and lung carcinoma may present CT findings of intracerebral hemorrhage (Deck et al. 1976; Gildersleeve et al. 1977; Solis et al. 1977; Enzmann et al. 1978a). Hemorrhaging metastases present with areas of increased density (60–80 Hounsfield units), but the density gradually reduces during the subsequent 10–14 days to an isodense or hypodense level due to a change in the composition of the clot (figs. 12.7 and 12.8).

Calcified metastases are rarely encountered except with osteogenic sarcoma, but the areas of increased density in such cases tend to be scattered rather than homogeneous. The actual density of such lesions as measured by CT will depend upon the size of the lesion and the density of the calcifications.

The Contrast-Enhanced Scan Most metastatic deposits demonstrate some degree of enhancement after an intravenous contrast medium is administered. In a series of 299 primary brain tumors and 115 metastatic tumors, Bardfeld and colleagues (1977) found that 92% of all supratentorial tumors and 89% of infratentorial tumors showed contrast enhancement (CE). Only one metastatic tumor failed to be enhanced.

Figure 12.6.

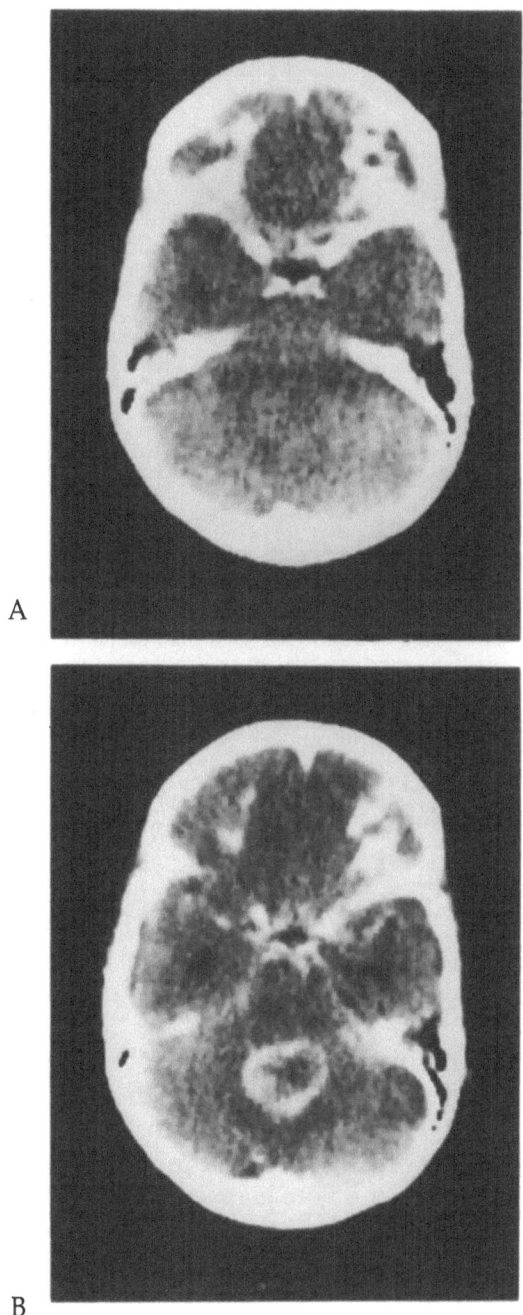

A

B

Isodense cerebellar metastasis from carcinoma of the colon. A. Precontrast study does not show the fourth ventricle. B. After intravenous contrast medium, the central cerebellar metastasis is clearly visible.

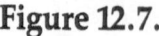

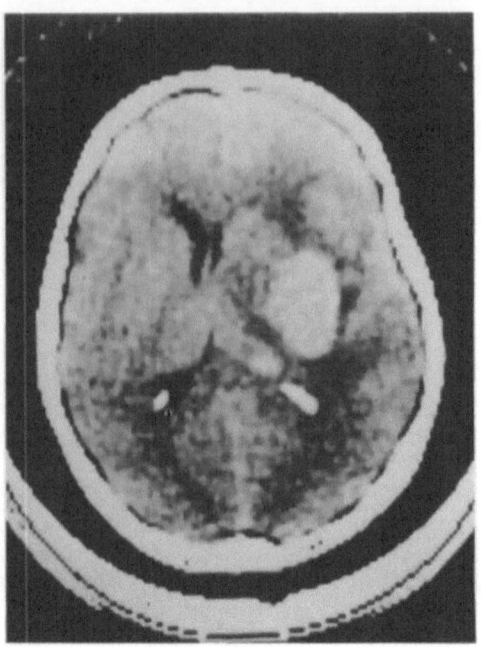

Hyperdense melanoma metastasis in the right basal ganglia. This hemorrhagic metastasis was not enhanced by contrast medium, but smaller, initially hypodense deposits visible on higher sections showed moderate contrast enhancement.

The incidence of CE is lower for melanoma metastases. Enzmann and others (1978a) found CE in 82% of lesions, but Solis and others (1977) found that only 27% of 14 melanoma metastases exhibited CE although additional lesions (presumably isodense before CE) were found in 36% of these patients.

Contrast medium distribution tends to be ring-like in most metastases—Constant and others (1977) found such a pattern in 50% of cases—but the degree of enhancement depends upon the initial density of the lesion, the volume of contrast material administered (the amount of iodine is the critical factor), and the time elapsed between the contrast administration and the scan. Hilal and Chang (1978) found that radiodense metastases showed less enhancement than radiolucent metastases and that meningiomas showed even greater enhancement than metastases although they were denser before contrast material administration.

Most metastases are more or less spherical in outline unless they are adjacent to the inner table of the skull or the falx. The tumor deposit is usually sharply demarcated by CE. Metastases arising from the dura or falx tend to have a flat base of attachment similar to meningiomas.

Figure 12.8.

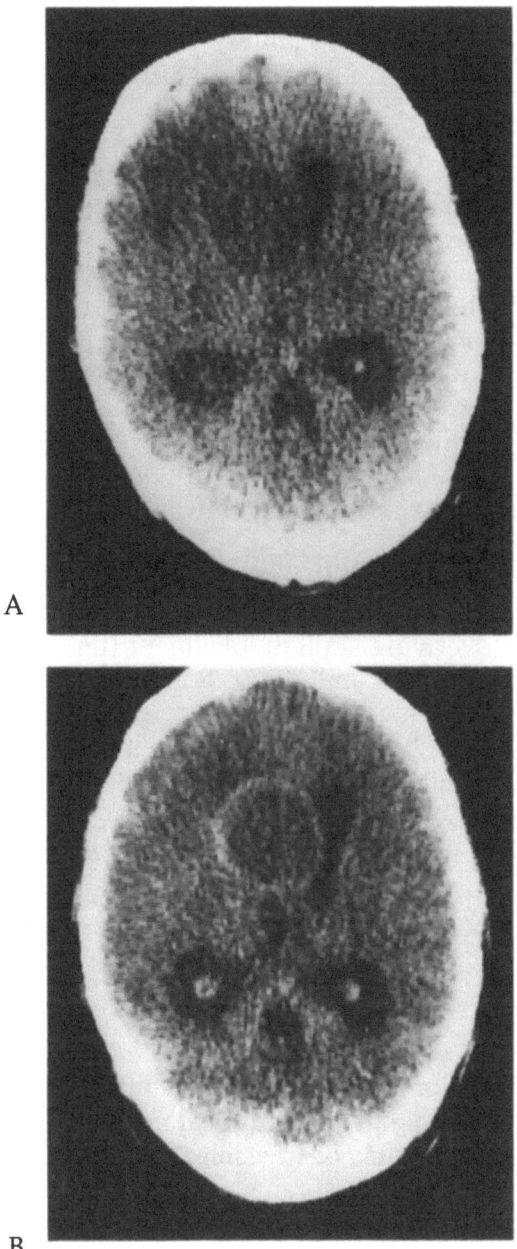

A

B

Hypodense hemorrhagic melanoma metastasis in the left frontal lobe with obstruction of the interventricular foramen. A. Precontrast study demonstrates a shift of the lateral ventricles to the right and obliteration of the left frontal horn. The trigones of each lateral ventricle are dilated. B. Ring-like enhancement of the metastasis is present after intravenous administration of contrast medium.

Multiple Metastases The presence of multiple contrast-enhancing lesions greatly increases the certainty of the diagnosis of metastatic disease. In a recent review of material at Memorial Sloan-Kettering Cancer Center, only 75 of 257 patients were found to have solitary lesions. Constant and others (1977) found a solitary metastasis in 13 of 68 patients, but Solis and others (1977), reviewing 15 cases of malignant melanoma, found 8 solitary lesions while seven had multiple deposits. Multiplicity of contrast enhancing lesions strongly suggests metastatic disease, but the diagnosis is not absolute: gliomas may be multicentric and abscesses and granulomas are sometimes multiple.

When metastases are multiple, they may be randomly scattered throughout the brain. Occasionally, a dominant metastatic deposit may be surrounded by satellite nodules suggesting that the deposits originated from a single tumor embolus which fragmented in a distal arterial branch. Fairly intense contrast enhancement may be seen in the compressed and deformed cerebral cortex adjacent to the dominant metastatic deposit. The mechanism of this phenomenon is not clear, but presumably it represents changes in the pial or subpial vasculature due to altered vasomotor control. The abnormal area fairly rapidly returns to normal after surgical resection of the metastasis.

Metastatic Lymphoma Patients with systemic lymphoma may eventually develop intracranial tumor deposits either in the epidural space, with or without overlying skull involvement (fig. 12.3), or in the parenchyma. The intraparenchymal deposits may resemble other metastases but tend to have ill-defined margins and relatively homogeneous contrast enhancement (fig. 12.9). Dubois and others (1978) have reported diffuse periventricular spread of tumor in a patient with diffuse histiocytic lymphoma. The appearance of metastatic lymphoma is similar to that seen in primary malignant lymphoma of brain and may resemble gliomas (Kazner et al. 1978).

Meningeal Carcinomatosis

Diffuse infiltration of the basal and convexity leptomeninges occasionally results in a characteristic appearance at CT. On the precontrast study the basal cisterns may be invisible, but after contrast medium injection an intense outline of the brainstem and gyri can be seen (fig. 12.10). Chronic meningitis due to tuberculosis may produce a similar appearance.

Although this appearance is almost pathognomonic, it is only seen occasionally. Enzmann and others (1978b) reviewed 42 patients with cytologic evidence of meningeal carcinoma in the cerebrospinal fluid. The CT was positive in less than 3% of patients with leukemia and lymphoma, 44% of patients with carcinoma, and 100% of patients with melanoma. Additional intraparenchymal metastases were identified in 18% and hydrocephalus in only 11%.

Figure 12.9.

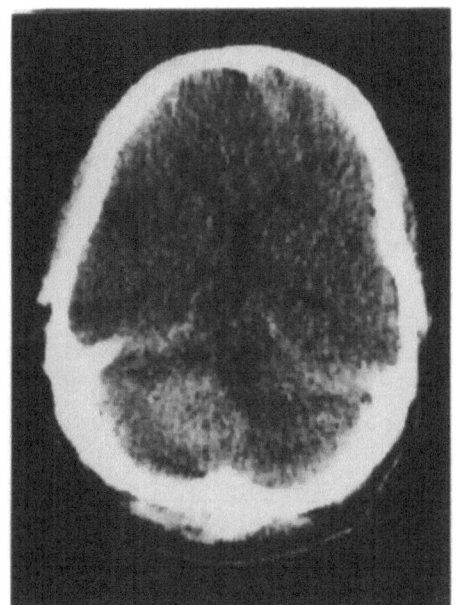

A

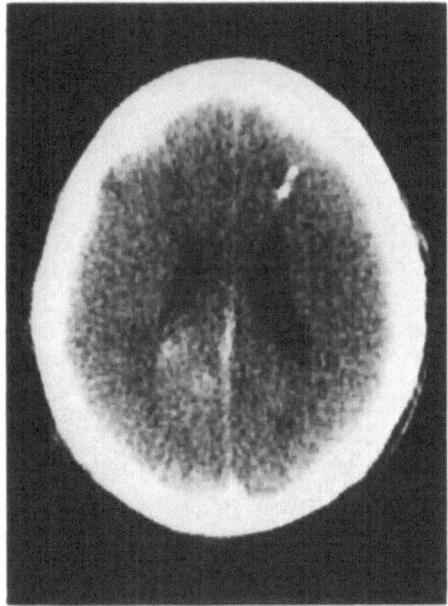

B

Multiple intracerebral deposits from widespread reticulum-cell sarcoma. A. Postcontrast section through the posterior fossa demonstrates a poorly defined, homogeneously enhanced mass in the left cerebellum. B. A section through the upper portions of the lateral ventricles demonstrates a second deposit in the roof of the left lateral ventricle near the splenium of the corpus callosum. A ventricular shunt is present in the right frontal lobe.

Figure 12.10.

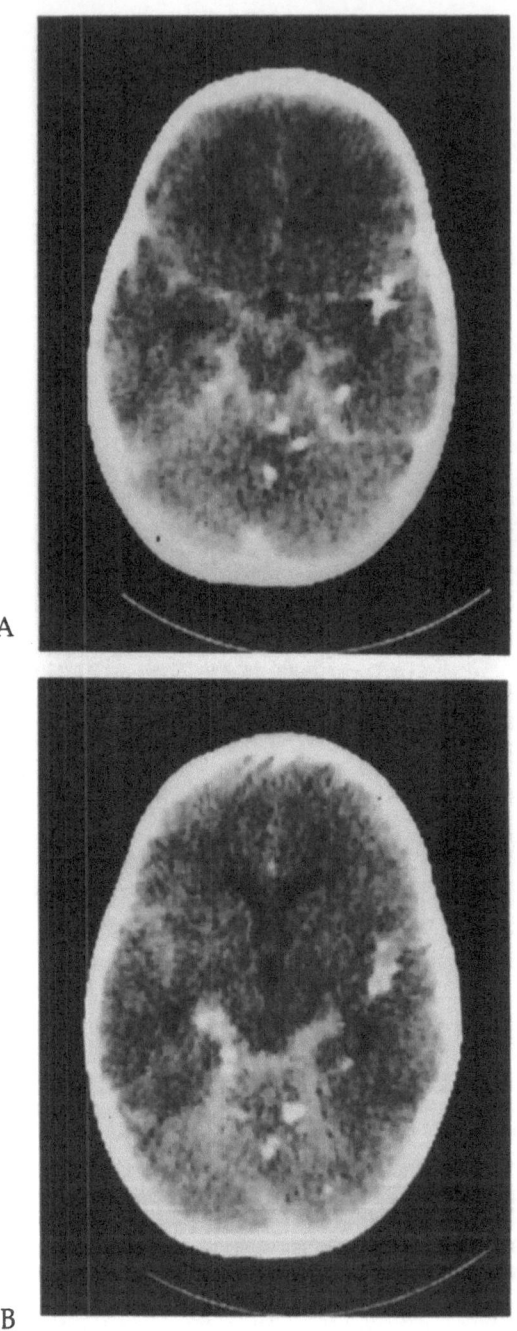

A

B

Meningeal carcinomatosis in a child with neuroblastoma. Note the intense contrast enhancement of the basal cisterns. A. Section through the cerebral peduncles. B. Section through the apex of the tentorium. Although the ventricles are normal in size, significant hydrocephalus developed several weeks later.

Differential Diagnosis of Metastases

Although the sensitivity (accuracy of detection) of computed tomography is extremely high, the specificity of the technique is lower. Primary gliomas, meningiomas, infarcts and abscesses may resemble metastatic tumors and should frequently be considered in the differential diagnosis of single or multiple intracranial mass lesions even in patients with known primary malignant tumors.

Progressive Multifocal Leukoencephalopathy   In patients who are subjected to severe immunosuppression from chemotherapy or in connection with organ transplantation, the development of areas of diminished density in the brain on CT without contrast enhancement may herald the presence of progressive multifocal leukoencephalopathy. The diagnosis can only be made with certainty by brain biopsy and viral culture (fig. 12.11) (Bosch et al. 1976; Lane et al. 1978).

Figure 12.11.

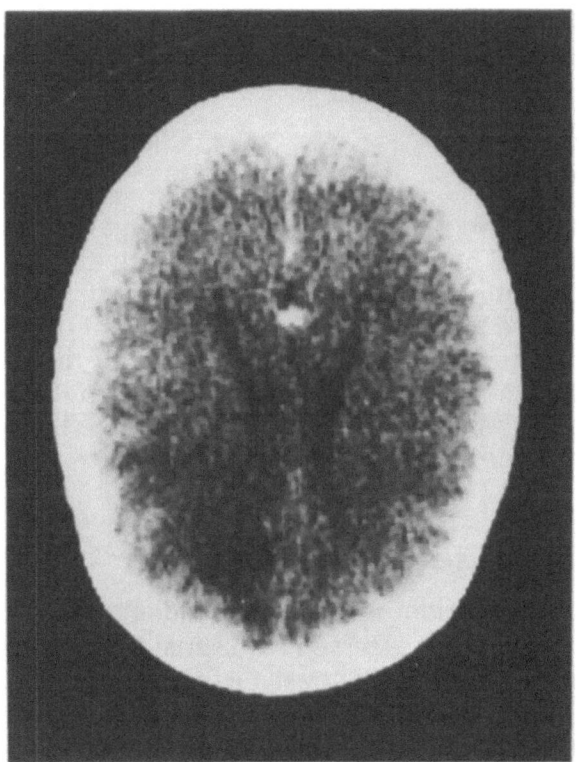

Progressive multifocal leukoencephalopathy in a patient with chronic myelogenous leukemia, immunosuppression following chemotherapy, and recent obtundation. The area of diminished density in the right frontal lobe showed no contrast enhancement but was used to guide a brain biopsy for electron microscopy and viral culture.

ACCURACY OF DETECTION

Computed tomography is superior to any other diagnostic modality for detecting the presence of metastatic deposits in the brain (Gawler et al. 1974; New et al. 1975; Pendergras et al. 1975). The importance of contrast enhancement has been emphasized by many workers. Bardfeld and others (1977) studied 47 patients with brain metastases: radionuclide scanning was positive in 94%; CT without contrast medium was positive in 89%; and CT with contrast was positive in 94%. CT was positive in two cases in which the radionuclide scan was negative and was clearly better in detecting multiple lesions. Buell and others (1978) found that CT was superior to radionuclide scanning for the detection of intracranial tumors with a detection rate (sensitivity) of 99% versus 91% and correct tumor type identification (specificity) of 76% versus 69%.

CT IN THE TREATMENT OF BRAIN METASTASES

CT provides a highly accurate and relatively innocuous method of evaluating the efficacy of various therapeutic modalities used for metastases (Pay et al. 1976).

Corticosteroids

The effects of corticosteroids on metastases may be seen on serial CT studies within 24–48 hours. There is a reduction in the volume of edemic fluid with a resulting diminution of the mass effect. Crocker and others (1976) demonstrated also that there was a significant decrease in contrast enhancement of the metastasis and a decrease in the accumulation of ^{99m}Tc-pertechnetate as demonstrated by emission tomography. It is possible that the administration of steroids prior to CT may mask the appearance of small metastases with minimal edema.

Radiation and Chemotherapy

The response of various metastases to radiation therapy and chemotherapy may be accurately assessed with serial CT studies (Hyman et al. 1978; Kretzchmar et al. 1978). Contrast medium is essential in such studies because there may be a concurrent diminution in edema and tumor size.

Radiosensitive tumors may show a progressive reduction in size with ultimate complete disappearance 4–6 months after irradiation. More commonly, unfortunately, the metastasis shrinks in size but then regrows to exceed its original size (figs. 12.12 and 12.13). Similar behavior may be seen after chemotherapy.

After radiation therapy, often 1–3 years later, enlargement of the cerebral ventricles and subarachnoid spaces may indicate the presence of brain atrophy due to irradiation.

Figure 12.12.

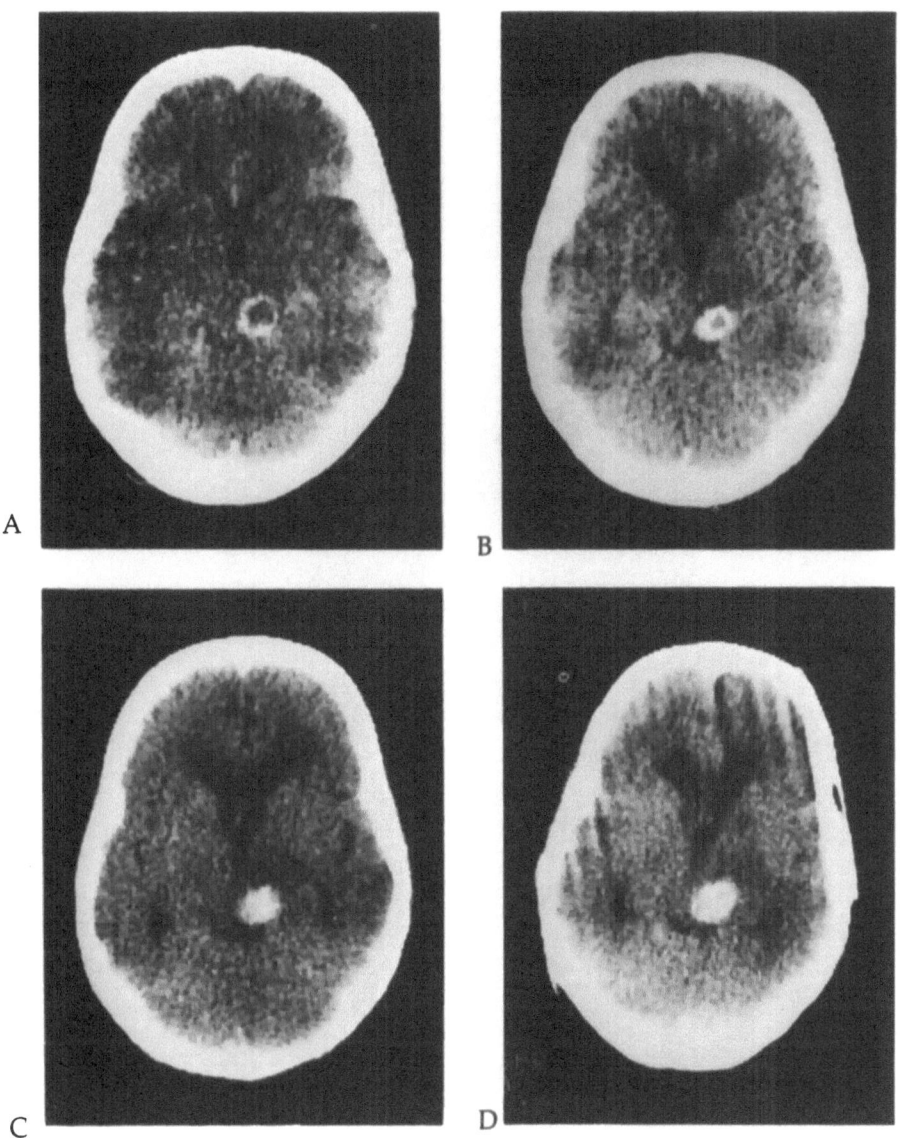

A

B

C

D

Right thalamic metastasis from carcinoma of the lung. The lesion demonstrates some response to radiation therapy, but it subsequently regrew and hydrocephalus developed. A. Initial study demonstrates a small mass with ring-like contrast enhancement in the posterior part of the right thalamus. B. Ten weeks later, after a course of radiation therapy, the metastasis is slightly smaller but shows more contrast enhancement and a thicker rim. There is hydrocephalus. C. Six months after the initial study the metastasis is slightly larger with uniform contrast enhancement. Marked hydrocephalus is present. D. Eight months after initial workup, the metastasis is even larger with surrounding edema, displacement of the third ventricle, and further ventricular enlargement.

Figure 12.13.

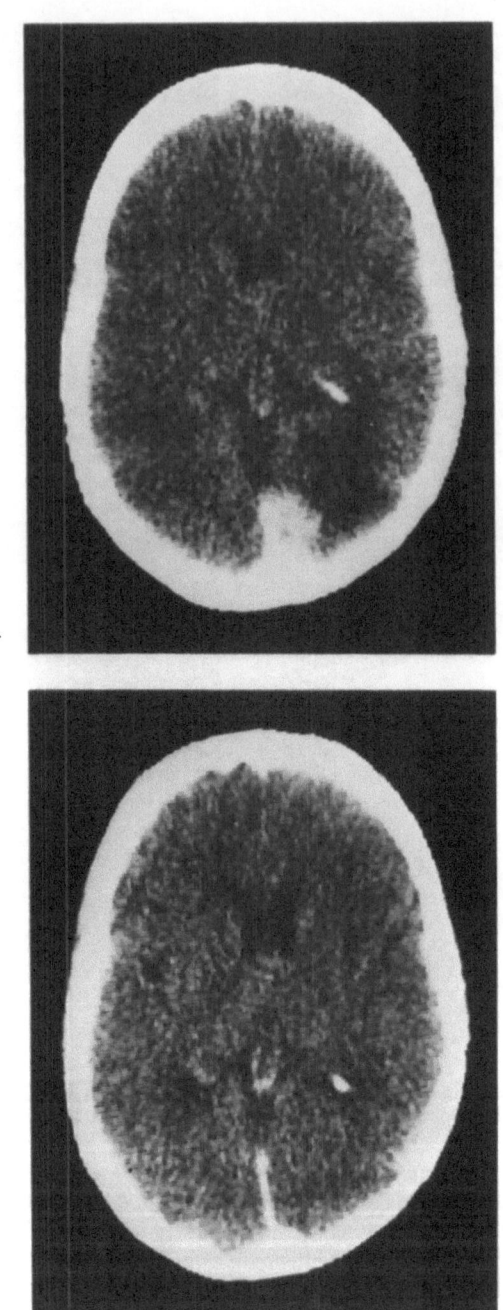

A

B

Carcinoma of the breast metastatic to the right occipital lobe with complete resolution after radiation therapy. A. Postcontrast section demonstrates a metastasis near the torcula with surrounding edema. B. Four months later, following radiation therapy, the metastasis and edema have completely resolved.

Surgery

Surgical management of cerebral metastases has become increasingly dependent on CT. Accurate localization of small metastases for surgical extirpation is now possible with the newer whole-body scanners. Various methods have been developed for establishing the precise location of a metastasis, but a method developed at Sloan-Kettering permits removal of small solitary subcortical deposits with a minimal disruption of the adjacent brain and a low morbidity.

The patient is placed in the scanner so sections are performed in either the standard axial or the coronal plane, depending on the site of metastasis. When the contrast-enhanced metastasis is seen on the CT image, an aluminum marker is placed on the scalp on a tangent to the deposit and the CT section is repeated (fig. 12.14). The precise depth of the deposit from inner table of the skull is measured on the CT scanner, and the scalp underlying the aluminum disc is marked. In the operating room, a small drill is passed through the scalp into the calvarium at the site of the marker. After the scalp is reflected, the drill hole in the calvarium is continued to the dura. After elevating the bone flap and dura, the precise position of the drill hole is transposed to the cerebral cortex where a small cerebrotomy to the required depth permits exposure and resection of the underlying metastasis.

Figure 12.14.

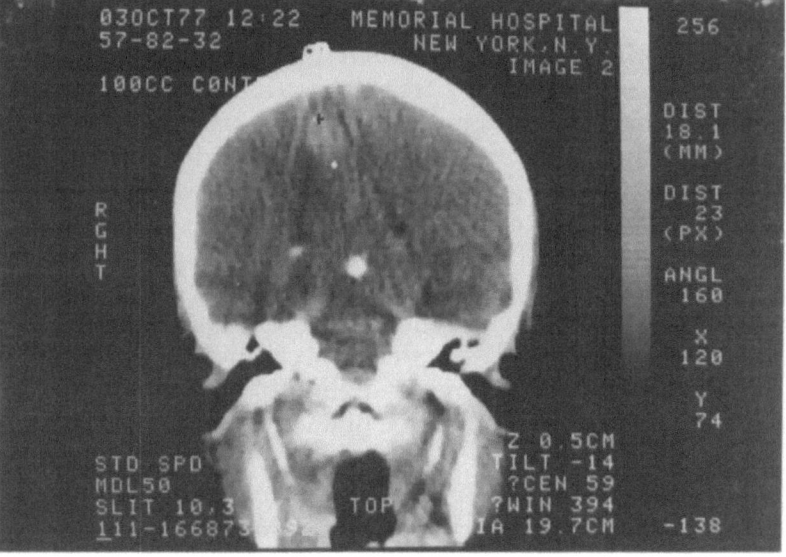

CT localization performed prior to surgical resection of a solitary parietal metastasis from malignant melanoma. A metal washer has been placed on the scalp perpendicular to the metastasis. The scalp is then marked, and in the operating room, a drill is used to mark the outer table of the calvarium prior to scalp elevation. The exact site for opening the cerebral cortex is then measured from the bone flap.

During the postoperative recovery period, CT has been extensively utilized to diagnose complications such as edema, hematoma, and infection. For 1–2 months after surgery CT evaluation of the tumor bed may be difficult. Occasionally areas of contrast enhancement apparently due to changes in the raw brain surface may lead to the erroneous diagnosis of residual tumor. Criteria for differentiating inflammation or healing from tumor are not available except that if followup CT examination after the first postoperative month demonstrates an enlarging contrast-enhancing component or an increase in brain edema, then residual tumor is likely (fig. 12.15 and 12.16).

CT AS A SCREENING PROCEDURE

The high sensitivity and safety of computed tomography makes it especially valuable for preoperative screening of patients with primary neoplasms that are likely to metastasize to the central nervous system. Jacobs and others (1977) have reported preoperative screening of 50 patients with lung carcinoma who were neurologically intact with normal plain skull films and normal radionuclide brain scans. They discovered 3 patients (6%) with occult brain metastases in the cerebellum or cerebral hemispheres. In addition they discovered one resolved cerebral infarct, one asymptomatic pituitary tumor, and 3 patients with significant cerebral atrophy.

The greater availability of CT scanning facilities certainly makes routine preoperative screening of all patients with lung carcinoma feasible although the cost effectiveness of such screening may be questioned. Screening of neurologically asymptomatic patients with metastatic disease in the lungs from other primary sites may also have to be considered in the future as complex chemotherapy regimens are used to control disseminated cancer. Many of the currently employed antineoplastic agents are relatively uneffective against brain metastases but extremely effective against deposits in other organs.

Primary Gliomas Gliomas will vary in their appearance depending on the degree of malignancy and vascularity. Low-grade astrocytomas may be isodense or hypodense with or without edema and mass effect. Contrast enhancement may be minimal, but calcifications may be present.

More malignant astrocytomas and glioblastoma multiforme are usually accompanied by a greater degree of edema and may show considerable contrast enhancement that is usually ring-like or nonhomogeneous and irregular in thickness. Although the appearance of a malignant glioma may be undistinguishable from that of a metastasis, a glioma often exhibits irregular finger-like extensions of the contrast-enhanced tumor along white matter bundles and fiber tracts.

Meningiomas, Acoustic Neurinomas and Chromophobe Adenomas Meningiomas may be distinguished from metastases by their usually homogeneous contrast enhancement and their attachment to the dura of the calvarium or falx. Additional changes in the underlying skull vault may support the diagnosis. Demonstration of a dural attachment of a

Figure 12.15.

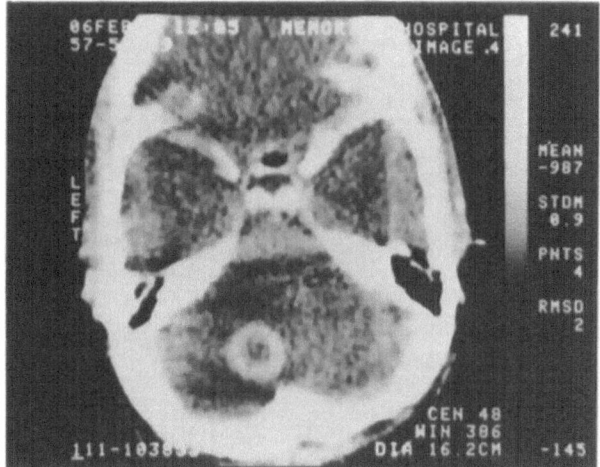

A

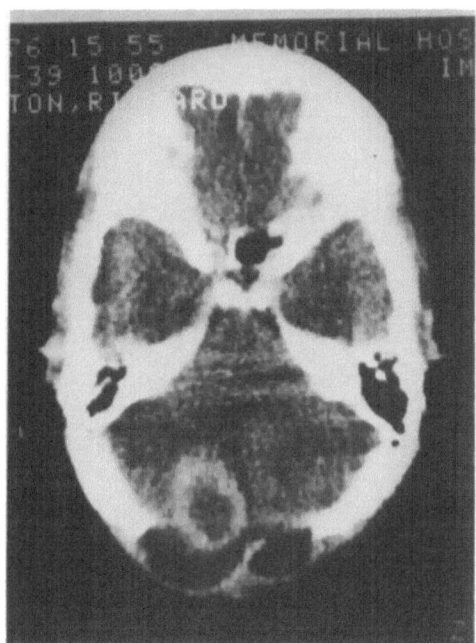

B

Hypernephroma metastasis in left cerebellum with tumor at the same site six weeks after apparently complete surgical resection. A. Typical contrast-enhanced metastasis in left cerebellum. B. Seven weeks after surgery, the patient demonstrates a large residual metastasis at the original site. Re-operation with complete resection of the metastasis resulted in a later CT scan that showed no residual tumor. Autopsy performed four months after the initial study revealed no evidence of tumor in the brain, but multiple metastases were present in the lung, skeleton, liver and the remaining left kidney. Death was due to septicemia and pneumonia.

Figure 12.16.

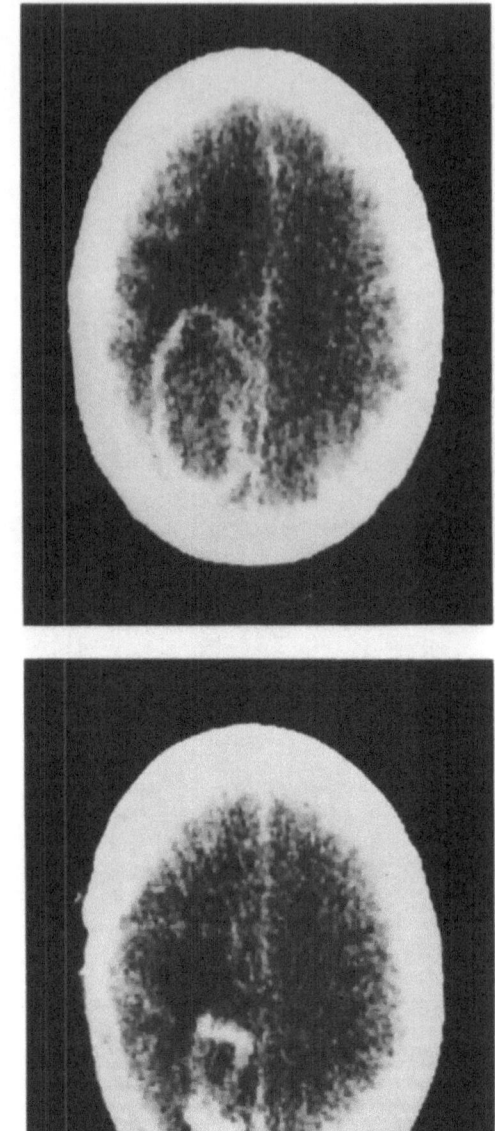

A

B

Left parietal metastasis from adenocarcinoma of the lung. Note the collapse of the rim after surgical resection. A. Large metastasis with rim-like contrast enhancement. B. Two weeks later, after surgical resection, the contrast-enhanced rim of the tumor is still present but has collapsed. Only the central portion of the tumor has actually been removed.

meningioma often requires special projections of CT scanning. For instance, for meningiomas on the high frontoparietal convexity, floor of the anterior or middle cranial fossae, or in the region of the sella, coronal CT sections may be invaluable. It is usually not possible to differentiate a meningioma from dural metastases or lymphoma unless additional calvarial or parenchymal lesions are present.

The location of certain tumors, such as acoustic neurinomas, meningiomas of the cerebellopontine angle (fig. 12.17) or tuberculum sella or chromophobe adenomas have relatively characteristic CT appearances, but occasional metastases closely mimic such tumors and make differentiation difficult. Plain radiographs may be useful for demonstrating characteristic changes such as enlarged internal acoustic canal (acoustic neurinoma), ballooned sella turcica (chromophobe adenoma), or hyperostosis of the tuberculum sellae (meningioma).

Cerebral Infarction   Cerebral infarcts occasionally occur in patients with disseminated cancer as a result of tumor emboli, pre-existent cerebrovascular disease, or abnormal coagulation states. The CT changes in cerebral infarction depend on the time interval between the outset of symptoms and signs, the size of the cerebral infarct, and the area of the brain that is involved.

Figure 12.17.

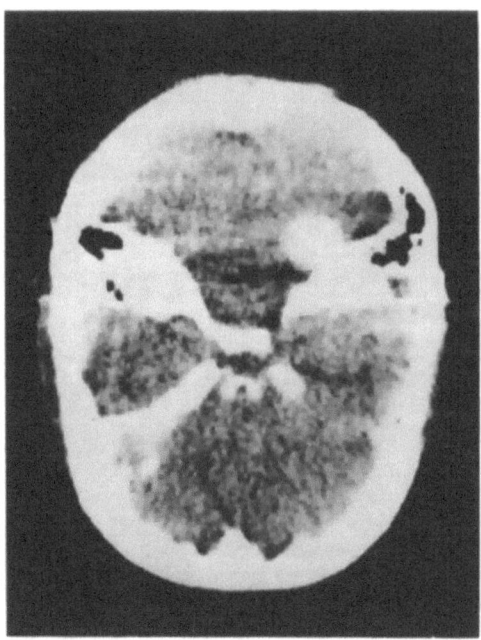

Hyperdense meningioma in the left cerebellopontine angle in a 76-year-old woman with carcinoma of the breast. The meningioma was found to be heavily calcified at autopsy.

Early changes of cerebral infarction, seen as early as 3 hours after the ictus, consist of an area of diminished density due to brain necrosis and edema often with a geographic area corresponding to the distribution of a single major cerebral vessel. Unlike the edema due to metastases, the diminished density may extend to the overlying cortex. Contrast enhancement is not usually seen initially but may become intense 10 days to 3 weeks after the ictus (fig. 12.17). The contrast enhancement characteristically involves the pial surface of the overlying brain and has a serpiginous outline, but it may also be seen at any site of collateral cerebral circulation such as the basal ganglia. Round or spherical areas of ring-like contrast enhancement as seen in metastases are not usually encountered after infarction (Kinkel and Jacobs 1976; Masdeu et al. 1977).

When the cerebral infarcts are more than 3 weeks old, contrast enhancement diminishes or disappears and the infarcted area shrinks leading to enlargement of the adjacent cerebral ventricle and subarachnoid space. A low-density fluid-filled cavity may develop centrally. Although cerebral infarcts may resemble metastases at certain times of their evolution (especially if the diagnosis is entertained because of the patient's history), serial CT scans at 2–3 week intervals are sufficiently characteristic to exclude other diagnoses.

Figure 12.18.

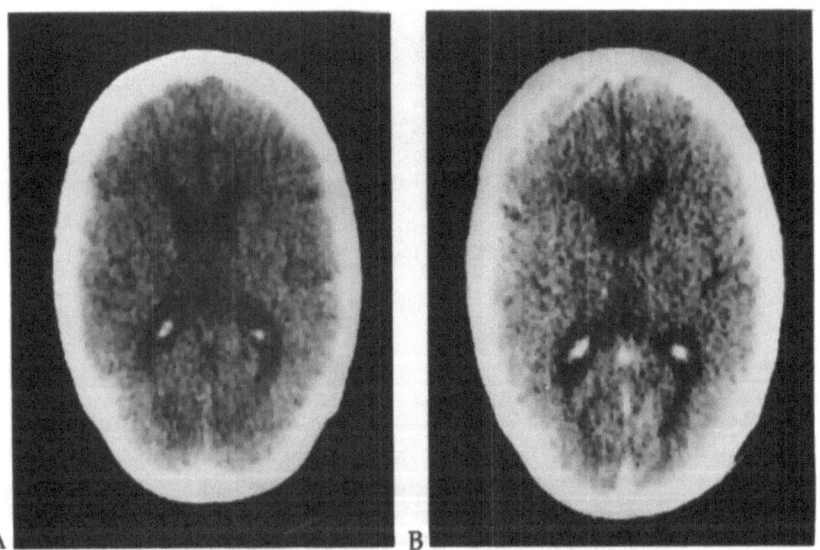

Bilateral occipital lobe infarcts in an elderly male with disseminated carcinoma of the prostate. A. Noncontrast study 10 days after the onset of symptoms demonstrates areas of decreased density at both occipital poles. There was no change after contrast administration. B. Contrast enhancement in the calcarine cortex is visible 4 weeks later. CT performed 2 months later showed no contrast enhancement but enlargement of the occipital horns and occipital sulci.

Cerebral Hemorrhage The early appearance of intracerebral hemorrhage is sufficiently characteristic to exclude other diagnoses, but the etiology of the hemorrhage (aneurysm, arteriovenous malformation or cryptic primary or metastatic tumor) may frequently be obscure. An intracerebral hemorrhage initially appears as a hyperdense (50–80 Hounsfield units), well-circumscribed mass. Rupture into the ventricles may result in a cast-like opacification of the cavity or simply fluid levels.

The density of a cerebral hemorrhage diminishes with time, and by 2–3 weeks of age the clot may be isodense and undistinguishable from the surrounding brain (Bergstrom et al. 1977). After several more weeks the hemorrhage appears hypodense (fig. 12.8). Contrast enhancement is not seen early but may appear 3–6 weeks later, at which stage it is ring-like and resembles a metastasis or abscess (fig. 12.19). The ring-like zone of contrast enhancement surrounds the hematoma which by this stage has become isodense or hypodense.

Abscesses and Granulomas Acute and chronic brain abscesses may be confused with metastases because of their similar appearance on CT and because of their frequent association with malignant disease, particu-

Figure 12.19.

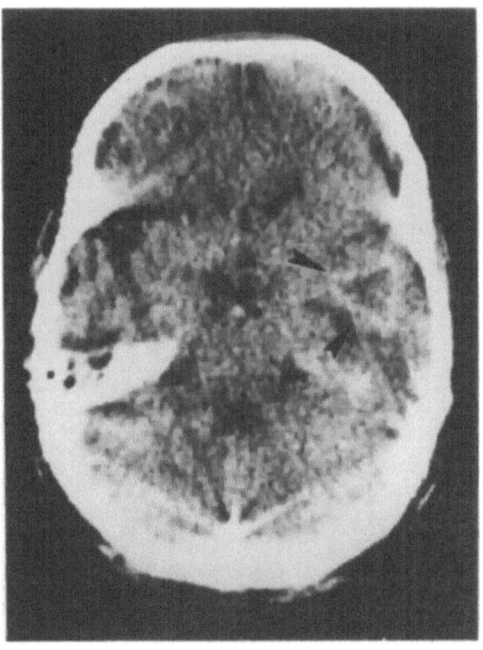

Resolving hematoma (arrows) of the right temporal lobe with rim-like contrast enhancement six weeks after the onset of the hemorrhage. This 60-year-old man with carcinoma of the lung was found to have a middle cerebral artery aneurysm by arteriography, explaining the hemorrhage.

larly in the lung. Chronic abscesses or granulomas due to fungus or tuberculosis may also present with simultaneous lesions in the lung and brain, further suggesting an erroneous diagnosis of malignant disease.

Abscesses, whether single or multiple, are usually oval or circular and hypodense with a ring-like contrast enhancement that may be uniform or nonuniform in thickness. Occasionally cavities may be multiseptate and rarely, an abscess may contain gas (Stevens et al. 1978).

Chronic granulomas may be hypodense, isodense or hyperdense with either ring-like or homogeneous contrast enhancement (Price and Danziger 1978). Frequently, craniotomy or needle aspiration is necessary to differentiate inflammatory lesions from metastases (fig. 12.20).

Radiation Necrosis and Drug-induced Leukoencephalopathy Injury to the brain from excessive radiation or from chemotherapeutic agents may result in changes that resemble metastases on computed tomography.

Radiation-induced necrosis of brain is characterized by a hypodense or isodense mass lesion with surrounding edema. The mass lesion almost always demonstrates contrast enhancement that may be ring-like or homogeneous (fig. 12.21) (Rottenberg et al. 1977; Mikhael 1978). The lesion can be differentiated from a recurrent tumor or abscess only by histologic examination (van Dellen and Danziger 1978).

Figure 12.20.

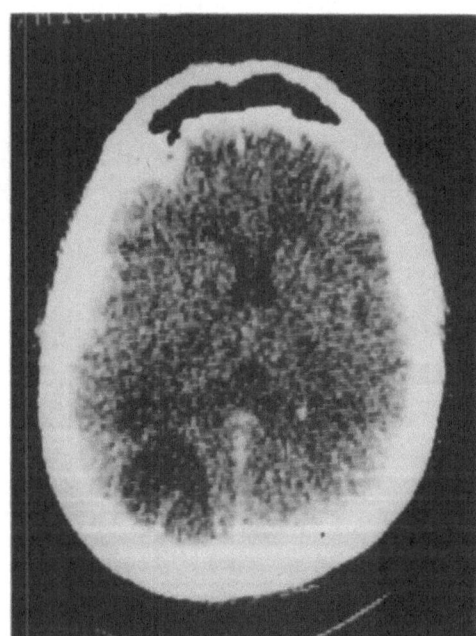

Actinomycotic abscess of the left parietal region in a 40-year-old male with hilar adenopathy on chest radiographs. An initial diagnosis of carcinoma of the lung could not be confirmed, but actinomyces was found in the abscess at craniotomy.

Figure 12.21.

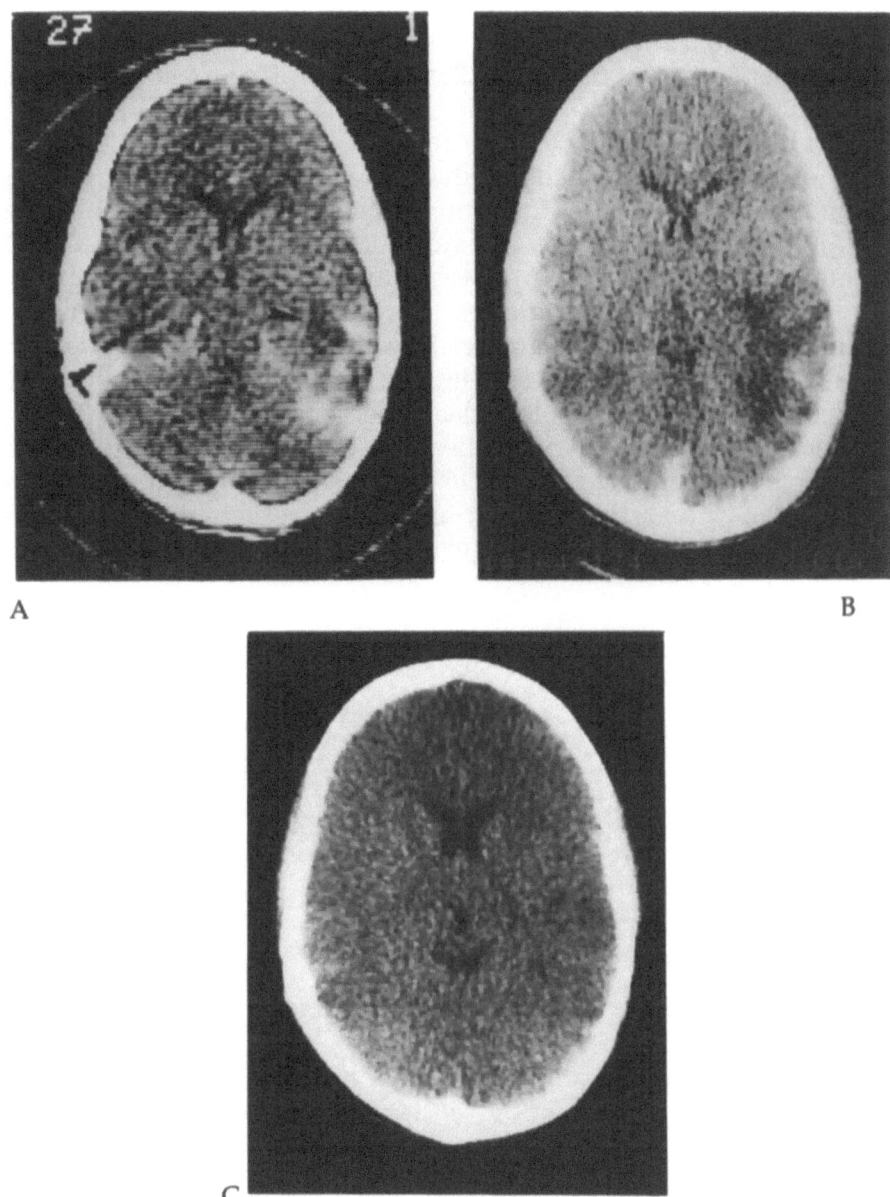

A

B

C

Radiation necrosis of the right temporal lobe after inadvertent administration of 10,000 R of beta radiation to an area of eosinophilic granuloma. A. Postcontrast study 6 months after irradiation demonstrates a low density area with some surrounding contrast enhancement (arrow) in the right temporal lobe. B. After 6 months a contrast-enhanced CT scan demonstrates an increase in edema. C. A third scan 8 months later or 20 months after irradiation shows that the appearances have returned to normal apart from slight ventricular enlargement.

Radiation or drug-induced leukoencephalopathy creates a localized or generalized diminution of the density of white matter of the cerebral hemispheres (fig. 12.22) with occasional mild ventricular enlargement and sulcal enlargement but without any contrast enhancement (Peylan-Ramu et al. 1977, 1978; Allen et al. 1978). The appearances may resemble edema due to metastatic deposits, but the absence of contrast enhancement excludes the latter.

Multiple Sclerosis During the active phase of multiple sclerosis, areas of diminished density with central ring-like areas of contrast enhancement may be seen (Cala and Mastaglia 1976; Aita et al. 1978; Sears et al. 1978). Such lesions may resemble metastases or abscesses, but they spontaneously disappear in 6–8 weeks (fig. 12.23).

Every day experience indicates, however, that a large number of often clinically significant metastases escape diagnosis by CT. Gawler and others (1974) found difficulty with lesions in the posterior fossa (brainstem and cerebellum) and were able to clearly demonstrate only 55%. Baker and Houser (1976) examined 3,500 patients of whom 348 had posterior fossa symptoms and signs. There were 16 erroneous diagnoses in the posterior fossa (4.6%) with 13 false-negative and 3 false-positive studies. Deck and others (1976) emphasized the role of artefacts in the posterior fossa due to movement or bone.

Figure 12.22.

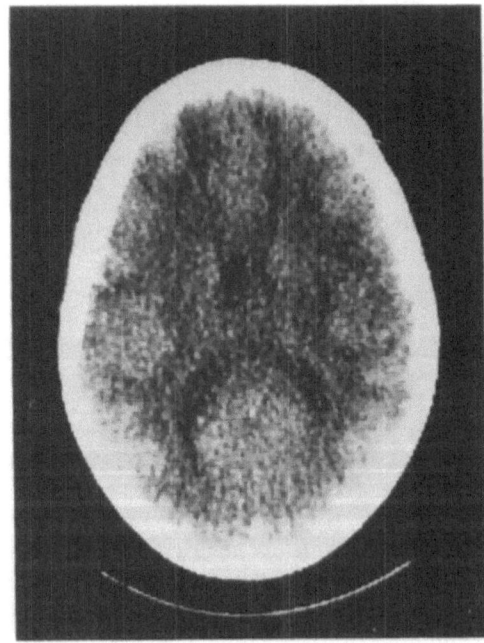

Methotrexate-induced leukoencephalopathy in a patient treated with high-dose systemic methotrexate and citrovorum factor rescue for osteogenic sarcoma of the femur.

Figure 12.23.

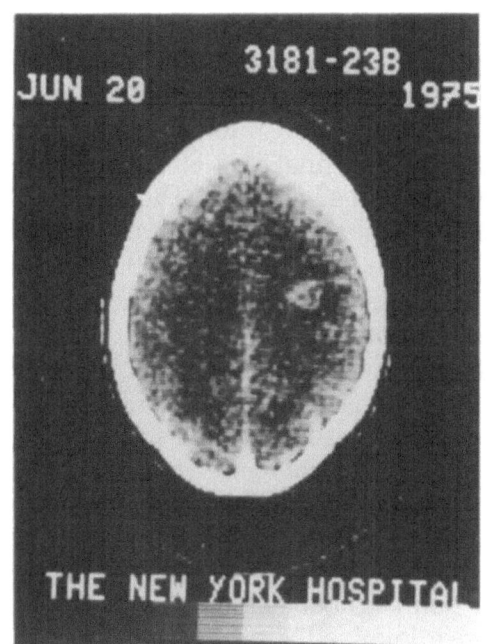

A

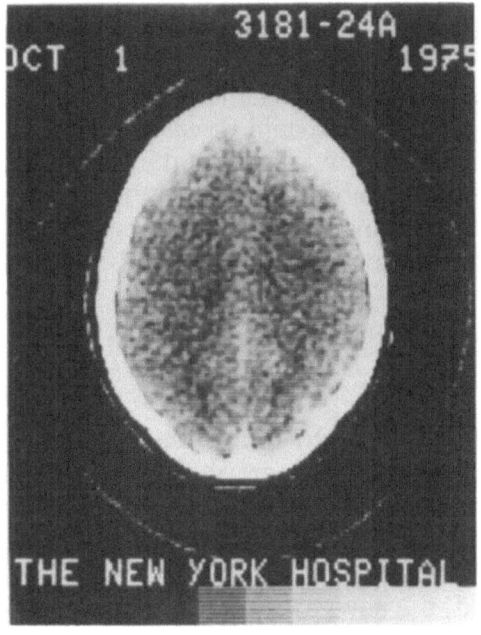

B

Multiple sclerosis with contrast enhancement and subsequent spontaneous resolution. A. Post-contrast study reveals a circular contrast-enhancing lesion resembling a metastasis. B. Three months later the CT appearances are normal.

To assess the true accuracy of CT scanning in the detection of intracranial disease, Messina (1977) compared the findings at autopsy with those at CT examination performed within 2 weeks to 2 months before death. Lesions at autopsy that could have significantly expanded or enlarged between the CT scans and death were excluded. False-negative CT studies (no CT evidence of metastases) occurred in 11% of patients studied with the upgraded 160 × 160 matrix EMI scanner and 27% of patients studied with the original 80 × 80 matrix machine. Brain metastases were found at autopsy in 47 patients. There were 143 metastases measuring more than 1 cm in diameter of which 42% were undetected on the CT examinations (although the studies on 160 × 160 matrix were better than the original 80 × 80 matrix).

Clearly then, although CT is superior to other modalities in detecting the presence of intracerebral metastases, it is not infallible. The chance of missing additional lesions is significant, and this is important when surgical removal of apparently solitary metastases is contemplated.

Various factors contribute to the errors in CT scanning. The quality of the scan depends upon the machine and the patient. Newer units with faster scanning times appear capable of greatly increased tissue-density resolution. Movement artefacts, a serious problem in seriously ill patients, may result in a nondiagnostic study, but with the new faster scanners, such artefacts are minimized. Certain metastases are missed because they are isodense and exhibit very little contrast enhancement. This phenomenon is common with hemorrhagic metastases due to melanoma or choriocarcinoma when the CT scan is performed during the isodense stage of the hematoma. A small number of metastases are obscured by the proximity of the lesion to the inner table of the skull vault or bone.

Metastases in the brainstem or cerebellum may remain undetected, even when they are causing significant symptoms and signs, because of their small size and the absence of surrounding edema. Such lesions may be more readily diagnosed with scanners that are capable of superior tissue-density resolution.

COMPLICATIONS OF CT SCANNING

Radiation Dosage

Although CT is relatively innocuous compared with cerebral angiography and pneumoencephalography, and the radiation dosage is not genetically or clinically significant in patients with proven neoplastic disease, the radiation dose to the cornea may be significant in young patients, particularly if they are subjected to frequent followup studies. As previously mentioned, the newer scanners are capable of delivering a radiation dosage of 4–10 rads to the area being studied and thus under certain circumstances, total dosage to the eye may reach 50–60 R. Detailed knowledge and training in the physical principles of CT scanning and radiation protection is essential to prevent unnecessary exposure of patients to such levels of radiation.

Contrast Material

The risks of anaphylactic reactions to intravenous administration of iodinated urographic agents are well known. Serious reactions, including death, occur with an incidence of 1 in 10,000 to 1 in 20,000 while less serious reactions are more common. With the use of large volumes of contrast materials, additional complications are occurring. At Memorial Hospital during the last 10 years there have been 10 episodes of focal or generalized seizures after the injection of a contrast medium. Although all patients have had CT evidence of a structural lesion to explain the seizure, the toxic effect of the contrast medium most certainly precipitated it.

Renal failure is becoming recognized as a serious but uncommon complication of contrast administration. Apparently it occurs in patients with minimal renal dysfunction and superadded dehydration. Administration of contrast media is therefore relatively contraindicated in any patient with elevated blood urea or creatinine.

REFERENCES

Aita, J. F. et al. Cranial C.T. appearance of acute multiple sclerosis. *Neurology* 28:251–255, 1978.

Allen, J. C. et al. Quantitative assessment of drug-induced leukoencephalopathy using computed tomography. *Neuroradiology* 16:44–47, 1978.

Baker, H. I., and Houser, O. W. Computed tomography in the diagnosis of posterior fossa lesions. *Radiol. Clin. North Am.* 14:129–147, 1976.

Bardfeld, P. A. et al. A comparison of radionuclide scanning and computed tomography in metastatic lesions of the brain. *J. Comput. Assist. Tomogr.* 1:315–318, 1977.

Becker, H. et al. Computed tomography in detecting calvarial metastases. A comparison with skull radiography and radionuclide scanning. *Neuroradiology* 16:504–505, 1978.

Bergstrom, M. et al. Variation with time of the alternation values of intracranial hematomas. *J. Comput. Assist. Tomogr.* 1:57–63, 1977.

Bosch, E. P.; Cancilla, P. A.; and Cornell, S. H. Computerized tomography in progressive multifocal leukoencephalopathy (letter). *Arch. Neurol.* 33:216, 1976.

Buell, U. et al. Computerized transaxial tomography and cerebral serial scintigraphy in intracranial tumors—rates of detection and tumor type identification. *J. Nucl. Med.* 19:476–479, 1978.

Butler, A. R., and Kricheff, I. I.: Non-contrast C.T. scanning: Limited value in suspected brain tumor. *Radiology* 126:689–693, 1978.

Cala, L. A., and Mastaglia, F. L. Computed tomography in multiple sclerosis. *Lancet* 1:689, 1976.

Constant, P. et al. Cerebral metastasis—a study of computerized tomography. *Comput. Tomogr.* 1:87–94, 1977.

Crocker, E. F. et al. The effect of steroids on the extra-vascular distribution of radiographic contrast material and technetium pertechnetate in brain tumors as determined by computed tomography. *Radiology* 119:471–474, 1976.

Deck, M. D. F.; Messina, A. V.; and Sackett, J. F. Computed tomography in metastatic disease of the brain. *Radiology* 119:115–120, 1976.

Dellen, J. R., van, and Danziger, A. Failure of computerized tomography to differentiate between radiation necrosis and cerebral tumor. *S. Afr. Med. J.* 53:171, 1978.

Dubois, P. J. et al. Subependymal and leptomeningeal spread of systemic malignant lymphoma demonstrated by cranial computed tomography. *J. Comput. Assist. Tomogr.* 2:218–221, 1978.

Enzmann, D. R. et al. Malignant melanoma metastatic to the central nervous system. *Radiology* 127:177–180, 1978a.

Enzmann, D. R. et al. Computed tomography in leptomeningeal spread of tumor. *J. Comput. Assist. Tomogr.* 2:448–455, 1978b.

Gawler, J. et al. Computer assisted tomography (EMI scanner). Its place in investigation of suspected intracranial tumors. *Lancet* 878:419–423, 1974.

Gildersleeve, N.; Koo, A. H.; and McDonald, C. J. Metastatic tumor presenting as intracerebral hemorrhage. Report of 6 cases examined by computed tomography. *Radiology* 124:109–112, 1977.

Hilal, S. K., and Chang, C. H. Specificity of computed tomography in the diagnosis of supratentorial neoplasms. *Neuroradiology* 16:537–539, 1978.

Hounsfield, G. N. Computerized transverse axial scanning (tomography). Part I: description of the system. *Br. J. Radiol.* 46:1016–1022, 1973.

Huckman, M. Clinical experience with the intravenous infusion of iodinated contrast material as an adjunct to computed tomography. *Surg. Neurol.* 4:297–318, 1975.

Hyman, R. A. et al. Computed tomographic evaluation of therapeutically induced changes in primary and secondary brain tumors. *Neuroradiology* 14:213–218, 1978.

Jacobs, L.; Kinkel, W. R.; and Vincent, R. G. Silent brain metastasis from lung carcinoma determined by computerized tomography. *Arch. Neurol.* 34:690–693, 1977.

Kazner, E. et al. Computer assisted tomography in primary malignant lymphomas of the brain. *J. Comput. Assist. Tomogr.* 2:125–134, 1978.

Kido, D. K. et al. Comparative sensitivity of C.T. scans, radiographs and radionuclide scans in detecting metastatic calvarial lesions. *Radiology* 128:371–375, 1978.

Kinkel, W. R., and Jacobs, L. Computerized axial tomography in cerebrovascular disease. *Neurology* 26:924–930, 1976.

Kramer, R. A.; Janetos, G. P.; and Perlstein, G. An approach to contrast enhancement in computed tomography of the brain. *Radiology* 116:641–647, 1975.

Kretzchmar, K. et al. The diagnostic value of C.T. for radiotherapy of cerebral tumors. *Neuroradiology* 14:245–250, 1978.

Lane, B.; Carroll, B. A.; and Pedley, T. A. Computerized cranial tomography in cerebral diseases of white matter. *Neuroradiology* 28:534–544, 1978.

Larson, E. B. et al. Impact of computed tomography on utilization of cerebral angiograms. *Am. J. Roentgenol.* 129:1–3, 1977.

Latchaw, R. E.; Gold, L. H. A.; and Tourje, E. J. A protocol for the use of contrast enhancement in cranial computed tomography. *Radiology* 126:681–687, 1978.

Masdeu, J. C.; Azar-Kia, B.; and Rubino, F. A. Evaluation of recent cerebral infarction by computerized tomography. *Arch. Neurol.* 34:417–421, 1977.

Messina, A. V. Cranial computerized tomography. *Arch. Neurol.* 34:602–607, 1977.

Mikhael, M. A. Radiation necrosis of the brain; correlation between computed tomography, pathology and dose distribution. *J. Comput. Assist. Tomogr.* 2:71–80, 1978.

New, P. F. et al. Computed tomography with the EMI scanner in the diagnosis of primary and metastatic intracranial neoplasms. *Radiology* 114:75–87, 1975.

Pay, N. T. et al. The usefulness of computed tomography during and after radiation therapy in patients with brain tumors. *Radiology* 121:79–83, 1976.

Pendergras, H. P. et al. Relative efficacy of radionuclide imaging and computed tomography of the brain. *Radiology* 116:363–366, 1975.

Peylan-Ramu, N. et al. Computer assisted tomography in methotrexate encephalopathy. *J. Comput. Assist. Tomogr.* 1:216–221, 1977.

Peylan-Ramu, N. et al. Abnormal C.T. scans of the brain in asymptomatic children with acute lymphocytic leukemia after prophylactic treatment of the central nervous system with radiation and intrathecal chemotherapy. *N. Engl. J. Med.* 293:815–818, 1978.

Price, H. I., and Danziger, A. Computed tomography in cranial tuberculosis. *Am. J. Roentgenol.* 130:769–771, 1978.

Rottenberg, D. A. et al. Cerebral necrosis following radiotherapy of extracranial neoplasms. *Ann. Neurol.* 1:339–357, 1977.

Sears, E. S.; Tindall, R. S. A.; and Zarnow H. Active multiple sclerosis enhanced computerized tomographic imaging of lesions and effects of corticosteroids. *Arch. Neurol.* 35:426–434, 1978.

Solis, O. J. et al. Intracerebral metastatic melanoma. C.T. evaluation. *Comput. Tomogr.* 1:135–149, 1977.

Stevens, E. A. et al. Computed tomographic brain scanning in intraparenchymal pyogenic abscesses. *Am. J. Roentgenol.* 130:111–114, 1978.

Wendling, L. R. et al. Transient, severe periventricular hypodensity after leukemic prophylaxis with cranial irradiation and intrathecal methotrexate. *J. Comput. Assist. Tomogr.* 2:502–505, 1978.

Weinstein, M. A.; Alfidi, R. J.; and Duchesnau, P. M. Computed tomography versus skull radiography. Guest editorial. *Am. J. Roentgenol.* 128:873, 1977.

13

Radionuclide Imaging of Cancer Metastases in the Brain

Richard S. Benua

Nuclear medicine contributes to the detection and management of cancer metastases in the brain by showing abnormal uptake of gamma-emitting nuclides by the tumors. The normal brain is delineated in such images because the traditional radiopharmaceuticals (human serum albumin, mercuhydrin, sodium pertechnetate, ^{99m}Tc-DTPA) do not pass the blood-brain barrier. Normal muscular, skeletal and glandular structures adjacent to the brain are visible and may contribute to identification of the true anatomic position of the metastases. Pertechnetate uptake in the choriod plexus and the salivary glands may be decreased by blocking with perchlorate or by using DTPA or glucoheptonate labeled with ^{99m}Tc. Both of these agents are excreted by glomerular filtration, and counting rates over the head for a given number of millicuries of either of them will be less than with pertechnetate at a fixed time after injection.

The target-to-nontarget (T/NT) ratio increases as the radiopharmaceutical is cleared from blood and other nontumor structures. Léveillé and coworkers (1977) have suggested that ^{99m}Tc-Sn-glucoheptonate, a modified corn syrup, may be metabolized by neoplastic tissue. Metabolic utilization would explain the increased T/NT ratio which has been observed at 2–6 hours after injection with this material but not with pertechnetate or DTPA. This may be an example of tumor detection by localization of a labeled metabolic substrate.

Other tumor-tissue precursors such as amino acids or thymidine labeled with positron-emitting nuclides of carbon, nitrogen or oxygen have been suggested for identifying brain metastasis. Skilled collaborators in the fields of physics, chemistry and biology will have to work together to produce such suitable radiopharmaceuticals for tumor detection in view of the time limits imposed by the short physical halflives of positron emitters.

Identification of small metastatic lesions within the brain also depends upon instrumentation. The spatial resolving power of the device will be crucial for separating two small lesions in close proximity. Krishnamurthy and others (1972) report negative brain scans in 5 of 15 patients with autopsy-proven metastases in the brain. The failure was mainly related to size, but site and pathology were also important in the failure to identify larger lesions. More sensitive detectors will be needed due to the statistical or random nature of radioactive disintegration, to limits on the patient imaging time, and to the amount of radiation which critical organs can tolerate.

Another problem in brain imaging is the separation of overlying scalp and skull metastases from intracranial disease. The tendency to develop multiple lesions in metastatic disease makes precise localization sometimes unreliable. The solution to calvarial interference may be a resort to tomographic reconstruction with either single-photon focused detectors or positron-emission tomographs analyzed by computer methods (Kuhl et al. 1976). (See also Chapter 14.) Dosimetric limits on photon availability in a reasonable time period are presently hampering these reconstructions.

The cost of metastasis detection will necessarily be weighed against the benefits to patients. Using standard radiopharmaceuticals ($20/dose) and conventional gamma cameras ($180/study), the expenditure for a radionuclide scan is presently less than computed tomography (CT). (See Chapter 12.) The cost of the cyclotron, of processing of the nuclide to a pharmaceutical, of the tomographic imaging device, and of the computer necessary for reconstruction may price sophisticated radionuclide scans well above present CT costs. Thus, the benefit to patient care will need to be great to justify the expenditure. Such an evaluation is best done by physicians responsible for the decision process for the patient. The conclusion reached will determine which sorts of studies are performed when brain metastases are suspected.

Standard radiographic procedures contribute much to clinical decisions. A neurologic skull series may differentiate intracranial metastases from skull neoplasms for one-third the price of a brain scan. The iodine-containing contrast agents, as usually required for CT identification of metastases (Fordham 1977), carries a small but finite risk of an anaphylaxis. The complications and discomfort of arterial puncture or subarachnoid air injection must be considered in the selection of diagnostic modalities.

Some published series at present are quoted to show that CT and RN are complementary. Christie and others (1976) found the RN 83%, CT 85% and both 89% correct in a series of brain tumors of unspecified type. Deck and collaborators (1976) found 30 instances of disagreement in 91 patients having both CT and RN scans within one month. In 6 the CT scan was correct, in 6 the RN was correct, 3 had skull metastases, and in 15 the discrepancies were unexplained. Other authors conclude that the CT alone is sufficient. New and others (1975) found positive CT exams in 24 patients with brain metastases whereas RN scanning missed one patient entirely and failed to show multiple disease in 3 others. Buell et al. (1978) found that CT identified 23 of 27 metastases in 16 patients, but RN scanning found only 17 of the 27. No lesions were detected on the RN scans which were not on the CT scans. CT accuracy is slightly better than the radionuclide (RN) scan for metastases according to Alderson and others (1977) although all 21 of his patients with brain metastases had positive CT and RN studies. Evens and Jost (1977) suggest that RN scanning need not be done after a positive CT, thus effecting a decrease in cost.

The use of RN scans for screening of asymptomatic cancer patients probably is not justified at this time regardless of the location of their primary tumor. Scans were positive in 17 of 26 patients symptomatic from brain metastases of lung cancer but in only 4 of 84 asymptomatic patients with a history of lung primaries (White et al. 1976). Muss and others (1976) found 11 positive RN studies in 37 symptomatic patients with a history of breast cancer, but only 1 positive among 79 asymptomatic breast cancer patients.

An RN scan may be considered in patients with a history of cancer when there are neurologic signs or symptoms and the CT examination is negative. An additional group for RN study would be symptomatic patients thought to be allergic to iodized contrast agents when the unenhanced CT examination is negative. Glucoheptonate labeled with ^{99m}Tc in larger than ordinary doses (>20 mCi) should be used with an immediate flow study and delayed imaging. The yield of additional metastases will be low, but occasionally otherwise undetected lesions will be identified to aid in the management of the patient. Dynamic studies of radionuclide flow may add information about vascular problems associated with the metastases.

The future of the radionuclide scan in evaluation of metastases to the brain is uncertain. Its use will be less as costs of medical care are limited by governmental regulation. It will be impossible to defend the use of RN imaging for screening patients without neurological signs and symptoms except in a few rare tumors such as oat-cell and choriocarcinoma. Improvements in the radionuclide scan will be costly.

New technologies leading to successful radionuclide brain scans will involve more specific radiopharmaceuticals which have a higher T/NT ratio. New agents which are metabolic precursors, their analogs, or antitumor antibodies may be developed to increase sensitivity and specificity. The radiolabels to be used on such new radiopharmaceuticals will depend on the instrumentation. Positron-emission tomography is a promising but expensive direction to look for improvement. Single-emission tomography is less expensive because neither cyclotrons nor rapid synthesis of compounds are required. Tomography of some type probably will be necessary. The present 1.5-cm limit on resolving power in tomography will be decreased, but more sensitive machines with high resolution will be very costly. Thus, the direction of radionuclide brain imaging may depend more on economics than upon science in the future.

REFERENCES

Alderson, P. O.; Gaido, M. H.; and Siegel, B. A. Computerized cranial tomography and radionuclide imaging in the detection of intracranial mass lesions. *Semin. Nucl. Med.* 7:161, 1977.

Buell, V. et al. Computerized transaxial tomography and cerebral serial scintigraphy in intracranial tumors, rates of detection and tumor type identification. *J. Nucl. Med.* 19:476, 1978.

Christie, J. H. et al. Computed tomographic and radionuclide studies in the diagnosis of intracranial disease. *Am. J. Roentgenol.* 127:171, 1976.

Deck, M. D. F.; Messina, A. V.; and Sackett, J. F. Computed tomography in metastatic disease of the brain. *Radiology* 119:115, 1976.

Evens, R. G., and Jost, R. G. The clinical efficacy and cost analysis of computed tomography and the radionuclide brain scan. *Semin. Nucl. Med.* 7:129, 1977.

Fordham, E. W. The complementary role of computerized axial transmission tomography and radionuclide imaging of the brain. *Semin. Nucl. Med.* 7:137, 1977.

Krishnamurthy, G. T. et al. Clinical value and limitation of Tc-99m brain scan, an autopsy correlation. *J. Nucl. Med.* 13:373, 1972.

Kuhl, D. E. et al. The Mark 10 system for radionuclide computed tomography of the brain. *Radiology* 121:405, 1976.

Leveille, J. et al. Tc-99m glucoheptonate in brain tumor detection an important advance in radiotracer techniques. *J. Nucl. Med.* 18:957, 1977.

Muss, H. B.; White, D. R.; and Cowan, R. T. Brain scanning in patients with recurrent breast cancer. *Cancer* 38:1574, 1976.

New, P. F. J. et al. Computed tomography with the EMI scanner in the diagnosis of primary and metastatic neoplasms. *Radiology* 114:75, 1975.

White, D. R.; Muss, H. B.; and Cowan, R. J. Brain scanning in patients with advanced lung cancer. *Clin. Nucl. Med.* 1:93, 1976.

14
Positron-
Emission
Tomography

Marcus E. Raichle

An understanding of disease processes in the human brain must ultimately be based on a knowledge of the underlying regional hemodynamic, metabolic, and biochemical changes. Although some such information is currently available from various animal models, the conflicting nature of these data often leaves many important questions unanswered and emphasizes the immense difficulty of developing and studying laboratory models of human disease. One obvious alternative is to develop a means by which the hemodynamic, biochemical and metabolic bases of cerebral disease can be safely studied sequentially in humans by using externally detected radiolabeled tracers.

Present methods of studying cerebral hemodynamics and metabolism in humans have serious shortcomings, but two significant developments have brought us closer to realization of this goal. First, the appearance within the medical environment of devices for nuclear bombardment, such as cyclotrons and linear accelerators, often coupled with ingenious techniques for rapid synthesis of radiopharmaceuticals, has provided radiopharmaceuticals suitable for in vivo hemodynamic and metabolic studies (Wolf and Redvanly 1977). The parallel development of appropriate mathematical models (Raichle et al. 1975) has provided the basis for practical algorithms that allow parameters of physiologic significance to be estimated from the data. Second, recent major developments in detection systems circumvent most of the disadvantages of conventional detection systems. These systems use the concept of emission tomography, which allows safe, quantitative, three-dimensional measurement of radioisotope distribution in tissue. This approach is analogous to quantitative tissue autoradiography.

Conventional nuclear medicine imaging utilizes either rectilinear scanners, scintillation cameras, or external scintillation probe systems. However, the quality of information obtained is seriously hampered by some physical characteristics of these conventional devices. First, representation of a three-dimensional object is compressed into a two-dimensional image with the radioactivity from heterogeneous tissue elements superimposed. Second, the field of view of the imaging collimator varies with the distance of the radiation detector from the object being imaged. Third, spatial distribution of the radiopharmaceutical in the object imaged is altered by attenuation of the gamma radiation in the tissues interposed between the source of radiation and the detector. The combined effect of the above characteristics severely precludes, except for specific favorable circumstances, accurate quantitative determination of the distribution of radioactivity.

Conventional detection systems have other unfavorable physical characteristics as well. Unperfused tissue in the detector field of view is not identified. Studies are generally restricted to the tissue served by the anterior and middle cerebral arteries on one side of the brain. Many current methods of studying cerebral hemodynamics and metabolism in vivo require the risk of internal carotid artery injections of radioisotopes, limiting the procedures to patients undergoing carotid catheterization for cerebral angiography.

Many problems of using conventional nuclear medicine to assess cerebral hemodynamics, biochemistry, and metabolism can be overcome by emission tomography in conjunction with positron-emitting radio-pharmaceuticals. Emission tomography is a technique that reveals the distribution of a previously administered radionuclide in any desired transverse section of the body. This is in contrast to transmission tomography (see Chapter 12), in which the image reflects the distribution of x-ray attenuation coefficients. The methods of data acquisition and image reconstruction in emission tomography are similar to those of transmission tomography. Conceptually, it is helpful to view emission tomography as analogous to quantitative tissue autoradiography with the added advantage of allowing in vivo studies (Phelps et al. 1975).

THEORETICAL BASIS FOR PET

Positron-emitting radionuclides are well suited for imaging by tomography because they give rise to annihilation radiation. Several radionuclides emit positrons, positively charged electrons, which are unstable and lose their kinetic energy in matter in a manner similar to that of electrons. When positrons come to rest, they interact with an electron. The two particles undergo annihilation, and the mass of the two particles is converted into two photons traveling at 180° from each other with an energy of about 511 keV. This is the annihilation radiation.

Annihilation radiation can be uniquely detected by two radiation detectors connected to a coincidence circuit, which records an event only if both detectors sense the annihilation photons simultaneously. This coincidence detection of annihilation radiation provides a method of so-called electronic collimation because the two detectors can record coincidence events only in the volume of space established by straight lines joining the two detectors. Thus, coincidence detection of the annihilation radiation provides a nearly uniform field of view (or sensitivity) in the region between the two detectors. Coincidence detection of annihilation radiation also permits easy accurate correction for the attenuation of radiation in tissues. In emission tomography the high energy of annihilation radiation (511-keV photons) allows greater tissue penetration and thus better detectability as compared to the 140-keV photons of ^{99m}Tc commonly used in gamma-ray emission tomography.

Two disadvantages of positron-emission tomography (PET) as compared to gamma-ray emission tomography are that PET is limited to positron-emitting radionuclides and that the total dose of radiation delivered to the patient by positron-emitting radionuclides includes both the annihilation radiation and the kinetic energy of the positrons. These problems are more than offset by the advantages obtained with positron-emitting radionuclides, however.

A number of PET systems are currently in use. Most of these systems have incorporated scintillation detectors. In its most simple form, a PET system consists of two detectors scanning the imaged object from different angles, but more detectors can be placed around the imaged object to improve the efficiency of radiation collection. The interested reader is referred to the following articles for detailed descriptions of the various instruments developed to date: Phelps et al. 1975; Chesler 1973; Budinger and Gullberg 1974; Hoffman et al. 1976; Brownell et al. 1977; Cho et al. 1977; Ter-Pogossian et al. 1978; Raichle et al. 1977.

APPLICATIONS OF PET

Cerebral Metabolism

Cerebral metabolism can be quantified by two approaches: using radiolabeled metabolic substrates as tracers, and using radiolabeled metabolic substrate analogs, which have blocking agents on the molecule to limit the extent of metabolism, as tracers.

The use of a radiolabeled metabolic substrate tracer to study metabolism is illustrated by our method of measuring regional cerebral glucose metabolic rate (CMRGlu) with emission tomography (Raichle et al. 1977, 1978). This approach is a modification of a technique previously described and validated (Raichle et al. 1975). The tomographic measurement of CMRGlu involves a 4-minute infusion of ^{11}C-glucose intravenously. By obtaining the time concentration history of the radioisotope in blood plus emission tomographs of the brain at the end of the infusion, CMRGlu is obtained with a mathematical model. In conjunction with the CMRGlu measurement, cerebral blood volume (CBV) is measured using the inhalation of ^{11}CO and PET. This measurement permits correction of the ^{11}C-glucose scan data for the ^{11}C-glucose present in the brain vascular compartment during the scan. By obtaining the brain images less than 10 minutes from the time of injection, the egress of labeled metabolites from the tissue is insignificant.

This approach to measuring metabolism using radiolabeled metabolic substrates as tracers has several important advantages. First, the tracer is biochemically identical to the compound being traced. Second, the method outlined above is relatively quick, thus permitting repeated measurements should they be required for evaluation of transient phenomena. Third, when only a relative mapping of regional rate of use is sought with an organ of interest, sampling of peripheral arterial blood is not necessary. Finally and most importantly, this method is not restricted to ^{11}C-glucose nor to the brain. This approach can be used with a wide variety of available radiopharmaceuticals utilized by the brain, heart, and other organs. There are a surprising number of positron-emitting radiopharmaceuticals for metabolic studies currently available (Wolf and Redvanly 1977).

Another approach to the study of cerebral metabolism is the use of radiolabeled metabolic substrate analogs. An example of this approach is the use of ^{18}F-2-fluoro-2-deoxy-D-glucose (^{18}F-FDG) to measure CMRGlu (Ido et al. 1977; Reivich et al. 1977). ^{18}F-FDG has been administered to humans and imaged with emission tomography to determine CMRGlu. This approach has the advantage of trapping the tracer in the tissue so the calculation of metabolic rates is not hampered by egress of labeled metabolites and free tracer in the tissue. However, these substrate analogs are not biochemically identical to the compound being traced. Therefore, corrections must be made in the tracer model for differences in transport properties and enzyme affinities, which vary among species (Sokoloff et al. 1977). These corrections may present an added difficulty when the organ of interest is diseased. Furthermore, only a few such compounds are available.

Cerebral Hemodynamics

A quantitative image of a vascular tracer in an equilibrium state is easily obtained with emission tomography. Thus, the measurement of cerebral blood volume (CBV) tomographically is relatively straightforward. CBV can be quantified noninvasively by using inhalation of [11]CO to label red blood cells (RBCs). When the labeled RBCs reach equilibrium, emission tomographic images of the ^{11}C-carboxyhemoglobin ([11]CO-Hgb) activity in the brain are obtained. At the same time venous blood samples are collected to calculate [11]CO-Hgb activity in the blood. With appropriate corrections for the density of blood, the brain tissue density, and the ratio of the mean tissue hematocrit of the brain to the large vessel hematocrit, CBV is calculated from the ratio of [11]CO-Hgb activity in the brain to the [11]CO-Hgb activity of the blood. With this method, an average CBV of 4.3 and 3.3 ml/100 gm for normal humans was found in emission tomographic scans obtained 4 and 8 cm above the orbitomeatal line (Raichle et al. unpublished data). Using a similar approach with ^{99m}Tc-labeled RBCs and gamma-ray emission tomography, CBV values of 2–4 ml/100 gm were found in tomographic sections obtained from various levels of the brain (Kuhl et al. 1975).

Accurate quantitative measure of cerebral blood flow (CBF) is not possible with present emission tomographic systems. Current emission tomographic systems do not have the capability of collecting statistically adequate data rapidly enough to make a dynamic tracer measurement. This factor precludes application to emission tomography of various tracer washout techniques currently used to measure CBF with external scintillation detection. Attempts to circumvent this difficulty are under way in a number of centers.

With current emission tomographic devices, accurate quantitative measurement of CBF will require development of an adequate technique that uses either steady-state infusion of a radiolabeled tracer or tissue trapping of a radiolabeled tracer to assure equilibrium during data collection. One PET approach to measuring regional CBF and oxygen metabolism uses tomographic imaging of the steady-state distribution of tracer in brain (Jones et al. 1976; Alpert et al. 1977). When ^{15}O-labeled CO_2 is inhaled, the label is rapidly transferred to water. Simple mathematical modeling permits one to relate the equilibrium quantity of ^{15}O-labeled water in a region of brain to the blood flow of that region. In a companion study the regional steady-state distribution of brain water formed while the subject breathes ^{15}O-labeled oxygen is imaged. The ratio of the two equilibrium images ($^{15}O_2 C^{15}O_2$) permits computation of the regional oxygen extraction fraction. The computed CBF and oxygen extraction fraction can be combined with the arterial blood oxygen content to yield the regional cerebral oxygen metabolism. Unfortunately, computation of CBF with this method is very sensitive to uncertainties in the brain tracer concentration due to the nonlinear nature of the blood flow equation. In addition, the ratio approach ($^{15}O_2 C^{15}O_2$) of assessing the regional oxygen extraction fraction requires images of very good statistical quality because errors in the calculation of either regional value are propagated in the resultant ratio. Also, use of the oxygen extraction fraction as an indicator of cerebral function is unclear because its value reflects both CBF and brain tissue oxygen metabolism. The development of very fast tomographic devices that would circumvent the above-mentioned difficulties in quantitative measurement of CBF are under study in many centers.

Tomographic imaging of ^{13}N-labeled ammonia ($^{13}NH_3$) at equilibrium has been proposed as an indicator of cerebral perfusion (Phelps et al. 1977), but labeled ammonia probably is not a suitable tracer for measuring this aspect of cerebral hemodynamics. The mechanism of ammonia uptake and trapping by the brain is not fully understood although metabolic factors undoubtedly play a role. The pH of the blood affects ammonia uptake by the brain. Furthermore, the uptake of ammonia by the brain seems to be affected by the brain capillary density. For this reason gray-white matter differences in ammonia uptake can be seen on emission tomographs of the brain. Brain ammonia uptake also changes with the volume velocity of blood flow but is not directly proportional to CBF. To compound the problem with ^{13}N-ammonia, the effects of cerebral pathology on ammonia uptake are not known. Thus, the equilibrium emission tomographs of $^{13}NH_3$

do not measure CBF and probably do not accurately measure cerebral perfusion. The usefulness of $^{13}NH_3$ probably will be limited to that of a qualitative scanning agent capable of demonstrating defects in cerebral perfusion.

Tissue Chemical Composition

Emission tomography provides quantitative measurement in vivo of brain-to-blood partition coefficients for various substrates. This approach is illustrated by our method of quantitatively measuring brain tissue acid–base status using ^{11}C-bicarbonate ($H^{11}CO_3^-$) and ^{11}CO-Hgb (Raichle et al. 1977). By obtaining equilibrium tomographs of these two radiopharmaceuticals, one can quantitatively measure the brain-to-blood partition coefficient for CO_2 (λCO_2). This allows determination of brain CO_2 content on a three-dimensional basis, which can then be used to calculate tissue pH. Values of brain CO_2 content in rhesus monkeys are in accord with previously described measurements of brain CO_2 content (Messeter and Siesjo 1971). This same approach, using appropriately labeled positron-emitting radiopharmaceuticals, can be used to measure in vivo parameters such as tissue lipid content, tissue water content, tissue drug concentrations, and the location of brain receptors and transmitters.

Blood-Brain Barrier

Gallium-68 in the form of ^{68}Ga-EDTA under normal conditions remains in the vascular spaces in the brain, but it accumulates in cerebral lesions where the blood-brain barrier is not intact. Thus, this positron-emitting radionuclide is useful in tomographic demonstration of blood-brain barrier defects to large protein molecules.

CONCLUSIONS

PET allows safe, quantitative three-dimensional measurement of radioisotope distribution in tissue. This approach, analogous to quantitative tissue autoradiography, offers the opportunity to study tissue metabolism, hemodynamics, and chemical composition with noninvasive methods in humans and animals in both normal and pathologic states. The potential of such a technique is obvious. The requirements for its successful implementation may not be so obvious. It may be clear to most that expensive machinery (cyclotrons, imaging devices, computers) is a necessary foundation, but not so clear that a critical mass of diverse human talents must be closely coordinated to make the full potential of PET a reality in the biomedical environment. Successful implementation of this technology will represent a true collaborative effort among physicists, chemists, mathematicians and biologists.

REFERENCES

Alpert, N. M. et al. Measurement of rCBF and rCMRO$_2$ by continuous inhalation of ^{15}O-labeled CO$_2$ and O$_2$. *Acta Neurol. Scand.* [*Suppl.*] 56:186–187, 1977.

Brownell, G. L. et al. Transverse section imaging of radionuclide distributions in heart, lung, and brain. In *Reconstruction tomography in diagnostic radiology and nuclear medicine*, eds. M. M. Ter-Pogossian et al. Baltimore: University Park Press, 1977.

Budinger, T. F., and Gullberg, G. T. Three-dimensional reconstruction of isotope distributions. *Phys. Med. Biol.* 19:387–389, 1974.

Chesler, D. A. Positron tomography and three-dimensional reconstruction technique. In *Tomographic imaging in nuclear medicine*, ed. G. S. Freedman. New York: Society of Nuclear Medicine, 1973.

Cho, Z. H.; Eriksson, L.; and Chan, J. A circular ring transverse axial positron camera. In *Reconstruction tomography in diagnostic radiology and nuclear medicine*, eds. M. M. Ter-Pogossian et al. Baltimore: University Park Press, 1977.

Ido, T. et al. Fluorination with F$_2$. A convenient synthesis of 2-deoxy-3-fluoro-D-glucose. *J. Org. Chem.* 42:2341–2342, 1977.

Hoffman, E. J. et al. Design and performance characteristics of a whole-body positron transaxial tomograph. *J. Nucl. Med.* 17:493–502, 1976.

Jones, T.; Chesler, D. A.; and Ter-Pogossian, M. M. The continuous inhalation of oxygen-15 for assessing regional oxygen extraction in the brain of man. *Br. J. Radiol.* 49:339–343, 1976.

Kuhl, D. E. et al. Local cerebral blood volume determined by three-dimensional reconstruction of radionuclide scan data. *Circ. Res.* 36: 610–619, 1975.

Messeter, K., and Siesjo, B. K. The intracellular pH in the brain in acute and sustained hypercapnia. *Acta Physiol. Scand.* 83:210–219, 1971.

Phelps, M. E. et al. Application of annihilation coincidence detection to transaxial reconstruction tomography. *J. Nucl. Med.* 16:210–224, 1975.

Phelps, M. E.; Hoffman, E. J.; and Raybaud, C. Factors which affect cerebral uptake and retention of ^{13}NH$_3$. *Stroke* 8:694–702, 1977.

Raichle, M. E. et al. In vivo measurement of brain glucose transport and metabolism employing glucose-^{11}C. *Am. J. Physiol.* 228:1936–1948, 1975.

Raichle, M. E. et al. Three-dimensional in vivo mapping of brain metabolism and acid-base status. *Acta Neurol. Scand.* [*Suppl.*], 56:188–189, 1977.

Raichle, M. E. et al. Measurement of regional substrate utilization rates by emission tomography. *Science* 199:986–987, 1978.

Reivich, M. et al. Measurement of local cerebral glucose metabolism in man with ^{18}F-2-fluoro-2-deoxy-d-glucose. *Acta Neurol. Scand.* [*Suppl.*] 56:190–191, 1977.

Sokoloff, L. et al. The (^{14}C) deoxyglucose method for the measurement of local cerebral glucose utilization: theory, procedure, and normal values in the conscious and anesthetized albino rat. *J. Neurochem.* 28: 897–916, 1977.

Ter-Pogossian, M. M. et al. A multislice positron emission computed tomograph (PETT IV) yielding transverse and longitudinal images. *Radiology* 128:477–484, 1978.

Wolf, A. P., and Redvanly, C. S. Carbon-11 and radiopharmaceuticals. *Int. J. Appl. Radiat. Isot.* 28:29–48, 1977.

Part 3
The Treatment
of
Brain Metastasis

15

Analysis of the Benefit of Palliation of Brain Metastases

Stanley E. Order

"Technical excellence is a standard; compassion is the intangible that distinguishes a physician"

The presentation of brain metastasis may occur in a variety of circumstances: a manifestation of progressively disseminated disease with headache or neurologic dysfunction; the concomitant presentation of brain metastasis and a primary lesion (often lung cancer); as a first sign of dissemination after a period of time with no evidence of disease. Regardless of these or other circumstances, the patient most often realizes the prognostic significance of such a finding. Analysis of the benefit of possible palliative treatment requires consideration of all of the issues. The patient, family, and physician have a direct role in decision making and each requires review. In addition, in a larger sense society plays an indirect role in the services and modalities available for patients both with potential cerebral metastasis as well as with active disease.

THE PATIENT'S VIEW

Patients respond to the first findings of cerebral metastasis with a spectrum of emotions: a sense of impending demise; the need for reassurance to continue life; the hope of reversal of severe neurologic deficits; and the desire for continued control over their life situations (table 15.1). For many patients, the desire to limit the time necessary for treatment and association with the hospital environment is also important. This latter point should be analyzed as well and perhaps is best described as the time-benefit ratio.

The emotional support needed to sustain a patient with a brain metastasis is neither taught nor analyzed with the convenience of common nomenclature in cancer therapy such as percentage of response and no evidence of disease. In our profession there is an assumption that emotional support always exists and may not be as critical as therapy. For individuals whose expected median survival is 75 days, however, serious

257

Table 15.1

PATIENT RESPONSE TO BRAIN METASTASIS

Sense of impending demise
Need for hope of reversal of symptoms
Feelings of loss of life control
Need for reassurance to continue life
Desire to limit therapy time and hospitalization

question may be raised concerning this assumption and the validity of the presumed support (Hendrickson and Gelber 1978).

MODALITY OF TREATMENT AND TIME-BENEFIT RATIO

In regard to the time-benefit ratio (time spent receiving treatment for relief of symptoms), introduction of various possible modalities may be considered (table 15.2). Surgical resection may be considered appropriate for special circumstances either without a certain diagnosis or in patients with a single metastasis and with the primary disease under control. In these circumstances exceptional results are sought but realized to be only remotely possible.

Surgery requires significant commitment of time and has an associated morbidity and mortality (Lang and Slater 1964). It should not be undertaken without careful discrimination. The suggestion of surgery for

Table 15.2

TECHNIQUE FOR TREATMENT OF BRAIN METASTASIS

Method	Time–Benefit Ratio	Complications	Risk–Benefit Ratio
Surgery	Prolonged	Morbidity, mortality	↑Risk
Steroids	Abbreviated	Dependence with steroid sequelae	Modest
Radiation single fraction	Abbreviated	Convulsions	↑Risk
Fractionated	Prolonged	—	Modest

single metastases from hypernephroma (a relatively radioresistant tumor) has not been clarified as yet (Stortebecker 1954). Steroid therapy has the distinct advantage of a more immediate response but is not well sustained when survival is prolonged. In addition, prolonged administration and dependency are associated with metabolic disruption and reduced resistance to infection. The time-benefit ratio may often be favorably reduced by immediate institution of steroid therapy or osmotic therapy with mannitol or other agents (Horton et al. 1971).

Radiation therapy may be used on an outpatient basis and requires a time commitment based on the single or fractionated dose to be used. Several publications have suggested that single, large doses (1,000 rads, whole-brain) yield equivalent results to fractionated courses of treatment (Hendrickson 1975; Shehata et al. 1974). My experience with such treatment has not indicated equivalent results, however; also convulsions have been noted, and sustained remission has not been satisfactory. Review of fractionation schemes has indicated that below 2,500 rads, significant benefit is not routinely achieved (Chu and Hilaris 1961). Fractionated courses above 2,500 rads yielded equivalent results, but a significant dose-response relationship has not been established. The dose (outside the current studies) commonly employed is 3,000 rads/10 fractions. The lack of a clear dose-response relationship suggests the possibility of reseeding and not simply recurrence as an explanation of the therapeutic plateau of radiation effectiveness.

THE PHYSICIAN'S ROLE

No one is more capable of analyzing patients' needs than the physician familiar with patients' courses, primary diseases, metastatic status, functional abilities, and emotional desires and perspectives (table 15.3). Against this background the physician must estimate the desire of patients to attempt to improve their physical status and the possibilities of such improvement.

Table 15.3

THE PHYSICIAN'S ANALYSIS

Functional status of patients
Emotional desires, needs, and perspective
Estimated duration of life
Probability of return of deficit
Time–benefit ratio

Evaluation of the primary tumor and other metastatic sites of disease and a Karnofsky functional status evaluation will aid in predicting the duration of survival. Evaluation of the neurologic functional status will identify the possible beneficial expectations of treatment (table 15.4). Should the comatose patient be reawakened? Is the neurologic impairment dense, irreversible, or possibly capable of resolution? Are other metastases causing significant symptoms overwhelming or controllable with the achievement of a reasonable quality of life?

In this regard the physician must also be cognizant of the results of therapy in order to determine possible patient benefit.

TREATMENT SITUATIONS

Various treatment alternatives for special circumstances are available and require the physician's decision:

(1) treatment of brain metastasis and concomitant primary tumor (lung cancer)
(2) retreatment
(3) treatment in advance of expected cranial metastasis (prophylaxis)
(4) new techniques of management of late stage disease

Table 15.4

A FUNCTIONAL CLASSIFICATION OF PATIENTS WITH BRAIN METASTASES

Class	Definition
I.	Intellectually and physically able to work; neurologic findings minor or not present.
II.	Intellectually intact and physically able to be at home although nursing care may be required; neurologic findings present but not a major factor.
III.	Major neurologic findings requiring hospitalization, medical care, and supervision.
IV.	Requires hospitalization and is in serious physical and neurologic state.

Concomitant Primary Tumor and Brain Metastasis

There are no distinct guidelines in the literature to indicate proper management of primary lung cancer with concomitant brain metastasis. Progression of the primary disease may lead to significant clinical symptoms with development of shortness of breath, hemoptysis, and local pain. The patient then requires additional treatment after previous treatment of a metastatic site and another sequence of visits to the Radiation Therapy Clinic. Utilization of the original visits to treat brain metastasis and the primary disease is worthwhile in my experience.

Retreatment

In an attempt to prolong remission from cranial metastasis, different radiation fractions were employed by the RTOG (Radiation Therapy Oncology Group), but no significant difference in duration of remission was noted (Hendrickson 1977). Therefore retreatment may have as its basis the recurrence of residual disease or the reseeding by primary disease in metastatic foci more susceptible to implantation. The schedule as well as total dose applied during retreatment of brain metastasis has been left to the discretion of the radiation therapist without an established literature for referral.

Treatment in Advance of Expected Metastasis

Prophylactic whole-brain irradiation in leukemia has been associated with a reduction in cranial leukemia (62% vs. 4.4%) and is an established technique (Hustu et al. 1973). In oat-cell cancer prophylactic irradiation reduces extension to the central nervous system (41% vs. 6.5%) although it does not influence survival (Bunn et al. 1977). Is it efficient to reduce the probability of cranial metastasis without influencing survival? We have adopted the treatment philosophy that patients in remission deserve prophylactic whole-brain irradiation by applying the philosophy of achieving the highest quality of life and disregarding the lack of effect on survival.

New Techniques of Management

Prophylaxis of anticipated cranial metastasis and treatment of active cranial metastasis could be approached by means other than direct irradiation. Recent interest in half-body irradiation for metastatic disease (Chapter 19) has led to clinical protocols which have the potential for cranial prophylaxis and concomitant treatment of metastatic disease in the upper half of the body. The complication of radiation pneumonitis has been reduced by lowering the total dose to 800 rads. This technique is now being explored in advanced malignancy (Prato et al. 1976).

An additional technique in advanced malignancy is autologous bone marrow graft following maximal cytotoxic reduction by chemotherapy and irradiation. The preliminary results with this approach are encouraging (Wharam et al., *in press*).

Philosophically, more aggressive prophylactic therapy in the presence of micrometastatic disease is a more attractive method of therapy than palliation of active disease if the risk-benefit ratio is acceptable.

SOCIETY

Today there is an acute sense of cost accounting for services. In addition, the so-called results desired are related to cure and productivity. What price is assigned to dignity and the quality of life? There is no cost-benefit ratio that can be anything more than humane when we consider a median survival of 75 days with intact cranial nerves, a functioning cerebellum, and the avoidance of convulsions and expressive aphasia.

ANALYSIS OF POTENTIAL BENEFIT

In an analysis of possible benefit from radiation treatment of brain metastasis, the shortened life expectancy (often 6 months or less) raises the first issue—time:

(1) time-benefit ratio, time spent in treatment versus potential time gained in benefit
(2) time to improve
(3) time of sustained improvement
(4) time of life remaining

The patient's status is the setting in which improvement is sought and includes the biologic activity of the cancer: status of primary tumor; extent of tumor dissemination; and extent of cranial metastasis. These factors may be influenced by intervention with additive therapy for generalized disease or brain metastasis such as steroids, chemotherapy, or hormonal therapy.

The RTOG used a linear logistic model to describe dependence of the frequency of improvement on the levels of all the covariates: initial performance status; extent of metastasis; primary site; status of primary; steroid treatment; and chemotherapy. This model, which assumes that the logarithm of the odds of improvement is a linear function of the covariates,[1] reveals only small differences in the magnitude of covariate influence.

---

[1] The model is expressed as $\log \{Px\} (1 - Px) = \alpha \beta x$ where β is now a vector of regression parameters (Hendrickson 1978).

In another phase of a similar study, a Cox model system was employed which described the dependence of survival on the covariates assuming a log of the hazard function.[2] Although statistical differences seemed to exist, the magnitude of the differences which are in terms of weeks of survival, are not impressive. Thus, analysis of the RTOG data indicates that none of the clinical and treatment factors listed previously seem to have a significant influence on incidence of improvement or survival.

All of these analyses utilized a neurologic function status (table 15.4) adopted from an older review which attempted to analyze the cumulative rate of improvement and survival by dividing percent surviving into percent still improved to determine at that point in time the percent alive and well at an interval as the palliative index (Order et al. 1968). This concept remains valid because it tests not how long a patient with metastasis lives, but the quality of life for the duration of life. For example, 3 months after treatment 64% were improved, 81% were alive and have a palliative index of 79%. The palliative index of 79% implies that 79% of all those patients alive at 3 months remain improved.

In the future, analysis of brain metastasis must be associated with a dramatic difference in duration of improvement in order to be convincing. Plans for the integration of radiation sensitizers in treatment schemes will be of interest, but an attack on micrometastatic disease concomitant with cranial irradiation deals more directly with the phenomenon of no significant dose-response relationship. Rather than more elaborate statistical review, consideration of concomitant malignant inhibition should be compared to cranial irradiation alone to see if a greater extension of time and improved quality of life could be achieved.

Suggestions for future study and analysis include shorter higher fractional doses of whole-brain irradiation in combination with radiation sensitizers, the use of new agents for cerebral edema (Bedikian et al. 1978), and effective systemic agents in randomized prospective studies. Analysis of benefit regardless of methodology will ultimately have to address the quality of life. For in brain metastasis (median survival of 75 days with an average of 2 weeks of treatment and a median time to improvement of 15 days), there is considerable room for improvement.

REFERENCES

Bedikian, A. Y. et al. Glycerol: a successful alternative to dexamethasone for patients receiving brain irradiation for metastatic disease. *Cancer Treat. Rep.* 62:1081–1083, 1978.

---

[2]$\log \lambda (\tau)\chi - \log \lambda \sigma (\tau) + \delta \chi$ where δ is a vector of the parameters (coefficients) associated with the levels of the covariates and $\lambda_0 (\tau)$ is an unknown function of τ.

Bunn, P. A., Jr. et al. Advances in small cell bronchogenic carcinoma. *Cancer Treat. Rep.* 61:333–342, 1977.

Chu, F. C. H., and Hilaris, B. B. Value of radiation therapy in the management of intracranial metastasis. *CA* 14:577–581, 1961.

Hendrickson, F. R. Radiation therapy of metastatic tumors. *Semin. Oncol.* 2:43–46, 1975.

Hendrickson, F. R. The optimum schedule for palliative radiotherapy for metastatic brain cancer. *Int. J. Rad. Oncol. Bio. Phys.* 2:165–168, 1977.

Hendrickson, F., and Gelber, R. Radiation Therapy Oncology Group. *Brain Metastasis Report* (1978).

Horton, J.; Baxter, D.; and Olson, K. The management of metastasis to the brain by irradiation and corticosteroids. *Am. J. Roentgenol.* 111:334–336, 1971.

Hustu, H. O. et al. Prevention of central nervous leukemia by irradiation. *CA* 32:585–596, 1973.

Lang, E. F., and Slater, J. Metastatic brain tumors: results of surgical and nonsurgical treatment. *Surg. Clin. North Am.* 44:865–872, 1964.

Order, S. E. et al. Improvement in the quality of survival following whole brain irradiation for brain metastasis. *Radiology* 94:149–153, 1968.

Prato, F. S. et al. The incidence of radiation pneumonitis as a result of single fraction upper half body irradiation. *CA* 39:71–78, 1976.

Shehata, W. M.; Hendrickson, F. R.; and Hindo, W. A. Rapid fractionation technique and retreatment of brain metastasis by irradiation. *CA* 34:257–261, 1974.

Stortebecker, T. P. Metastatic tumors of the brain from a neurosurgical point of view: follow up study of 158 cases. *J. Neurosurg.* 11:84–111, 1954.

Wharam, M. D. et al. Systemic irradiation for selected stage IV and recurrent pediatric tumors: tolerance to therapy and interval results. *Int. J. Rad. Oncol. Bio. Phys.* (*in press*).

16

The Memorial Hospital Experience

Florence Chu

In the late 1940s the members of the Department of Radiation Therapy at Memorial Hospital began to treat patients with brain metastases. At that time the literature contained scanty information regarding the beneficial effects of irradiation for intracranial metastases. Since there was insufficient experience to guide us, we had to proceed cautiously. It was decided that the whole brain needed to be irradiated because intracranial metastases are most frequently multiple. It also seemed wise to begin with small doses in order to avoid the risk of increasing the intracranial pressure.

The technique developed consisted of whole-brain irradiation through two opposed lateral fields using 250-kVp x-rays. Daily treatments consisting of a 50 or 100 rads midplane dose was given for the first 3 or 4 days, depending on the condition of the patient. In the absence of any symptoms and signs of increased intracranial pressure, the dose could be increased by 50 rads daily until it reached 350–400 rads. The total dose was usually 3,000 rads delivered in 3–4 weeks.

The first report on the results of radiation therapy of brain metastases from our department was by Chao, Phillips, and Nickson in 1954. A consecutive series of 38 cases treated between January 1949 and June 1953 was evaluated. Of these, palliation of neurologic symptoms and signs resulted in 24 patients, a response rate of 63%. Based on these beneficial effects there was justification to recommend palliative radiation therapy for brain metastases.

Because of the encouraging preliminary results of brain irradiation for metastases, the staff of the Department of Radiation Therapy treated an increasing number of such patients. Our second report on the experience with irradiation for brain metastases was by Chu and Hilaris in 1961. A series of 218 patients with intracranial metastases from various primaries treated between January 1954 and June 1958 was evaluated. Carcinoma of the breast and carcinoma of the lung were the most frequent primary sites. An analysis of the overall results of treatment showed that 35 patients did not complete the prescribed course of radiation therapy due to rapid progression of generalized cancer or death. An additional 12 patients were lost to followup so that the response to radiation therapy could not be evaluated. The remaining 158 patients completed the prescribed course of treatment and were available for evaluation. Of this group, 123 (78%) showed improvement of neurologic symptoms and signs. The mean duration of improvement was 5 months (the longest being 27 months). If the patients with incomplete treatment or lost to followup were also considered as failures, the overall response rate was 57% (123 of 218).

In this same study it was found that a total dosage of more than 2,750 rads, delivered over a period of about 3 weeks, appeared to give better palliation than did radiation of less than 2,750 rads. Therefore, we continued to use a dose of 3,000–3,500 rads delivered in a period of 3–4 weeks. It was also found that the majority of patients died of advanced cancer, or other causes without evidence of recurrence of intracranial disease. When recurrence of intracranial symptoms did occur, palliation could be achieved with a second course of irradiation.

Worthwhile palliation seen in the majority of the patients so treated indicated clearly to us that total-brain irradiation is an effective approach to the management of patients with advanced cancer. In most instances the amelioration of symptoms and signs of neurologic dysfunction was dramatic and gratifying. Some patients went back to work and lived a useful life for several months or longer.

A third report by Nisce, Hilaris and Chu (1971) on radiation therapy of brain metastases covered a period from 1961 through 1967. There were a total of 560 patients treated. During this time two major changes were made. First, there was a gradual change in the modality, 250 kVp x-ray to megavoltage therapy; and second, the use of corticosteroids was introduced in about 1962. The use of corticosteroids prior to radiation therapy almost invariably produced immediate and sometimes dramatic improvement of neurologic symptoms. These improvements were short-lived, however, and radiation therapy was necessary to control the intracranial tumors. Originally low initial radiation doses of 50–100 rads were given, but with the adjuvant use of corticosteroids, the initial doses were increased to 200–250 rads. It was possible to increase the total dose to 3,500–4,000 rads in 3–4 weeks with the advent of megavoltage therapy and the use of steroids.

In this series worthwhile palliation was obtained in 54% of the total 560 patients and 80% of the 376 patients who completed the planned course of irradiation and were available for evaluation. The mean duration of remission was 5 months and the median duration, 3 months. The longest duration was 5 years.

From a review of the overall experience and an analysis of the results of irradiation of 816 patients from our 3 series, a pattern appeared to have emerged. Approximately one-fifth (20%) of the patients with brain metastases do not complete the prescribed course of radiation therapy because their general status deteriorates rapidly. Most of these patients die of their disease within a short period of time. Approximately one-half of all patients and three-fourths of those who receive a full course of irradiation benefit from it. The addition of corticosteroids, the change from orthovoltage irradiation to megavoltage irradiation, and the increase of the total tumor dose from 3,000 rads in 3–4 weeks to 3,500–4,000 rads in 3–4 weeks did not materially change the overall results. The use of megavoltage irradiation and adjuvant corticosteroids reduced radiation reactions and facilitated administration of irradiation. However, there was no influence on the overall response rate or duration of response when compared to 250 kVp irradiation without adjuvant corticosteroids. We continue to advocate total-brain irradiation to a dose of 3,000–3,500 rads in 3–4 weeks.

During the ensuing years other changes have occurred. Orthovoltage radiation therapy has been totally eliminated, and all patients are treated with megavoltage. A Neurology Service was established in the Department of Medicine in 1967. The Service was later expanded to an independent department, under the leadership of Dr. Jerome Posner, allowing for better services in diagnosis, patient care and followup. In addition, there was increased communication and exchange of stimulating ideas between the members of the Neurology and Radiation Therapy Departments. Newer and better diagnostic procedures such as radionuclide brain scans and CT scans also became available, minimizing the chances of making a false-positive or false-negative diagnosis.

A few different time-dose fractionation schemes were tried. One of the schemes involved a high-dose, short-duration course of radiation therapy. The rationale was to salvage some of the patients who ordinarily would die of brain metastases before the conventional course of therapy could be completed. Short-course therapy also shortens the hospitalization of patients with a limited life expectancy.

The rapid high-dose course (1500 rads in 2 treatments over 3 days) was employed at Memorial Hospital from May 1970 through December 1973 to treat most patients with known brain metastases from all primary sites. In a report by Young, Posner, Chu and Nisce (1974), the results of treatment of 83 patients receiving rapid course were compared retrospectively with a group of 79 patients treated conventionally (approximately 3,000 rads in 15 treatments over a period of 3 weeks). Neurologic improvement occurred in 57% of patients in the rapid-course group and 62% in the slow-course group. The rapid-course radiation resulted in a shorter duration of remission and higher complication rates than the slow course. Complications included acute cerebral herniation, headaches, nausea and vomiting, and fever. This regimen of 750 rads × 2 over 3 days was subsequently abandoned.

Unfortunately, the results of brain irradiation have not changed materially over the years. We are still getting an overall response rate of about 60% for an average duration of 5–6 months. This seeming lack of obvious improvement in results does not deter our efforts in searching for better methods of treatment. Currently we are using an unorthodox schedule developed mainly by Dr. Jae Ho Kim. This consists of a priming dose of 500 rads for 3 daily doses after which the patient is given 4 days rest and then receives a daily dose of 300 rads for 8 treatments. A total dose of 3,900 rads is delivered over a period of 2.5 weeks, which is equivalent to about 6,300 rads delivered in 5 weeks using conventional daily fractionations. The new fractionated schemes were designed on the basis of clinical and cellular radiobiologic considerations. The use of initial high fractional dose should facilitate a rapid tumor cytolysis so that the subsequent fractionated irradiation is more effective. The 4-day rest interval is introduced to enhance the tumor reoxygenation process so as to minimize the cell population in an hypoxic state. All patients receive corticosteroids. Patients seem to tolerate this schedule well. The results of treatment will be evaluated in the near future. We will also be designing new protocols which will probably involve either hyperfractionation or radiation sensitizers.

I believe this workshop on brain metastasis and subsequent book are particularly timely and meaningful. A group of interested oncologists shared their experiences and ideas, discussed this problem in depth, and more importantly, pooled their resources to plan further investigative studies. We need innovative ideas to improve the results of treatment. Cerebral metastases complicate advanced cancer in about 15–20% of patients. These metastatic lesions are associated with devastating physical, emotional and nursing problems. Thus, whatever palliation does occur and whatever improvements in the results of treatment, either in terms of the response rate or duration of response, or both, are extremely worthwhile.

REFERENCES

Chao, J. H.; Phillips, R.; and Nickson, J. J. Roentgen-ray therapy of cerebral metastases. *Cancer* 7:682–689, 1954.

Chu, F. C. H., and Hilaris, B. S. Value of radiation therapy in the management of intracranial metastases. *Cancer* 14:577–581, 1961.

Nisce, L. Z.; Hilaris, B. S.; and Chu, F. C. H. A review of experience with irradiation of brain metastasis. *Am. J. Roentgenol.* 111:329–333, 1971.

Young, D. F. et al. Rapid-course radiation therapy of cerebral metastases: results and complications. *Cancer* 34:1069–1076, 1974.

17

The Hahnemann
Experience

Luther W. Brady
Deepchand Bajpai

The incidence of metastatic disease of the central nervous system represents about 1–5% of all cancers (see Chapter 1). The incidence of metastatic intracranial disease is increasing but still remains a rarity in children. The common primary sites are bronchus (31–34%), breast (13–39%), gastrointestinal tract (16%), kidney (8%), skin (7%), and thyroid (4%). Metastatic tumors of the central nervous system are multiple in 70% of the patients afflicted and are likely to coexist with metastases to other sites (86–93% of patients).

Metastases in the course of malignancy are of three essential types: (1) metachronous metastases where the primary lesion has been successfully controlled and months to years later a focus is found at a distant site (7–14% of all brain metastases); (2) precocious metastases where the metastatic lesion is the first sign of cancer with no detectable evidence of the primary source (5–10% of all brain metastases); (3) synchronous metastases where a solitary metastatic lesion and a defined primary cancer present simultaneously (80–85% of brain metastases). The frequency of solitary metastatic lesions to the brain and central nervous system varies considerably. They are a function of the type of experience being analyzed, whether at surgery or necropsy.

Brain metastasis is a disabling and dramatic clinical event in the evolution of malignant dissemination. It is definitely life-threatening and emotionally debilitating because the loss of mental acuity and motor functions are symptoms which are poorly handled by patients and families. In addition, brain metastases can affect the whole life style of a patient, compromising ambulation and personal care. Treatment of such patients can improve the clinical status to a degree that they can spend the remainder of their lives in a satisfactory manner and continue to take care of themselves.

Among the most notable achievements in radiotherapy for palliation of metastatic disease is the treatment of brain metastases. Palliation in these situations is viewed by patients and their families with considerable relief because with appropriate management, symptoms resolve and the neurologic signs improve. In some situations the neurologic improvement is maintained until the patient succumbs to systemic disease. The mainstay of the treatment of intracranial metastatic disease has been radiation therapy. It is preferable to surgery when the primary neoplasm is not

269

under control and there are widespread metastases elsewhere in the body. A noteworthy fact nevertheless remains: the treatment will have little influence on the ultimate course of the disease or the duration of the patient's survival. Support of this contention emerges from an in-depth study of the patients seen at Hahnemann Medical College and Hospital, representing the experience of a clinical team dealing with problems of metastatic intracranial malignancy. The widespread persistence of a nihilistic attitude toward the treatment of brain metastases by radiation technique is inappropriate.

METHODS

We reviewed 343 consecutive patients with intracranial metastatic disease seen from 1961–1977, patients ranged from 25–82 years with a median of 55 years. There were 222 males and 121 females; 281 patients were white and 62 patients were black (table 17.1). The most common primary site was the lung (210 patients, 61.2%). About 51 patients (14.8%) had primary sites in the breast. The gastrointestinal tract and genitourinary tract accounted for many of the remainder, and 4.08% had an unknown primary site (table 17.2).

The most commonly encountered presenting symptoms were hemiplegia, hemiparesis, and headaches with dizziness and vertigo, convulsions, visual disturbance and memory loss. The symptoms in general reflected the location of the tumor. The incidence of metastases varied from 68.2% in the cerebrum to 4.4% in the cerebellum and 27.2% in multiple sites (table 17.3).

Kindt (1964) and Allen (1967) have pointed out a definite predilection for metastases to lodge along the posterior aspect of the Rolandic fissure near the junction of the temporal, parietal, and occipital lobes. In large measure tumors were located within the distribution of the middle cerebral artery. A possible explanation is that the location is related to the principles of bloodflow in the arteries. In general there was no preponderance of lesions either to the right or the left side.

Table 17.1

INTRACRANIAL METASTATIC MALIGNANCY
RACE, AGE AND SEX OF 343 PATIENTS
(1961–1977)

Age	Sex		Race	
	Male	Female	Black	White
25–82 years				
(Median 55 yr.)	222	121	62	281

Table 17.2

INTRACRANIAL METASTATIC MALIGNANCY
SITE OF PRIMARY LESION
(1961–1977)

	Number of Patients	Percentage
Lung	210	61.2
Breast	51	14.8
Gastrointestinal	15	4.3
Leukemia	10	2.9
Head and neck	8	2.3
Hodgkin's	7	2.04
Non-Hodgkin's lymphoma	3	0.8
Kidney	7	2.04
Prostate	3	0.8
Bladder	1	0.2
Testes	1	0.2
Multiple myeloma	4	1.1
Melanoma	5	1.4
Mesothelioma	2	0.5
Mycosis fungoides	1	0.2
Ovary	1	0.2
Unknown	14	4.08
TOTAL	343	100

Table 17.3

INTRACRANIAL METASTATIC MALIGNANCY
PRESENTING SYMPTOMS AND SIGNS
343 PATIENTS
(1961–1977)

	Number of Patients	Percentage of Total
Hemiparesis and hemiplegia	136	39.6
Headache	135	39.3
Dizziness and vertigo	72	20.9
Convulsions	45	13.1
Memory loss	43	12.5
Visual disturbance	58	16.9
Cranial nerve deficits	26	7.5
Disorientation	16	4.6

The diagnosis was established on the basis of a careful history and diagnostic studies including roentgenograms of the skull (displacement of the pineal gland or other indirect evidence of increased intercranial pressure yielded positive studies in 40 patients). Brain scans were positive in 249 patients, computed tomography in 30 patients, and arteriograms in 55 patients. A few cases of clinical suspicion of intracranial metastases were not documented by diagnostic modalities, but on the basis of neurologic deficits a course of radiotherapy was directed to the whole brain especially if the primary tumors were lung or breast (table 17.4).

A small number of patients (27.2%) demonstrated multiple intracranial metastatic lesions. This may simply reflect the fact that the data are based on observation intravitam. One would expect a much higher incidence of multiple lesions if the brain itself were to be examined pathologically since lesions which do not manifest clinically or radiographically are frequently evident at necropsy (table 17.5).

The treatment program was carried out on all patients with external beam therapy with the intent to irradiate the entire brain through two parallel opposed fields. This approach was adopted in view of the hematogenous dissemination of the disease and the anticipated multiplicity of intracerebral lesions. The calculated tumor dose was estimated at the

Table 17.4

INTRACRANIAL METASTATIC MALIGNANCY DIAGNOSIS

	Number Positive
Radionuclide scanning	249
CT scanning	30
Skull radiography	40
Arteriography	55
Craniotomy	25

Table 17.5

INTRACRANIAL METASTATIC MALIGNANCY
LOCATION OF DOMINANT METASTASIS AS DETERMINED
BY RADIONUCLIDE SCANNING
(1961–1977)

	Number of Patients	Percentage of Total
Parietal	72	24.4
Frontal	50	17.0
Fronto Parietal	27	9.1
Temporal	18	6.1
Cerebellum	13	4.4
Parietooccipital	25	8.5
Parietotemporal	9	3.06
Multiple	80	27.2
TOTAL	294	100

midplane of the brain and was 4,000 rads in a median elapsed time of 28 days until 1972. From 1973–1977 we treated 114 patients with external beam radiation to the whole brain. We have used four different time-dose fractionations during this time in collaboration with the RTOG. These include 2,000 rads in 1 week (13 patients), 3,000 rads in 3 weeks (10 patients), 3,000 rads in 2 weeks (41 patients), and 4,000 rads in 4 weeks (25 patients). Reviewing our patients with these different dose fractionations, we found two treatments (3,000 rads in 2 weeks and 4,000 rads in 4 weeks) to yield comparatively similar results relative to control of disease. None of the dose fractionations improved survival, but a majority of the patients responding to the whole-brain irradiation with good to excellent response received the above mentioned treatment schedules. We have now been using 3,000 rads in 2 weeks as our standard policy in conjunction with steroids. Supervoltage radiation techniques are utilized with parallel opposing fields.

Steroid therapy was administered to 256 patients during the treatment program with external beam radiotherapy. We used either dexamethasone or prednisone; the usual dose was 16 mg of dexamethasone or its equivalent in prednisone given in a divided dose over a 24-hour period. We did not document specific neurologic improvement, but there was improvement in all symptoms. In fact the best symptomatic improvements were noted in those who had most severe symptoms in terms of mental confusion, lethargy and headache.

We believe that, as noted by others, steroids mainly act by decreasing the edema around the metastases (see Chapter 23). After the relief of symptoms, the steroids were tapered off to nothing. No definite pattern was followed in decreasing the steroids. We did not give doses higher than 16 mg over a period of 24 hours even in those patients who did not show adequate response to the steroid medication in conjunction with radiotherapy. We did not encounter any significant complications relative to steroid medication such as abdominal discomfort, steroid myopathy, insomnia, or tremors, but the side effects of steroids in the face of neurologic symptoms are difficult to evaluate. No patient required interruption of treatment due to radiation edema. All exhibited epilation at completion of treatment but hair regrew in survivors within 4–5 months.

In 19 patients re-treatment with a second course of radiation therapy was administered for recurrence of symptoms. All these patients were again evaluated by careful history, clinical examination and diagnostic tests. They showed excellent to good response in the initial treatment with radiotherapy in conjunction with steroid medication. The dose level for re-treatment was calculated at a tumor dose of 2,500 rads in a median elapsed time of 3 weeks. We did not encounter any significant problems in terms of re-treatment, which on two occasions was as early as 3 months.

Craniotomy was carried out in 25 patients prior to institution of radiation therapy, but in no instance tumor removal was judged to be complete. All the patients were subjected to a full course of postoperative external beam radiotherapy. All patients who presented with convulsions either general or focal were given phenytoin (300–400 mg) in divided doses. No patients received prophylactic phenytoin medication.

RESULTS

The median survival of 303 patients who completed the projected course of radiation therapy for intracranial metastatic disease was 5 months from completion of the radiation therapy. During radiation therapy 40 patients died but in no instance could death be attributed directly to the radiation therapy.

An excellent response to treatment was defined as complete disappearance of symptoms with the restoration of intellectual and physical capability of resuming work; it was achieved by 114 patients (38%) with the median survival in this group of 6 months. A good response was defined as good return of function with some limitations in activity and minimal neurologic deficits. In this category 83 patients (28%) were identified with a median survival of 4.5 months. A fair response to treatment was characterized by persistent debilitating symptoms albeit with some return of function: 52 patients (18%) exhibited this degree of response with a median survival of 2 months. A persistent incapacitating deficit with minimal improvement characterized a poor response to treatment. Twenty patients (6%) had a poor response and their median survival was 1.5 months. Failure to improve in any recognizable respect occurred in 28 patients with a median survival of 1 month. Six patients stopped treatment on their own decision or that of the primary physician (table 17.6).

The best median survival was obtained in brain metastases from carcinoma of the breast (6 months) and lymphoma (4 months). Poor survival was noted in metastases from carcinoma of the lung: a median of 3.5 months. Metastases from other primaries did not represent statistically significant numbers to suggest any definite conclusions (table 17.7).

There are eight patients still alive from one to four years after completion of radiotherapy: two had lymphoma metastases; two had breast primaries; one had metastases from an unknown primary; one each had multiple myeloma, lung cancer, and ovarian cancer.

CONCLUSIONS

Radiation therapists encounter a high proportion of patients with metastatic deposits in the central nervous system for whom treatment is deemed appropriate. The symptoms caused by the cerebral metastases themselves; the general condition of the patient; the number and size of other metastases; the site and histiologic nature of the primary lesion; and previous treatment are all relevant factors in considering the most advisable form of treatment.

Table 17.6

INTRACRANIAL METASTATIC MALIGNANCY
MEDIAN SURVIVAL AFTER COMPLETION OF TREATMENT
ACCORDING TO RESPONSE
(1961–1977)

	Number of Patients (%)	Median Survival (months)
Excellent	114 (38)	6 (1–48)
Good	83 (28)	4.5 (1–24)
Fair	52 (18)	2 (1–11)
Poor	20 (6)	1.5
None	28 (9)	1
Total	297 (100)	5
Expired on Treatment	40	
Stopped Treatment	6	
TOTAL	343	

Table 17.7

INTRACRANIAL METASTATIC MALIGNANCY
MEDIAN SURVIVAL AFTER COMPLETION OF TREATMENT
ACCORDING TO PRIMARY SITE
(1961–1977)

Primary Site	Number of Patients	Median Survival (months)
Lung	210	3.5
Breast	51	6

Our experience suggests that although in unselected patients radiation therapy cannot result in cure, good or excellent palliative results may be obtained in a remarkably high percentage of cases. The ultimate effect with regard to the prolongation of life may be negligible because the average duration of life in untreated patients approximates 3 months versus 5 months in the treated group. Unfortunately neither the degree nor the duration of relief of symptoms is predictable in individuals; even in some apparently hopeless cases, unexpectedly good to excellent results have been obtained and in some instances have lasted as long as 48 months.

In 230 patients (75%) there was no clinical evidence of regrowth of tumor involving the brain. This observation favors the utilization of radiation therapy in patients with metastatic intracranial deposits particularly in those considered not suitable for definitive neurosurgical intervention but whose death from generalized disease is not imminent.

On the basis of these data, palliative radiation therapy for intracranial metastases appears justified. Relief of symptoms and lessening of disability afford major benefit in the terminal care of such patients.

REFERENCES

Allen, M. B., Jr.; Dick, D. A.; and Hightower, S. S. The value and limitations of brain scanning. A review of 401 consecutive cases. *Clin. Radiol.* 18:19–27, 1967.

Aronson, S. M.; Garcia, J. H.; and Aronson, B. E. Metastatic neoplasms of the brain: their frequency in relation to age. *Cancer* 17:558–563, 1964.

Bouchard, J. Radiation therapy of metastatic intracranial tumors. In *Radiation therapy of tumors and diseases of the nervous system*, ed. G. H. Gletcher. Philadelphia: Lea and Febiger, 1966.

Bowen, R., Jr.; Knapp, J. R.; and Collins, V. P. Radiotherapy of cerebral metastases. *Texas State J. Med.* 61:894–898, 1965.

Chao, J.; Phillips, R.; and Nickson, J. J. Roentgen-ray therapy of cerebral metastases. *Cancer* 7:682–689, 1954.

Chu, F. C., and Hilaris, B. B. Value of radiation therapy in the management of intracranial metastases. *Cancer* 14:577–581, 1961.

Diamond, H. D. Hodgkin's disease: neurologic sequelae. *Missouri Med.* 54:945–955, 1957.

Jelliffe, A. M., and Thompson, A. D. The prognosis in Hodgkin's disease. *Br. J. Cancer* 9:21–36, 1955.

Kindt, G. W. The pattern of location of cerebral metastatic tumors. *J. Neurosurg.* 21:54–57, 1964.

King, D. F.; Moon, W. J.; and Brown, N. Corticosteroid drugs in the management of primary and secondary malignant cerebral tumors. *Med. J. Aust.* 2:878–881, 1965.

Lang, E. F., and Slater, J. Metastatic brain tumors. Results of surgical and nonsurgical treatment. *Surg. Clin. North Am.* 44:865–872, 1964.

Murphy, W. *Radiation therapy*. Philadelphia: W. B. Saunders, Co., 1967.

O'Connel, J. E. The place of surgery in intracranial metastatic malignant disease. *Proc. R. Soc. Med.* 57:1159–1164, 1964.

Pool, J. L.; Ransohoff, J.; and Cornell, J. W. The treatment of malignant brain tumors, primary and metastatic. *N. Y. State J. Med.* 57:3983–3988, 1957.

Richards, P., and McKissock, W. Intracranial metastases. *Br. Med. J.* 1:15–18, 1963.

Vieth, R. G., and Odom, G. L. Intracranial metastases and their neurosurgical treatment. *J. Neurosurg.* 323:375–378, 1965.

Windeyer, B. Metastases in the central nervous system: treatment by radiotherapy and chemotherapy. *Proc. R. Soc. Med.* 57:1153–1159, 1964.

18

RTOG Experience and New Concepts

William M. Wara
Frank R. Hendrickson

The appropriate treatment for patients with brain metastases remains controversial because palliation and improvement in quality of life are the therapeutic goals rather than patient survival or ultimate course of disease. Therefore, the treatment regimen should be designed to offer the maximum response with the most economic use of time for the patient.

To investigate this problem and to provide the most efficient solution, the Radiation Therapy Oncology Group (RTOG) conducted two randomized trials between January 1971 and February 1976 to determine the effectiveness of various time-dose fractionation schemes for palliation of patients with brain metastases. Previous reports of these studies have been published (Hendrickson 1977; Kramer, *in press*) with an extensive analysis of results by Borgelt and others (*in press*); this presentation summarizes the data and provides new concepts for future studies.

Factors which must be assessed in evaluating patient response to irradiation are multiple and complex: primary site and primary site control, age, extent of generalized metastases, initial neurologic status, general functional status, improvement of function, duration of improvement, and corticosteroid use.

MATERIALS AND METHODS

The general functional and neurologic status for patients reviewed have been divided into the classes listed in table 18.1. The most frequent symptoms were headache, motor loss and impaired mentation. Other predominant symptoms included lethargy, cranial nerve abnormality, cerebellar dysfunction, sensory loss, and seizures.

In the first study (1971–1973), 993 patients were entered and randomly assigned to one of four treatment regimens: 3,000 rads/2 weeks, 3,000 rads/3 weeks, 4,000 rads/3 weeks, or 4,000 rads/4 weeks. The use of corticosteroids was not a controlled variable but was recorded and evaluated. Patients were stratified according to site of the primary lesion (lung, breast, other) and the presence or absence of metastases to sites other than brain was recorded.

279

Table 18.1

A. GENERAL PERFORMANCE STATUS

Class	Description
1	No symptoms
2	Symptoms but ambulatory
3	In bed up to 50% of the time
4	In bed more than 50% of the time
5	100% bedridden

B. NEUROLOGIC FUNCTION

Class	Description
1	Able to work; neurologic findings minor or absent
2	Able to be at home although nursing care may be required
3	Requires hospitalization and medical care with major neurologic findings
4	Requires hospitalization and in serious physical or neurologic state (includes coma)

Treatment response was evaluated by periodic reassessment of general and neurologic function and by neurologic testing and radionuclide brain scans. Duration of all endpoints was measured from the date of randomization. In the first study 84% of patients completed the planned course of irradiation, while 6% died during treatment.

The second study (1973–1976) was designed to evaluate other time-dose fractionation regimens. The criteria for entry, stratification and randomization were essentially the same as for the first study. The doses employed were 2,000 rads/1 week, 3,000 rads/2 weeks, and 4,000 rads/3 weeks. A total of 1,001 patients were entered: 88% completed their treatment regimen and 5% died during therapy.

In both studies approximately 60% of patients presented with metastases from lung primaries and 15% from breast primaries (table 18.2). The patients of the second study had a slightly worsened overall average neurologic status although no difference in response to chemotherapeutic or steroid management could be discerned (Borgelt et al.). Patients with

Table 18.2

PATIENT PROFILE BEFORE THERAPY

	1971–1973 Primaries			1973–1976 Primaries		
	Lung	Breast	Total	Lung	Breast	Total
Number of Patients	560	166	910	507	146	902
Neurologic Function						
Class			*Percentage of Total*			
1	15	17	14	16	14	16
2	47	48	46	39	36	39
3	34	30	35	39	46	40

Columns don't include class IV therefore doesn't total 100%.

primary breast disease were more frequently controlled, while lung cancer patients developed brain metastases earlier in the course of disease, consistent with previously reported patterns (Montana et al. 1972; Nisce et al. 1971; Order et al. 1968; Posner 1977).

RESULTS

Neurologic Function

The overall incidence of improvement in neurologic function (improvement to a higher performance class) was 47% in the first study and 52% in the second. Patients presenting with a poorer initial neurologic status had a higher response rate (60–70%) than those with a better initial evaluation (35–40%) (table 18.3).

Within the specific categories, no time-dose fractionation relationship was observed in the first study. In the second study patients with an initial neurologic function of 1 had a significantly longer time to progression of disease when treated with 4,000 rads/3 weeks ($p = 0.05$). This trend was reversed for patients with greater neurologic impairment with only 50% of these patients neurologically stable at time of death.

Corticosteroids did not appear to influence status or survival in these patients although this was an uncontrolled variable. Ambulatory patients had a higher response rate as did patients in whom brain was the only metastatic site. Neither status or origin of the primary disease nor chemotherapeutic intervention appeared to influence the response (table 18.3).

Table 18.3

PATIENTS WITH IMPROVEMENT IN NEUROLOGIC FUNCTION
EVALUATED IN RELATIONSHIP TO ORIGINAL STATUS AND HISTOLOGY

	Initial Neurologic Function			
	Class 2		Class 3	
	First Study	Second Study	First Study	Second Study
	Percentage Showing Improvement			
Lung	38	37	62	72
Breast	38	32	66	66
Ambulatory	42	39	76	88
Nonambulatory	22	23	58	67

Neurologic Symptoms

Headache, motor loss, and impaired mentation were improved in 60–82% of all patients evaluated. The treatment regimens did not differ in ability to palliate these symptoms. Patients presenting with motor loss had the lowest complete response rate (table 18.4).

General Status and Survival

Improvement in general status correlated highly with improvement in neurologic status: 80% of those who improved neurologically also showed improvement in general status.

Overall median survival was 18 weeks in the first study and 15 weeks in the second study with no significant difference noted among the various radiation regimens. Ambulatory patients survived longer (21 weeks median) versus nonambulatory patients (12 weeks). Patients with primary breast cancer survived longer (21 weeks median) than those with primary lung cancer (16 weeks) (Borgelt et al. *in press*).

Lung cancer patients whose only metastatic disease involved brain survived longer than those with disseminated disease. Patients who responded neurologically had a longer post-treatment survival (table 18.5). Of all patients evaluated, 75–80% were palliated with improved or stable neurologic state. No difference could be demonstrated between the different time-dose fractionation regimens.

Table 18.4

SPECIFIC SYMPTOM RELIEF

	First Study		Second Study	
	Complete Response	Overall	Complete Response	Overall
		Percentage of Patients		
Headache	52	82	69	82
Motor Loss	32	74	37	61
Impaired Mentation	34	71	52	69
Cerebellar Dysfunction	39	75	50	64
Cranial Nerve Deficit	40	71	44	59

Table 18.5

MEDIAN SURVIVAL

Status	Median Survival	
	Lung Primary	Breast Primary
Initial Neurologic Function 2		
Improved to NF* 1*	27 weeks	29 weeks
No improvement	11 weeks	16 weeks
Initial Neurologic Function 3		
Improved to NF 1	27 weeks	45 weeks
Improved to NF 2	13 weeks	10 weeks
No improvement	3 weeks	4 weeks

*NF = neurologic function.

DISCUSSION

These two studies confirm the efficacy of whole brain irradiation using conventional fractionation schemes which have previously been reported. The initial neurologic and general patient status predict patient response and survival (Chao et al. 1954; Order et al. 1968; Posner 1977).

Approximately 50% of patients in the two studies showed improved neurologic symptoms with patients presenting in initially poorer condition having a higher response rate. As seen in table 18.3, ambulatory patients had a smaller percent of their group improving than did nonambulatory patients. No statistical difference was noted between any of the treatment regimens when patients were properly stratified according to site and other prognostic variables.

Because these studies suggest that patients who present with a primary tumor metastatic only to brain may fare better, a current RTOG protocol (1976–1978) seeks to evaluate higher radiation doses (5,000 rads/4 weeks vs. 3,000 rads/2 weeks) to determine whether protracted treatment benefits this selected subpopulation of patients with brain metastases.

New protocols are being formulated and activated in an effort to lengthen survival based upon combinations of radiation therapy with other treatment modalities. A planned RTOG protocol to evaluate the hypoxic cell radiosensitizer, misonidazole, with 600-rad fractions given twice a week for 3 weeks along with the sensitizer will be opened shortly for patient entry. Pilot studies underway at the University of California at San Francisco (UCSF) in a small group of patients treated with daily fractionated BCNU and irradiation have shown improved results over historic controls. A combination of the two treatment designs might be even more advantageous.

The original RTOG studies have shown that more rapid treatment regimens can be as effective as more conventional fractionation. However, many patients continue to fail with progressive disease within the central nervous system, making imperative the continued evaluation of new treatment regimens to offer greater palliation and longer control of brain metastases.

REFERENCES

Borgelt, B. et al. The palliation of brain metastases: final results of the first two studies by the Radiation Therapy Oncology Group. *Int. J. Radiat. Oncol. Biol. Phys (in press)*

Chao, J. H.; Phillips, R.; and Nickson, J. J. Roentgen-ray therapy of cerebral metastases. *Cancer* 7:682–689, 1954.

Chu, F. C. H., and Hilaris, B. B. Value of radiation therapy in the management of intracranial metastases. *Cancer* 14:577–581, 1961.

Hendrickson, F. R. Radiation therapy of metastatic tumors. *Semin. Oncol.* 2:43–46, 1975.

Hendrickson, F. R. The optimum schedule for palliative radiotherapy for metastatic brain cancer. *Int. J. Radiat. Oncol. Biol. Phys.* 2:165–168, 1977.

Hindo, W. A. et al. Large dose increment irradiation in treatment of cerebral metastases. *Cancer* 26:138–141, 1970.

Horton, J.; Baxter, D. H.; and Olson, K. B. The management of metastases to the brain by irradiation and corticosteroids. *Am. J. Roentgenol.* 111:334–336, 1971.

Kramer, S. Therapeutic trials in the management of metastatic brain tumors by different time/dose fraction schemes of radiation therapy. *J. Natl. Cancer Inst.* (*in press*)

Montana, G. S.; Meacham, W. F.; and Caldwell, W. L. Brain irradiation for metastatic disease of lung origin. *Cancer* 29:1477–1480, 1972.

Nisce, L. Z.; Hilaris, B. B.; and Chu, F. C. H. A review of experience with irradiation of brain metastasis. *Am. J. Roentgenol.* 111:329–333, 1971.

Order, S. E. et al. Improvement in quality of survival following whole-brain irradiation for brain metastases. *Radiology* 91:149–153, 1968.

Posner, J. B. Management of central nervous system metastases. *Semin. Oncol.* 4:81–91, 1977.

19

The Princess Margaret and Ontario Cancer Foundation Experience

Peter J. Fitzpatrick
Colin W. Keen

Brain metastases develop as a lethal complication in 1–5% of all cancers (Brady et al. 1974). Their appearance heralds a poor prognosis associated with profound neurologic, intellectual and physical defects. Patients require extensive support, and with palliative treatment about two-thirds will improve to some degree. The improvement is often brief and negligible, however, with few patients being rehabilitated to a normal existence. In order to determine optimum care and make meaningful conclusions, several groups of patients treated at the Ontario Cancer Institute since 1971 were studied. This chapter includes data from two retrospective and one randomized prospective study. Every attempt was made to study only patients with intracerebral metastases and without skull lesions. Because metastases are frequently multiple, it has been Institute policy for many years to irradiate the whole brain. Different doses and fractions of radiation were used according to the whims of individual physicians: 1,000 rads in a single exposure, 2,000 rads in 5 exposures in 5 days, and 3,000 rads in 10 exposures in 2 weeks were the common regimens.

Formation of Treatment Policy

A cancer is considered potentially curable when an appreciable percentage of all patients survive over 5 years. Within such cancers, early detection yields the highest cure rates, and treatment is designed to eradicate all disease in the treated area permanently. Few cancers that have metastasized to distant organs are curable by any means and treatment is considered palliative. Here the patient's general condition, age and fate if untreated are paramount in forming a treatment plan. The primary tumor, its natural history, the site and size of metastases, and their multiplicity, resectability and radiosensitivity are reviewed.

Palliation never justifies the reactions of radical treatment, and the cost from the patients' standpoint must be considered. The guidelines for successful palliation, set down by the late Miss Margaret Todd over 40 years ago, are difficult to improve.

(1) Prolongation of life only in a symptom-free condition. The ultimate period of distressing symptoms must not be lengthened.

(2) The relief or prevention of symptoms such as pain, discharge, hemorrhage or starvation pending dissemination of the disease with its sequel, and easier death.

(3) Temporary arrest of growth which, without prolonging life, replaces gradually increasing distress with a short period of relief followed by a much more rapid decline.

(4) The psychologic effects of a simple treatment which relieves symptoms and postpones the patient's realization of the inevitable.

Palliative Radiotherapy

Radiotherapy has great value in completing the aims of successful palliation. The radiation dose, field size and fractionation vary with the size, site, and radiosensitivity of the metastasis. These factors are modified by the patient's general condition.

Soon after the discovery of x-rays and radium, it became apparent that repeated use of these agents over a number of days produced better results than a single exposure alone. By trial and error the therapeutic ratio between a lethal tumor dose and normal tissue tolerance was established for different tumors at different sites. Although advances in radiobiology have revealed some of the actions of ionizing radiation at the cellular and subcellular levels, most courses of radiotherapy rest on an empirical basis.

Many tumors extensively infiltrate surrounding tissues and others metastasize to the regional nodes, and irradiated areas have to be large to encompass the cancer. This big volume limits the radiotolerance of normal tissues and prevents some tumors from being radiocurable. The therapeutic index can be increased by reducing the dose of radiation, however, and repeating it over several days or weeks. For palliation a single or a short sharp course of irradiation is needed to produce immediate symptomatic relief especially when the patient has only a short time to live. This approach can be repeated if necessary with minimum inconvenience to the patient and a considerable saving in support resources.

Metastases, frequently multiple and widespread, require repeated courses of treatment for different problems. To deal with this situation total-body irradiation and half-body radiotherapy were developed (Fitzpatrick and Rider 1976). With these techniques many metastases can be palliated at one time. With half-body irradiation it is possible to deliver up to 1,000 rads in a single exposure to one half of the body. Radiobiologic evidence suggests that a single dose of 800 rads has a cell lethality of 99.5%

or better, and theoretically with a tumor having a doubling time of 3 months a remission of approximately 30 months may be anticipated.

Clinical experience has shown that 1,000 rads produces better and longer palliation than 300 rads. This dose of irradiation is roughly equivalent to 2,000 rads given in 5 fractions in 5 days or 3,000 rads given in 10 fractions in 2 weeks. The reason is that cells given a sublethal dose of radiation have the power of recovery and so the total dose with fractionated radiation must be higher to achieve the same cell kill. Faster tumor regression follows a big dose, but the associated side effects often limit this approach.

In order to compare the killing of cells with different doses, fractionation and time of radiation, Ellis (1971) developed the nominal single dose (NSD) concept. Other factors including the radiobiologic effectiveness (RBE) and quality of radiation are involved, and so the NSD formula and equivalent dose in rets is a useful working arrangement (fig. 19.1).

Symptomatic brain metastases can be palliated by radiotherapy. Because of the poor prognosis and variables associated with patient and tumor, some of the Ontario Cancer Institute experience may help to define optimal care.

CLINICAL EXPERIENCE

Since 1974 three studies on brain metastases, two retrospective and one prospective, have been completed. Some patients in the two retrospective studies were reviewed twice. Metastases from 24 primary tumors

Figure 19.1.

NOMINAL SINGLE DOSE (Ellis)

$$NSD = \frac{D}{T^{0.11} \times N^{0.24}}$$

Rad.	#	Ret
1000	1	1000
2000	5	1097
3000	10	1291
4000	20	1350

The nominal single dose concept is a way of comparing the biologic effectiveness of different schemes of radiation (Ellis 1971).

were identified, the commonest arising from the breast or lung. We decided to analyze data on the breast and lung metastases separately with the other tumors being grouped together because of small numbers at any one site.

All patients were irradiated with a simple parallel pair technique on a cobalt 60 unit in the supine position (fig. 19.2). The whole brain was treated to a midplane dose of 1,000 rads in a single exposure, 2,000 rads in 5 exposures in 5 days, or 3,000 rads in 10 treatments in 2 weeks (fig. 19.3).

Figure 19.2.

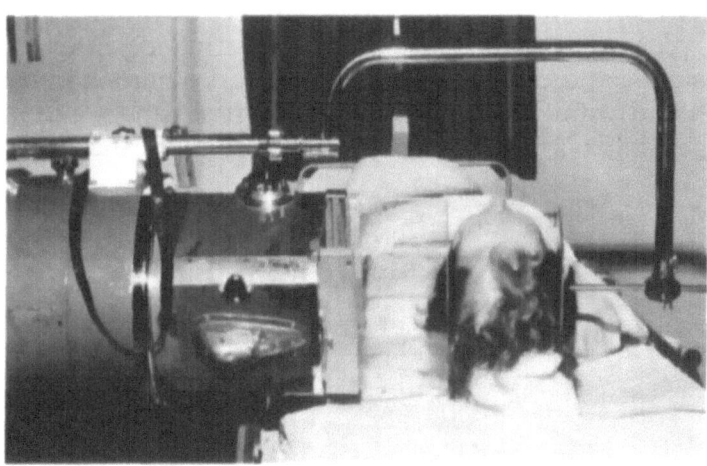

This patient's whole brain is being irradiated.

Figure 19.3.

Irradiation brain metastases
Usually multiple - Tx whole brain
^{60}Co / 20 x 15 cm
MPD 1000/1 2000/5 3000/10

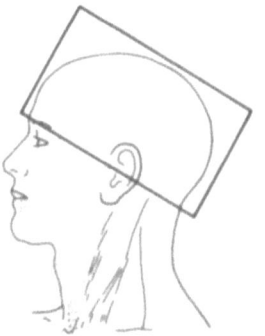 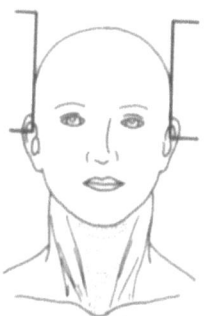

Radiation technique and dose schedules used in these studies.

There was no firm policy on the administration of steroids; patients treated with them prior or concomitant with radiotherapy were those with the greatest defects, probably an index of raised intracranial pressure.

Multivariate analyses were performed in attempt to define benefits in the many different clinical situations and establish treatment policies.

In each case the age, general condition, initial treatment, and subsequent treatment were reviewed with special attention to the extent of metastatic disease and the probable prognosis. Brain metastases were recorded by site and number (single or multiple). In addition to the clinical examination with detailed neurologic and intellectual assessment, x-rays, radionuclide scans, and when available, information obtained at craniotomy were used in the assessments. Retrospectively numbers were assigned and recorded to the patient's overall performance, intellectual and neurologic status, and extent of nursing care and other support needed before and after treatment (fig. 19.4). The length of benefit and survival, both measured in days, and control or progression of cancer were listed elsewhere.

Figure 19.4.

TREATMENT BENEFIT ASSESSMENT

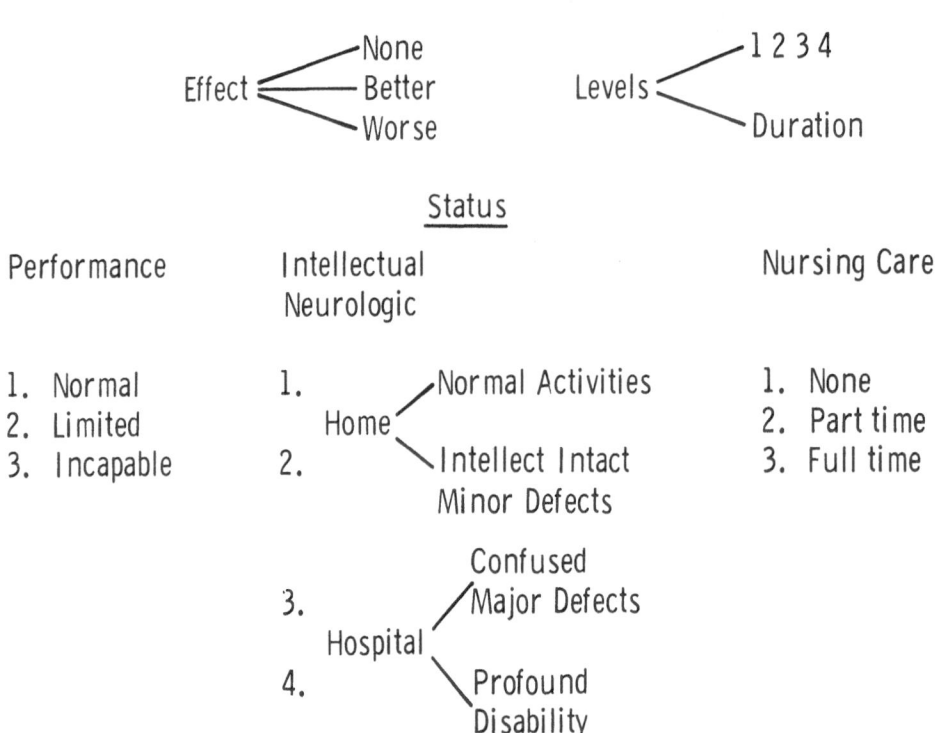

Parameters and scales used to assess the benefits of treatment.

FIRST RETROSPECTIVE STUDY

The 354 consecutive patients with brain metastasis treated between 1971 and 1974 were reviewed. In addition to brain metastases some of these patients had skull metastases which were responsible for their problems. Lung and breast were the common primary tumors with melanoma a distant third (fig. 19.5).

Although in most cases steroids, usually dexamethasone (4 mg tid), was used only in patients with greatly increased intracranial pressure and severe neurologic deficits, we attempted to assess their value. No advantage was found in breast or lung patients with any dose regimen although we had thought that steroids helped in large single-dose treatments (figs. 19.6 and 19.7).

Figure 19.5.

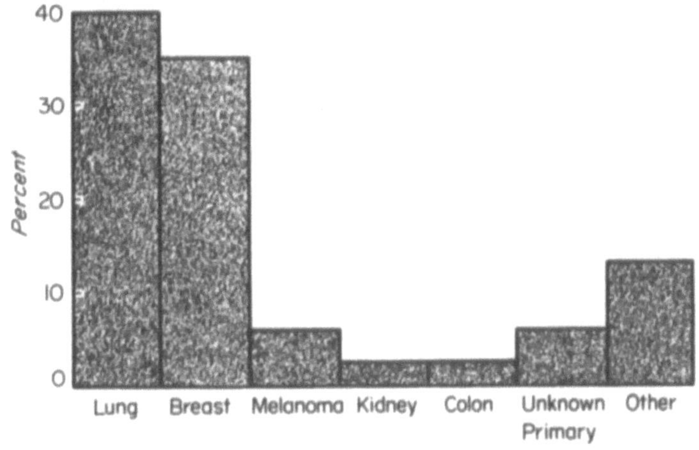

Distribution of primary cancers among 354 patients with brain metastases.

Figure 19.6.

AVERAGE SURVIVAL IN WEEKS

Fractions	With Steroids	Without Steroids	Total
1	11.5	27.8	20.8
5	22.1	24.3	23.5
10	19.8	33.0	28.4
	19.0	29.0	25.4

Cerebral metastases from breast cancer. Dexamethasone (Decadron) (12–16 mg/day) did not influence the survival time.

Figure 19.7.

AVERAGE SURVIVAL IN WEEKS

	With Steroids	Without Steroids	Total
1 Fraction	12	12.5	12.4
5 Fractions	20	12.2	15.2
10 Fractions	20	17.7	19.0
	18.2	13.8	15.6

Cerebral metastases from lung cancer. Dexamethasone (Decadron) (12–16 mg/day) did not influence the survival time.

The median survivals for lung and breast patients were 12 and 22 weeks, respectively, although a few patients lived over 2 years (figs. 19.8 and 19.9). Alternatively, 75% of breast and lung patients had died by 31 and 22 weeks after treatment. Retreatment is disappointing, but a comparable response was found in the 50% of patients who lived longer than 6 months.

Figure 19.8.

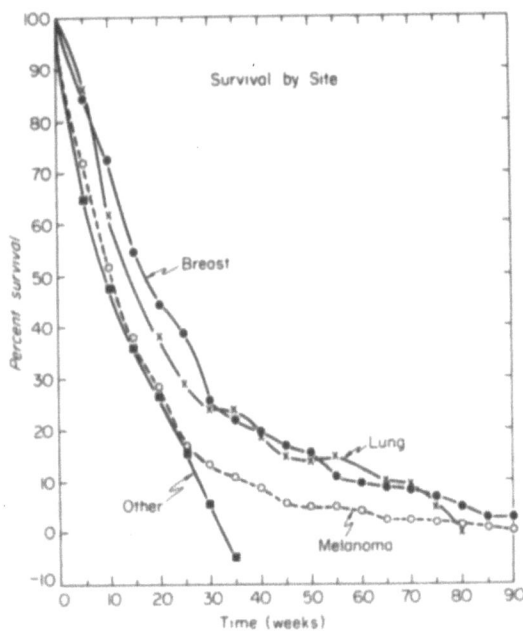

Actuarial survival of 354 patients with brain metastases regardless of treatment modality.

Figure 19.9.

CEREBRAL METASTASES : SURVIVAL BY SITE

	Average	Range in Weeks
Lung	15.6	0 - 84
Breast	25.3	0 - 129
Melanoma	22.7	0 - 97
Kidney	14.7	0 - 23
Unknown	12.6	0 - 32
Other	18.3	0 - 78

Survival times for 354 patients with brain metastases treated by irradiation.

SECOND RETROSPECTIVE STUDY

These 282 patients, all with brain metastases and treated since 1971, were randomly selected from the computer files. Some patients were included in the previous study. The 24 primary tumors which were identified were stratified into lung, breast and other groups (fig. 19.10).

Figure 19.10.

BRAIN METASTASES 282 PATIENTS

		Rad
	38	1000
Breast 146	60	2000
	48	3000
	33	1000
Lung 93	32	2000
	28	3000
	10	1000
Other (22 Diff. tumours) 43	16	2000
	17	3000

The spectrum of primary tumors and treatment of patients in the second retrospective study.

Lung Cancer

The treatment and results in 93 patients are summarized in figures 19.11 and 19.12. Random samples of 10 patients in each of the 3 treatment groups and those who survived longer than 6 months were analyzed in detail. The median age was 59 years and survival after treatment about 3 months. All dose regimens produced similar results. Two-thirds of patients achieved improvement in neurologic and intellectual deficits for a short period, but the overall performance status and nursing requirements did not change. The benefits achieved lasted for only one-third of their remaining life, even for those patients who lived longer than 6 months. All patients had multiple intracerebral metastases with rampant cancer elsewhere that required additional palliation.

Breast Cancer

This group of 146 patients fared a little better than the lung patients (fig. 19.13). The slightly longer overall survival of 5.5 months reflects the difference in the natural history of the tumor rather than a measure of therapeutic response. Detailed analysis of the overall lung results proved of little value, and so only a random sample of ten patients with breast cancer surviving longer than 6 months was undertaken (fig. 19.14). Two-thirds of the patients had a significant improvement in their neurologic status, but their overall performance status did not improve to the same extent. This was due to the progression of extracerebral disease in the period after brain irradiation. Most patients had multiple brain metastases, and we could not identify the factors affecting the extent or duration of response. In general, a patient in good overall condition with minimal disease in the brain and elsewhere achieved the best palliation. A profound neurologic deficit was a poor prognostic sign and no such patient survived 2 years.

Other Primary Cancers

The results from 22 different primary tumors arising from the gingiva, tongue, esophagus, stomach, cecum, colon, rectum, pancreas, kidney, bladder, penis, thyroid, skin (including melanoma), cervix, uterus, ovary, prostate, testicle, bone, muscle or lymph nodes were grouped together (figs. 19.15 and 19.16). Overall, the measurable benefits were nil although useful palliation was recorded for a short while in some patients.

RANDOMIZED PROSPECTIVE CLINICAL TRIAL

In 1977 Harwood and Simpson published this study which compared results with doses of 3,000 rads in 2 weeks with a single dose of 1,000 rads. These patients with minimal disease had not received brain irradiation or

Figure 19.11.

Rad.	Pts.	Med. Surv. Days
1000	33	82
2000	32	125
3000	28	100

LUNG   93 PTS.

Pts.	Rad.	Performance		Intellect Neurologic		Nursing Care		Benefit Days
		B	A	B	A	B	A	
10	1000	2	2	3	1	3	3	14
10	2000	3	3	3	2	3	3	30
10	3000	2	2	2	2	2	2	60
Alive > 6 Mths 2 3 3	1000 2000 3000	3	3	3	2	3	3	75
Benefit		0		+		0		+

Patients with primary lung cancer and cerebral metastases. Both survival and symptomatic relief with any treatment was poor. (A = after treatment; B = before treatment.)

Figure 19.12.

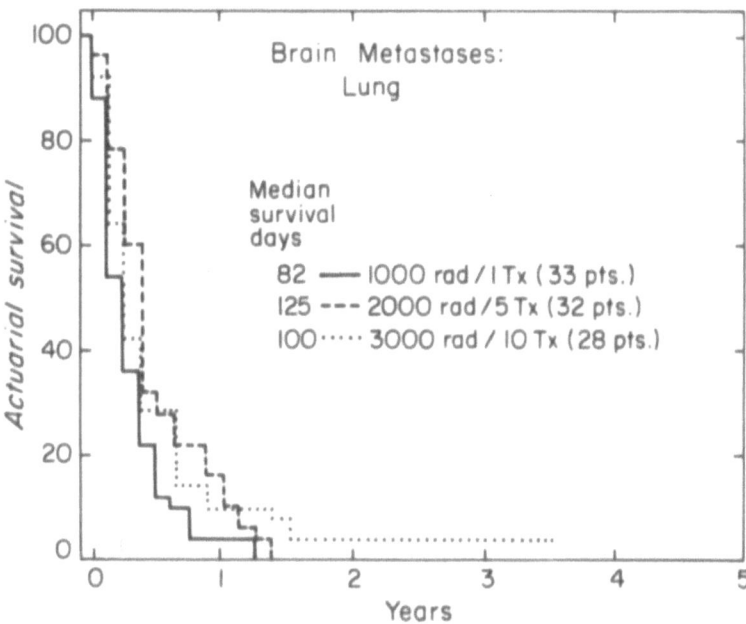

Kaplan-Meier actuarial survival curve for lung cancer patients with cerebral metastases. This method is useful when patient numbers are small. The poor results are obvious.

Figure 19.13.

Rad.	Pts.	Med. Surv. Days
1000	38	175
2000	66	101
3000	48	184

BREAST   146 PTS.

	Pts.	Rad.	Performance		Intellect Neurologic		Nursing Care		Benefit Survival Days	
			B	A	B	A	B	A		
Alive	4	1000	3	2	3	1	2	1	480	570
> 6 Mths	3	2000	2	1	3	1	2	1	840	840
	3	3000	2	2	2	2	2	2	660	750
Benefit			+		+		+		++	

Patients with primary breast cancer and cerebral metastases. There was no significant advantage in any treatment schedule. Responses were better in patients who survived 6 months or longer.

Figure 19.14.

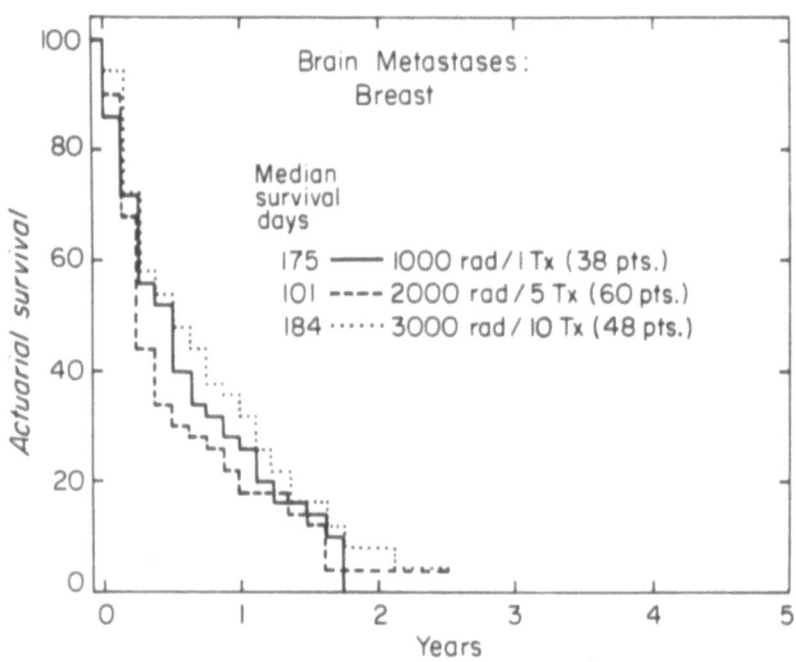

Kaplan-Meier actuarial survival curve demonstrates the rapid attrition of patients with breast cancer and cerebral metastases.

Figure 19.15.

Rad.	Pts.	Med. Surv. Days
1000	10	52
2000	16	91
3000	17	136

OTHER   43 PTS.
(22 Diff. Tumours)

Pts.	Rad.	Performance		Intellect Neurologic		Nursing Care		Benefit Days
		B	A	B	A	B	A	
5	1000	2	2	3	3	3	3	14
5	2000	2	2	1	1	2	2	30
5	3000	2	2	2	2	3	2	70

Alive > 6 Mths	Not Assessed			
Benefit	0	0	0	0

Irradiation produced no measurable benefit in 15 random patients with primary tumors other than breast or lung.

Figure 19.16.

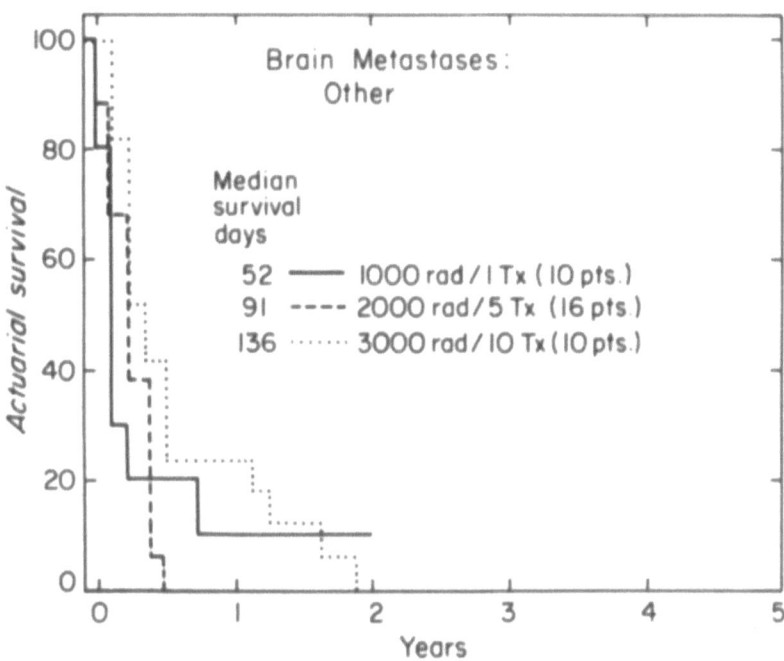

Kaplan-Meier actuarial survival curve for 22 other tumors confirms the poor prognosis.

chemotherapy during the preceding 3 weeks. Patients were stratified similarly to those in the other studies with steroids used only to relieve increased intracranial pressure.

The median survival in days was 132 and 121 for those treated with
1,000 and 3,000 rads (p = 0.082) (fig. 19.17). Among the patients treated
with a single 1,000 rads, 47% developed acute complications including
increased headache, nausea and vomiting, an increased neurologic deficit
or fall in the level of consciousness. 27% of patients treated with fractionated irradiation developed these symptoms. This difference, not statistically significant, did not influence survival (p = 0.254).

No deaths were attributed to the treatment although 2 patients died
before completing irradiation. Seventy percent of patients died from brain
metastases, including 75% of lung patients, 40% of the breast patients,
and 90% among the other group. The median survival among their level 1
and level 2 (neurologic and intellectual status) patients, respectively, was
170 and 183 for doses of 1,000 rads and 80 and 103 days for doses of 3,000
rads.

A second course of cerebral irradiation was generally less effective
with only 4 of 11 patients obtaining a similar response to the initial treat-

Figure 19.17.

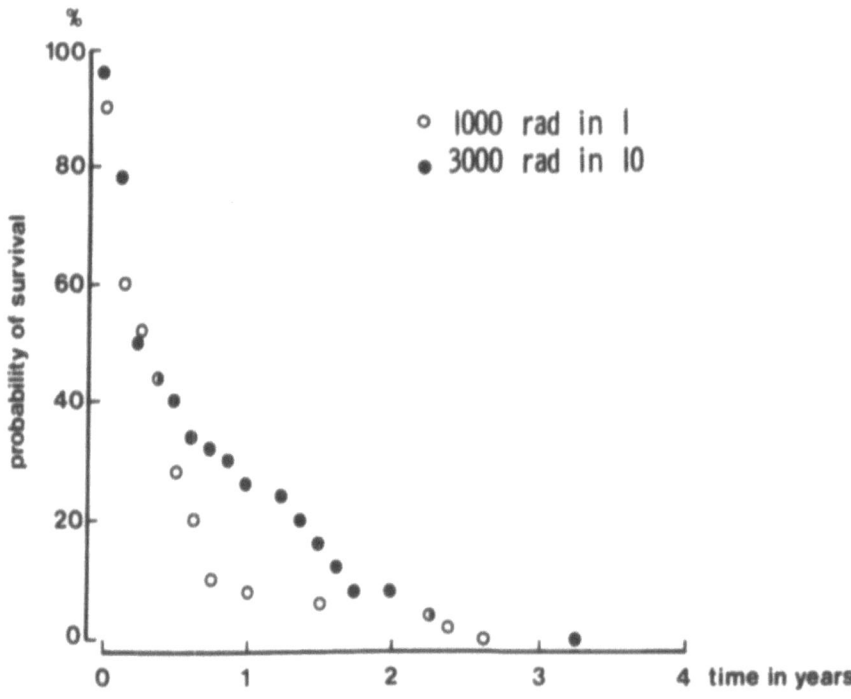

*In this randomized prospective study there was no significant difference in
survival. (Harwood and Simpson 1977.)*

Table 19.1

THE DEGREE OF IMPROVEMENT AFTER IRRADIATION

Dose (rads)	Number of Fractions	Marked Improvement (No.)	(%)	Slight Improvement (No.)	(%)	Total (No.)	(%)
1000	1	(19/51)	37	(10/51)	20	(29/51)	57
3000	10	(14/50)	28	(18/50)	36	(32/50)	64
		$p = 0.441$		$p = 0.101$		$p = 0.603$	

ment. Improvement followed in just over half of the patients, but there was no significant difference between the 1,000 and 3,000 rad groups (table 19.1).

DISCUSSION AND CONCLUSIONS

After brain metastases develop, death is inevitable. Our three studies confirm the appalling prognosis for patients with brain metastases which has not improved in 20 years. They also support the concept of concentrated irradiation in palliation (Hindo et al. 1970; Shehata et al. 1974; Dutreix et al. 1971; Abbo 1976). Prospective RTOG studies failed to show any difference in results with dose schedules varying from 3,000 rads in 2 weeks to 4,000 rads in 1 month (Hendrickson 1977). Their response rates and survival times were similar to ours. Although we could not quantitate it, we have the strong impression that symptoms are abated more rapidly with a single or 5-day fractioned course of irradiation. Higher doses with longer protraction are unwarranted because of the poor survival of these patients.

One-half to two-thirds of the patients died as a complication of their brain metastases, but nearly all of them had progressive cancer elsewhere requiring additional palliative treatment. The natural history and aggression of the primary cancer dictates prognosis and each patient's care should be individualized. Survival can be predicted from these covariants and the patient's neurologic deficit at the time of treatment.

Intracerebral metastases were nearly always multiple and frequently associated with skull lesions. Those patients with a solitary lesion who underwent craniotomy, had tumor excised, and were then irradiated achieved the best palliation; however, few patients were suitable for this approach. We did not assess the influence of the site of metastases on prognosis.

In measuring (putting numbers) to different responses and support requirements, vagueness in the medical notes together with marginal improvements made them difficult to evaluate. The prognosis was clearly related to the primary tumor, the extent of metastatic disease, and the patient's functional level at the time of treatment. Among the lung patients, although many responses were recorded, we could only quantitate benefit in the neurologic and intellectual states and that only lasted for one-third of the patient's remaining life. There was no advantage to any one radiation technique, and most patients spent their last days in the hospital. Similar unsatisfactory results were obtained in the other patient group. Some breast patients fared better than others, living in reasonable health for 2–3 years. Among these, 60 patients (41%) survived longer than 6 months, and as a group they did better in every respect than those patients with lung or other tumors. This again reflects the natural history of the primary cancer.

Although a short, sharp course of irradiation brings more rapid improvement and puts less strain on the radiotherapy staff and facilities, it did not reduce stay in the hospital or the level of nursing care required. We attempted a cost-effectiveness analysis in this respect, but the dollar savings with 1 or 5 treatments compared to 10 treatments or more were small. These patients present a heavy nursing burden, and most remained in expensive acute hospital beds because of the shortage of chronic care facilities. The major costs in dollars relate to hospitalization and the support services.

Cost-effectiveness is difficult to evaluate because although most costs in dollars are identifiable there is no unit to measure benefit (Fitzpatrick 1974). Benefits are both quantitative and qualitative: they are physical, psychological, temporal (an extra month of life), and financial. Specifically they include cure, increased survival time, reduced disability, relief of symptoms, and ability to live a normal life. In our retrospective assessments we only used three of four categories with a treatment response moving a patient into a higher group. The results for palliation were both disappointing and short lived.

Optimum care may be defined as treatment which provides the maximum benefit to the patient at the minimum cost. In a group whose life expectancy is measured in weeks, protracted treatment schedules have no place. Immediate benefits are very similar whether 1, 5, or 10 fractions are used. There is some suggestion that with 5 or 10 fractions there is a lower relapse rate, but it was impossible to measure. We suggest that when patients have a poor prognosis, either in terms of histology or extent of disease, then 1 fraction of 1,000 rads is probably optimum treatment. Conversely, in patients whose disease is running a more chronic course, 2,000 rads in 5 fractions appears to be optimum. With few exceptions a repeat course of irradiation is a waste of time. The best care for any one patient rests, as always, on making an individual decision and taking all medical and humanitarian factors into account. This is normal, good clinical practice and particularly relevant in palliative treatment. Doctors and nurses must remain willing to maintain supportive care when the glamorous but misleading concept of cure has departed and to help a patient toward a dignified death (Hawkins 1974).

Because of the difficulties in defining cost-effectiveness in treatment, especially in advanced cancer, we suggest the concept summarized in the term *net human benefit* (NHB) (G. M. Morrison, personal communication). Our computer spewed out a welter of statistics, which we tried to digest, but the poor results are not the end of these studies. The human factors and individual personal benefit make it impossible to put a price tag on the preterminal care of patients. What are the effects of a fatal disease with distressing symptoms and debilitating treatment on the mind? What are the social consequences of this hapless situation? Voltaire wrote, "Doctors pour drugs of which they know little, for diseases of which they know less, into human beings of whom they know nothing." This is not altogether the case today, but we still find it hard to measure and record treatment benefits.

SUMMARY

Since 1974 two retrospective and one randomized prospective study on brain metastases have been completed. Over 500 patients with 24 different primary tumours, the most common being lung and breast, were subject to multivariate analysis. Treatment consisted of total brain irradiation with 1,000, 2,000 or 3,000 rads in one, five or ten exposures. Steroids were only used to combat raised intracranial pressure. The prognosis was poor and similar for all treatment groups. The median actuarial survival for lung, breast and other patients was 100, 170 and 100 days although a few patients lived over one year. The performance, neurologic and intellectual status, and the nursing care required before and after treatment was measured. With few exceptions the only real benefit was in improved neurologic and intellectual levels which lasted for one-half of the patient's remaining life. Optimum treatment for patients with a poor prognosis is 1,000 rads in a single exposure and for the others 2,000 rads in five daily fractions.

REFERENCES

Abbo, A. W. Brain metastases and possibilities of their treatment, with special reference to single-session whole-brain irradiation. *Radiol. Clin.* 45:443–452, 1976.

Brady, L. W. et al. Radiation therapy for intracranial metastatic neoplasia. *Radiol. Clin. Biol.* 43:40–47, 1974.

Dutreix, J. et al. Concentrated irradiation. *Ann. Clin. Res.* 3:9–15, 1971.

Ellis, F. Nominal standard dose and the Ret. *Br. J. Radiol.* 44:101–108, 1971.

Fitzpatrick, P. J. Cost-effectiveness in cancer. *Can. Med. J.* 3:652, 1974.

Fitzpatrick, P. J., and Rider, W. D. Half-body radiotherapy. *Int. J. Radiat. Oncol. Biol. Phys.* 1:197, 1976.

Harwood, A. R., and Simpson, W. J. Radiation therapy of cerebral metastases. A randomized prospective clinical trial. *Int. J. Radiat. Oncol. Biol. Phys.* 2:1091–1094, 1977.

Hawkins, N. V. Conclusion for workshop on palliation. Centennial Conference on Laryngeal Cancer, Toronto, 1974.

Hendrickson, F. R. The optimum schedule for palliative radiotherapy of metastatic brain cancer. *Int. J. Radiat. Oncol. Biol. Phys.* 2:165–168, 1977.

Hindo, W. A. et al. Large dose increment irradiation in treatment of cerebral metastases. *Cancer* 26:138–141, 1970.

Shehata, W. M.; Hendrickson, F. R.; and Hindo, W. A. Rapid fractionation technique and retreatment of cerebral metastases by irradiation. *Cancer* 34:257–261, 1974.

20

The Southern California Permanente Medical Group Experience: Functional Results

Harvey Gilbert
A. Robert Kagan
John Wagner
Kaspar Fuchs
Herman Nussbaum
Aroor R. Rao

Brain metastasis usually signals the beginning of a downhill course. Return to unimpeded normal functioning is not common and, if present, is usually of short duration. The median survival after treatment is 3–6 months. Many authors dealing with this subject have used median survival or initial improvement as a measure of the success of their therapeutic intervention. Frequently these parameters do not indicate the usefulness of the treatment advocated. Is improvement of a few days duration worthwhile? Is patient survival for 6 months (4 months of which are in bed and helpless) useful? Is there any measure of quality of survival in a functional sense that can be universally acceptable? Are there any prognostic factors such as the primary site, presenting functional status, disease-free interval, type of presenting symptoms, site of cerebral metastasis, or presence of other non-neurologic metastatic disease that might give us a clue as to the success with radiation therapy?

The following chapter attempts to answer some of these questions.

METHODS

Ninety patients treated by radiation therapy in our Southern California Permanente Medical Group Regional Radiation Therapy Department were reviewed with special attention to treatment regimen, functional status (before therapy and monthly thereafter until death), primary tumor site, disease-free interval, and the presence of extraneurologic visceral or bony disease. Many patients with brain metastasis at our institution are

303

either not referred or denied treatment because of advanced disease. This is demonstrated by the fact that only 29 of 90 patients had evidence of extraneurologic disease at the time whole-brain irradiation was started.

Radiation Therapy

All patients were treated with supervoltage radiation therapy to the whole brain. Three dose-time regimens were used: (1) 3,000–4,000 rads over 3–4 weeks; (2) 2,000 rads in 5 fractions over 1 week; (3) 2 doses of 650 rads each in 48 hours with a repeat in 3 weeks. The reason for using these three regimens was to find the dose-time relationship which would produce optimum benefit with least disruption of life patterns to the patient. Most patients received dexamethasone or prednisone as needed. The patients were followed mainly by history and physical examination.

Success in Therapy

A good response to therapy was defined as maintenance of a functional level III or greater for at least 2 consecutive months after initiating therapy (table 20.1). The reason for selecting functional level III was that a patient at that level or above would have some measure of self-sufficiency. In some instances the onset of improvement did not occur immediately.

Survival

Survival was measured in two ways. The first measurement was from the time of first metastasis until death (no matter where the metastasis was). The second measure of survival was from the beginning of radiation therapy for brain metastasis until death.

Free Interval

This is the time from first diagnosis of the primary disease until the first metastasis.

RESULTS

Patients were evaluated in three separate groups based on the primary tumor site (tables 20.2, 20.3, and 20.4). There were 55 patients with lung cancer, 21 patients with breast cancer, and 14 patients with miscellaneous primary tumors treated for metastatic brain disease. The miscellaneous group comprised patients with the following histologic types:

Table 20.1

FUNCTION SCALE

Level*	Definition	Help Needed	
		Financial	Physical
I	Patient is fully functional and is able to make a living in former position or another easily acquired	No	No
II	Patient is functional but not able to work	Yes	No
III	Patient takes care of personal needs and is functionally ambulatory but requires outside help at least 50% of the time. Stays in bed much of day but can get up for personal hygienic functions	Yes	Part-time
IV	Patient requires full-time help whether bedridden or not.	Yes	Full-time

*Level I, II, and III = high group
 Level IV = low group

colon (2), melanoma (2), unknown primary (6), renal (1), adrenal (1) and prostate (2).

Lung Cancer

There were 25 patients who presented as functional III or greater (high group). Of these 22 or 88% achieved a good response (table 20.2). Among the 30 patients who presented in functional class IV (low group), only 17% achieved a good response. The median free interval was the same in both groups.

Two measures of survival were obtained. First, the length of time from onset of any metastasis (brain or other) until death was determined and the median calculated for each group. Also a median survival was calculated from the onset of brain metastasis until death. The median survival from first metastasis was 7 months in the high group and 4 months in the low group. The survival from brain metastasis was 6 months in the high group and 3 months in the low group. More than 88% of all patients in both groups died due to neurologic disease. The presence of visceral

Table 20.2

SURVIVAL AND SUCCESS OF RADIATION: LUNG PRIMARY

Functional Status	Number of Patients	Percentage of Total	Median* Free Interval	
			% <6 mos.	% >6 mos.
High Group	25	45	17	8
Low Group	30	55	23	7

*Free interval = time from diagnosis of the primary to first metastasis.
†Survival from first metastasis = time to death from first metastasis.

disease did not seem to vary between the high and low groups but was significantly longer than for the lung cancer patients.

Breast Cancer

Among the breast cancer patients, 10 presented as functional III or greater (high group = level I, II, or III). Of these, 8 or 80% achieved a good response (table 20.3). There were 11 patients who presented in functional class IV (low group); of these, 2 or 18% achieved a good response. The median free interval was approximately the same in both groups. The me-

Table 20.3

SURVIVAL AND SUCCESS OF RADIATION: BREAST PRIMARY

Functional Status	Number of Patients	Percentage of Total	Median* Free Interval	
			% <6 mos.	% >6 mos.
High Group	10	48	2	8
Low Group	11	52	—	11

*Free interval = time from diagnosis of the primary to first metastasis.
†Survival from first metastasis = time to death from first metastasis.

Quality of Response Good Response		Survival From First Metastasis	Survival From Brain Metastasis to Death	Deaths From Brain Metastasis
Number	Percentage	Mediant (Range)	Median (Range)	
22	88	7 mos. (1–16 mos.)	6 mos. (1–16 mos.)	22 (88%)
5	17	4 mos. (1–14 mos.)	3 mos. (1–14 mos.)	29 (97%)

dian survival from first metastasis was 15 months in the high group and 9 months in the low group. The survival from brain metastasis was 7 months in the high group and 3 months in the low group. More than 70% of all patients in both groups died due to recurrent brain metastasis.

Miscellaneous Tumors

Miscellaneous primary tumors were present in 14 patients (table 20.4). Of these, 5 patients presented a high status and 3 (60%) had a good response. Among the 9 patients who presented with low status 4 patients

Quality of Response Good Response		Survival From First Metastasis	Survival From Brain Metastasis to Death	Deaths From Brain Metastasis
Number	Percentage	Mediant (Range)	Median (Range)	
8	80	15 mos. (3–44 mos.)	7 mos. (3–36 mos.)	8 (80%)
2	18	9 mos. (1–30 mos.)		8 (73%)

Table 20.4

SURVIVAL AND SUCCESS OF RADIATION: MISCELLANEOUS PRIMARIES

Functional Status	Number of Patients	Percentage of Total	Median* Free Interval	
			% <6 mos.	% >6 mos.
High Group	5	36	3	2
Low Group	9	65	3	6

*Free interval = time from diagnosis of the primary to first metastasis.
†Survival from first metastasis = time to death from first metastasis.

Table 20.5

PATIENT PRESENTING WITH EXTRANEUROLOGIC DISEASE

Status	Number of Patients	Site	Survival From First Metastasis to Death
High Scale	9	2 Larynx 5 Breast 2 Prostate	19 mos. (4–44 mos.)
Low Scale	15*	4 Lung 7 Breast 2 Gastrointestinal 2 Other	11 mos. (4–30 mos.)
TOTALS	24		13 mos. (4–44 mos.)

*One patient lost to follow up.

(44%) attained a good response. The median free interval was slightly longer in the high group. More than 60% of patients ultimately died of neurologic disease induced by tumor. Median survivals from first metastasis and first brain metastasis were 6 months and 4 months respectively in the high presenting group and 6 months and 5 months respectively in the low group.

Quality of Response Good Response		Survival From First Metastasis Mediant (Range)	Survival From Brain Metastasis to Death Median (Range)	Deaths From Brain Metastasis
Number	Percentage			
3	60	6 mos. (3–19 mos.)	4 mos. (1–12 mos.)	3 (60%)
4	44	6 mos. (3–20 mos.)	5 mos. (3–16 mos.)	9 (100%)

	Survival From First CNS to Death	Death From CNS Metastasis	Good Response to Therapy
	6 mos. (1–36 mos.)	4 (44%)	7 (78%)
	5 mos. (2–16 mos.)	11* (78%)	5 (33%)
	5 mos. (1–36 mos.)	15 (65%)	12 (50%)

Extraneurologic Metastases

Extraneurologic metastases were present at diagnosis of brain metastasis in 24 patients (table 20.5). Of these, 9 patients presented in a high category (2 lung, 5 breast, and 2 prostate), and 7 patients (78%) in the high group achieved a good response. There were 15 patients (4 lung, 7 breast, 2 colon, and 2 other) who presented in a low status and only 5 (33%) of these had a good response. Median survival from first metastasis and first neurologic metastasis were 19 months and 6 months respectively in the high-status patients and 11 months and 5 months respectively in the low-status patients. Only 44% of the patients with extraneurologic metastases in the high functional group died due to neurologic disease compared to 78% of those in the low functional category.

Long term Survivors

Of 25 lung cancer patients with a high (level I, II, or III) functional status, there were 5 patients who lived 12–16 months from their first brain metastasis, but of 30 lung cancer patients with a low status, only one lived for more than 12 months (14 months) (table 20.6). Of 10 patients with breast cancer and a high status, 4 patients lived 12–36 months. Of the 11 patients with breast cancer presenting with a low status, only 2 patients lived 12 months. Of the 5 high patients in the miscellaneous group, one patient lived 12–16 months.

Dose of Radiation Therapy

No particular benefit was seen with one dose-time relationship over another. The major predictor of good response was the presenting functional status and not dose or time of radiation. Two 650-rad sessions produced some acute febrile reactions and headache. We now use 2,000 rads in one week, leaving the patient on dexamethasone during the treatments.

DISCUSSION

A comprehensive review of the literature reveals a median survival of 3–6 months after radiation therapy for intracerebral metastasis with or without steroids. Only 10% of these treated patients are alive at the end of one year. Our median survival was similar, but our survival time was related more to presenting functional status rather than the primary site or recurrence-free interval to first metastasis. Long-term survival (12 months or greater) was also related to the initial functional status.

Useful Responses to Treatment

Several articles have reported a 60–80% worthwhile response but the length of response was not noted (Order et al. 1968; Hendrickson 1977; Harwood and Simpson 1977). Others have reported 80% of patients who presented with a high status had a reasonable chance (> 80%) of a useful

Table 20.6

LONG-TERM SURVIVORS—TIME FROM FIRST BRAIN METASTASIS

Site of Primary Tumor	Functional Karnofsky Status	Number of Patients	Number of Survivors 12 mos. or more	Percentage of Total
Lung	High	25	3–12 mos. 2–15 mos.	20
	Low	30	1–14 mos.	<3
Breast	High	10	1–12 mos. 1–15 mos. 1–20 mos. 1–36 mos.	40
	Low	11	2–12 mos.	18
Miscellaneous Tumor	High	5	1–16 mos.	20
	Low	9	1–12 mos.	11

response (Chu and Hilaris 1961; Nisce et al. 1971). Unlike Order and Chu and colleagues (1961, 1968), we could not show a significant good response rate in patients with low neurologic function (tables 20.4 and 20.5), which would be similar but not identical to our low subgroups arising in breast, lung and miscellaneous primary sites. Few of our patients were amenable to primary surgical resection.

Our 90 patients reviewed here are subject to the natural selection process inherent in a group referred and treated in a department of radiation therapy. There are certainly patients whom we did not see and some whom we saw but did not treat. This would indicate that the radiation patients presented in this clinical investigation are a more favorable group than one would find by reviewing all patients with cerebral metastases.

Quality of Life

We realize that the length of survival and level of functioning that is considered worthwhile varies significantly among clinicians. Few of our patients ever achieved complete normalcy after their brain metastases. Therefore, what level and length of functioning should we anticipate as a good response? We feel that the minimum definition of a good response is functional III (level I, II, or III) or better for 2 months or longer.

Any patient not achieving or maintaining this functional level for 2 months in our view probably has not truly benefited by treatment. The psychological trauma and morbidity that these patients sustained during therapy, especially the female patients, tended to lower their quality of life. In addition, some of those patients presenting with extraneurologic disease (table 20.5), who lived more than one year after radiation and who died of painful nonneurologic disease, in many ways also were not benefited. Survival and initial improvement in cerebral metastases in the neurologic functional class does not tell the entire story.

The Great Equalizer

If one looks at survival alone, the key is that once brain metastases develop (tables 20.2 and 20.3), the length of survival is the same no matter what the primary site. However, the quality of survival and its duration depends on the presenting functional status.

CONCLUSIONS

(1) Patients with brain metastases have the same survival from the time of treatment of brain metastases regardless of the primary site (after correction for initial performance status).

(2) The success of therapy depends mainly on the presenting functional status. Among patients with a high status (Level I, II, or III) 80% achieve a good response, and 20% of those with a low status (level IV) achieve a good response. Most long-term survivors (> 12 months) present with a high status. A good response is considered remaining in level I, II, or III for 2 or more months.

(3) No apparent difference in response was noted for any particular dose-time relationship.

(4) At the present time the functional status is the best scale for measuring the quality of life and predicting the response to management. However, a better language to describe the quality of life in patients with metastatic disease is urgently needed.

(5) It is apparent in the era of dexamethasone that functional status should be measured after instituting this medication. Certainly if the neurologic deficit does not reverse on dexamethasone then the likelihood of significant improvement with radiation is extremely low.

REFERENCES

Chu, F. C. H., and Hilaris, B. S. Value of radiation therapy in the management of intracranial metastases. *Cancer* 14:577–581, 1961.

Harwood, A. R., and Simpson, W. J. Radiation therapy of cerebral metastases: a randomized prospective clinical trial. *Int. J. Radiat. Oncol. Biol. Phys.* 2:1091–1094, 1977.

Hendrickson, F. R. Optimum schedule for palliative radiation therapy for metastatic brain cancer. *Int. J. Radiat. Oncol. Biol. Phys.* 2:165–168, 1977.

Nisce, L. Z.; Hilaris, B. S.; and Chu, F. C. H. A review of experience with irradiation of brain metastases. *Am. J. Roentgenol.* 111:329, 1971.

Order, S. E. et al. Improvement in quality of survival following whole brain irradiation for brain metastasis. *Radiology* 91:149–153, 1968.

21
Clinical Effects of Radiation on the Adult Nervous System

Myron Wollin
Robert A. Kagan
Harvey A. Gilbert
Herman Nussbaum
Paul Y. M. Chan
Aroor R. Rao

The dose-time events that cause clinical injury and morphologic lesions to the spinal cord and brain are similar. Radiation injury to the central nervous system requires relatively intensive radiation (table 21.1) (Lindgren 1958; Rottenberg et al. 1977; Abbatucci 1978). It is reasonable to assume that a high proportion of individuals who incur some degree of histologic damage to the brain, for example, the cerebral hemispheres, have no detectable clinical syndrome. It is highly unlikely that this clinically silent morphologic damage in the irradiated brain occurs in the irradiated spinal cord. Therefore, it follows that so-called radiation myelitis may be used as a model for analyzing the probability of radiation injury to the central nervous system.

A further reason for analyzing radiation myelitis, is that one must have numerous injured and noninjured individuals if one is to demonstrate the radiation dose that causes injury (Kagan et al. 1973). This information is available for radiation myelitis but not for cerebral necrosis.

Finally there are difficulties in trying to assess objectively the effects of radiation on the brain in patients with intracranial (Rubenstein 1970) and extracranial (Rottenberg et al. 1977; Kagan et al. 1971) malignancies. A precise analysis concerning radiation injury to the brain must account for the presence of concomitant infection, residual surgical effects, chemotherapy, and tumor regrowth. These knotty histopathologic problems are easier to analyze in the spinal cord because striking changes in blood vessels and white matter are more likely due to the effects of radiation (Brown and Kagan 1978). Nonetheless, vascular, toxic, and demyelinating lesions unrelated to cancer or related to the remote effects of cancer on the nervous system must be considered in the differential diagnosis.

Nearly one-third of clinically injured patients show injury within one

314

Table 21.1

PUBLISHED TOLERANCE OF THE CENTRAL NERVOUS SYSTEM
TO SUPERVOLTAGE RADIATION—SPINAL CORD
AND BRAIN (COMPOSITE TABLE)

Number of Fractions of Irradiation Per Patient Treated	Volume of Nervous System* Irradiated		
	Over ⅔	One-Half	Less Than ⅓
10	3,500	4,000	4,500
15	4,000	4,500	5,000
25	4,500	5,250	5,750

*For the brain, more than ⅔ of brain volume, ½ of brain volume, and less than ⅓ of brain volume. For the spinal cord, over ⅔ applies to more than 10 cm of spinal cord irradiated; ½ applies to 5–10 cm of spinal cord irradiated; less than ⅓ applies to less than 5 cm of cord irradiated.

year of receiving radiation therapy. It is indeed puzzling and fortunate that the brain and spinal cord of a large number of irradiated patients with cancer of the head and neck or thorax receive the published tolerance doses (table 21.1) and that the incidence of clinical damage is rare. However, analysis of clinical data does partly indicate that the size of the daily dose, total dose, and overall treatment time is important for analyzing certain types of morbidity, such as irradiation myelitis. Unfortunately when one attempts to test normal tissue injury expressed as a power function against clinical information, the correlation is far from being all-inclusive (Wollin and Kagan 1976).

An evaluation of clinical injury such as irradiation myelitis suggests broadly that there are three classes of results:

(1) Patients in whom the injury or noninjury does not appear to be dependent on the radiation dose within the range of doses commonly used.
(2) Patients in whom the effects appear to occur when a threshold dose is exceeded independently of the time over which the dose is given.
(3) Patients in whom the proportion of injury and noninjury can be affected significantly by a choice of dose, time and fraction number.

This chapter reviews irradiation myelitis and identifies which of the above three classes applies to the findings.

MATERIALS AND METHODS

The clinical literature contains 143 patients with radiation myelitis for whom dose-time fractionation information is given. In addition, similar information was found in the literature for those patients who received radiation to the thoracic or cervical spinal cord and who did not get radiation myelitis. Because of the different radiobiologic effect of megavoltage and 250 kVp, the latter doses were increased by 15%.

No attempt was made to take bone absorption into account. If a range for the spinal cord dose was given, the highest was used. If any treatment was given in one fraction, this patient was not used. If no fraction number but the total time was given, 5 days/week was assumed. Patients who received radiation under hyperbaric oxygen were excluded.

The data was analyzed using three different biologic models: nominal standard dose (NSD) (Ellis 1967); biological index of reaction (BIR) (Wollin and Kagan 1976), and equivalent dose (ED) (Wara et al. 1973). Myelopathy of the thoracic and cervical cord were analyzed separately.

The extent to which dose determines outcome can be calculated by a statistical test called point biserial correlation (RPB) (Bruning and Klintz 1968). Ideally, the higher the dose is, then the greater the biologic effect is. The test does not require grouping of data into various dose levels but is calculated point by point. A perfect correlation could give an RPB of +1; an RPB of 0 shows no correlation. We used Student's t test to determine the level of significance in order to rule out chance correlation because of small sample size.

If the RPB is squared and multiplied by 100, the resulting value is called the coefficient of determination (RPB^2) (Bahn 1972). The RPB^2 can be considered as giving a percentage estimate of how dose changes the clinical outcome: the number of complications and morbidity or of cures or failures depends on dose. An RPB^2 of 30% indicates that at least 30% of the clinical outcome must be explained by dose, time, and fractionation. If dose and technique are the major factors determining outcome, then the RPB^2 approaches 100%. An RPB^2 of 10%, however, means that 90% of the outcome is determined by factors other than dose, such as biologic factors inherent in the tumor or the host.

RESULTS

Table 21.2 lists the dose-time data for the 55 patients with radiation vasculomyelopathy of the cervical spinal cord. Table 21.3 lists the dose-time fractionation data for the 88 patients with myelopathy of the thoracic spinal cord. Table 21.4 summarizes the point biserial correlation analysis of the myelopathy patients. Abbatucci (1978) is listed separately because his data is precise and uniform. The correlation of dose with injury is small, between 1 and 5%, but this low percentage correlation with biologic dose is highly significant (p = .025–0.0005) and very real. The correlation between dose and injury is valid whether one looks at Abbatucci's series

Table 21.2

DOSE TIME FRACTION IN PATIENTS WITH IRRADIATION
VASCULOMYELOPATHY OF THE CERVICAL SPINAL CORD IN
ORDER OF INCREASING NSD

T Days	N Fractions	Dose in Rads	References
58	41	4,000	Fogelholm et al. 1974
47	42	4,085	Jellinger and Sturm 1970
59	42	4,600	Eyster and Wilson 1970
10	16	3,040	Palmer 1972
51	38	4,500	Dynes and Smedal 1960
27	23	3,750	Wara et al. 1973
42	31	4,600	Pallis et al. 1961
17	14	3,530	Boden 1948
18	17	3,800	Jellinger and Sturm 1970
47	34	5,000	Eyster and Wilson 1970
59	44	5,510	Palmer 1972
56	40	5,450	Reagan et al. 1968
51	38	5,400	Reagan et al. 1968
38	27	4,860	Wara et al. 1973
29	16	4,170	Palmer 1972
68	49	6,000	Dynes and Smedal 1960
17	14	3,820	Boden 1948
17	14	3,820	Boden 1948
42	25	5,000	Wara et al. 1973

Table 21.2 (Continued)

T Days	N Fractions	Dose in Rads	References
24	11	4,000	Henry et al. 1969
56	40	6,000	Reagan et al. 1968
52	39	6,000	Dynes and Smedal 1960
32	26	5,200	Atkins and Tretter 1966
42	18	5,110	Abbatucci 1978
40	36	6,050	Jellinger and Sturm 1970
48	18	5,400	Abbatucci 1978
46	18	5,400	Abbatucci 1978
44	18	5,400	Abbatucci 1978
42	18	5,400	Abbatucci 1978
42	18	5,400	Abbatucci 1978
42	18	5,400	Abbatucci 1978
42	18	5,400	Abbatucci 1978
42	18	5,400	Abbatucci 1978
47	34	6,400	Reagan et al. 1968
50	40	6,720	Jellinger and Sturm 1970
17	14	4,705	Boden 1948
10	9	4,000	Reagan et al. 1968
31	24	6,000	Reagan et al. 1968
17	14	4,950	Boden 1948
17	14	4,950	Boden 1948
46	18	5,940	Abbatucci 1978

Table 21.2 (Continued)

T Days	N Fractions	Dose in Rads	References
44	18	6,000	Abbatucci 1978
61	40	7,920	Jellinger and Sturm 1978
37	32	7,290	Jellinger and Sturm 1978
32	23	6,705	Lampert and Davis 1964
20	15	5,880	Malamud et al. 1954
32	23	7,000	Pallis et al. 1961
28	20	6,820	Jellinger and Sturm 1970
17	14	5,950	Boden 1948
43	32	8,117	Reagan et al. 1968
17	14	6,120	Boden 1948
29	21	7,290	Jellinger and Sturm 1970
35	26	8,700	Pallis et al. 1961
28	20	8,035	Jellinger and Sturm 1970
28	20	8,220	Jellinger and Sturm 1970

Table 21.3

DOSE TIME FRACTION IN PATIENTS WITH IRRADIATION
VASCULOMYELOPATHY OF THE THORACIC SPINAL CORD IN
ORDER OF INCREASING NSD

T Days	N Fractions	Dose in Rads	References
13	10	2,040	Atkins and Tretter 1966
79	50	3,719	Maier et al. 1969
43	24	3,582	Byfield 1972
64	46	4,390	Maier et al. 1969
85	50	4,650	Maier et al. 1969
72	50	4,650	Maier et al. 1969
72	50	4,653	Maier et al. 1969
68	48	4,701	Maier et al. 1969
36	27	3,840	Maier et al. 1969
29	22	3,660	Maier et al. 1969
83	50	5,060	Maier et al. 1969
50	37	4,558	Maier et al. 1969
87	50	5,300	Maier et al. 1969
26	19	3,690	Maier et al. 1969
7	2	1,900	Atkins and Tretter 1966
7	2	1,900	Atkins and Tretter 1966
7	2	1,900	Atkins and Tretter 1966
7	2	1,900	Atkins and Tretter 1966
32	23	4,120	Maier et al. 1969

Table 21.3 (Continued)

T Days	N Fractions	Dose in Rads	References
40	29	4,730	Reagan et al. 1968
21	10	3,480	Atkins and Tretter 1966
21	15	3,870	Locksmith and Powers 1968
21	16	3,950	Locksmith and Powers 1968
26	12	3,800	Atkins and Tretter 1966
28	21	4,410	Pallis et al. 1961
18	15	3,890	Locksmith and Powers 1968
21	16	4,070	Locksmith and Powers 1968
26	10	3,740	Palmer 1972
95	39	6,000	Dynes and Smedal 1960
55	40	5,700	Eyster and Wilson 1970
23	6	3,300	Wara et al. 1973
25	12	4,000	Atkins and Tretter 1966
30	14	4,250	Palmer 1972
57	41	6,000	Dynes and Smedal 1960
39	28	5,310	Maier et al. 1969
54	39	6,000	Dynes and Smedal 1960
35	15	4,550	Atkins and Tretter 1966
51	8	4,090	Palmer 1972
59	27	5,600	Lambert 1978
51	38	6,000	Dynes and Smedal 1960

Table 21.3 (Continued)

T Days	N Fractions	Dose in Rads	References
37	26	5,342	Reinhold et al. 1976
49	36	6,000	Dynes and Smedal 1960
49	36	6,000	Dynes and Smedal 1960
27	19	4,850	Locksmith and Powers 1968
23	13	4,370	Locksmith and Powers 1968
43	30	5,800	Lambert 1978
14	3	2,960	Atkins and Tretter 1966
42	30	6,000	Bhavilai 1974
29	8	4,200	Coy et al. 1969
45	29	6,100	Den Hoed-Sijtsema et al. 1971
25	8	4,200	Coy et al. 1969
59	37	6,700	Wara et al. 1973
23	8	4,200	Coy et al. 1969
55	37	6,700	Wara et al. 1973
55	36	6,753	Wara et al. 1973
44	29	6,282	Reinhold et al. 1976
48	19	5,782	Reinhold et al. 1976
41	29	6,300	Den Hoed-Sijtsema et al. 1971
26	20	5,500	Den Hoed-Sijtsema et al. 1971
37	27	6,174	Reinhold et al. 1976
43	30	6,515	Reinhold et al. 1976
26	20	5,609	Reinhold et al. 1976

Table 21.3 (Continued)

T Days	N Fractions	Dose in Rads	References
43	31	6,633	Reinhold et al. 1976
35	25	6,186	Reinhold et al. 1976
40	30	6,562	Reinhold et al. 1976
30	23	6,000	Reagan et al. 1968
33	24	6,161	Reinhold et al. 1976
40	29	6,700	Den Hoed-Sijtsema et al. 1971
43	28	6,700	Den Hoed-Sijtsema et al. 1971
24	6	4,350	Wara et al. 1973
47	30	6,895	Reinhold et al. 1976
18	12	5,000	Dynes and Smedal 1960
64	23	6,727	Reinhold et al. 1976
30	27	6,500	Den Hoed-Sijtsema et al. 1971
43	29	6,884	Reinhold et al. 1976
27	20	6,000	Den Hoed-Sijtsema et al. 1971
61	26	7,000	Wara et al. 1973
46	30	7,091	Reinhold et al. 1976
42	28	6,912	Reinhold et al. 1976
30	24	6,500	Den Hoed-Sijtsema et al. 1971
37	24	6,700	Den Hoed-Sijtsema et al. 1971
42	18	6,354	Reinhold et al. 1976
55	22	6,953	Reinhold et al. 1976
40	18	6,453	Reinhold et al. 1976

Table 21.3 (Continued)

T Days	N Fractions	Dose in Rads	References
35	20	6,600	Den Hoed-Sijtsema et al. 1971
41	29	7,394	Reinhold et al. 1976
35	26	7,600	Den Hoed-Sijtsema et al. 1971
51	46	10,000	Jellinger and Sturm 1970

Table 21.4

RELATIONSHIP OF BIOLOGIC DOSE TO PATIENTS WITH RADIATION
VASCULOMYELOPATHY USING THE POINT BISERIAL CORRELATION METHOD

	Myelopathy	Controls	NSD $N^{0.24}T^{0.11}$	BIR $T^A N^B$	ED $N^{0.377}T^{0.058}$
Thoracic and Cervical* RPB^2	143	508	2.2%	0.3%	2.2%
p			0.0005	N.S.†	0.0005
Thoracic‡ RPB^2	88	100	0.3%	2.5%	2.1%
p			N.S.†	0.025	0.025
Cervical§ RPB^2	55	408	4.1%	1.1%	3.0%
p			0.0005	0.025	0.0005
Abbatucci (1978) RPB^2	11	212	1.0%	5.4%	3.3%
p			N.S.†	0.0005	0.005

*Abbatucci 1978; Wara et al. 1973; Lambert 1978; Bhavilai 1974; Jellinger and Sturm 1970; Henry et al. 1969; Pallis et al. 1961; Dynes and Smedal 1960; Fogelholm et al. 1974; Eyster and Wilson 1970; Locksmith and Powers 1968; Boden 1948; Reinhold et al. 1976; Malamud et al. 1954; Atkins and Tretter 1966; Byfield 1972; Lampert and Davis 1964; Maier et al. 1969; Reagan et al. 1968; Coy et al. 1969; Palmer 1972; Den Hoed-Sijtsema et al. 1971.

†Not significant.

‡Den Hoed-Sijtsema et al. 1971; Palmer 1972; Coy et al. 1969; Reagan et al. 1968; Maier et al. 1969; Byfield 1972; Atkins and Tretter 1966; Reinhold et al. 1976; Locksmith and Powers 1968; Eyster and Wilson 1970; Dynes and Smedal 1960; Pallis et al. 1961; Jellinger and Sturm 1970; Bhavilai 1974; Lambert 1978; Wara et al. 1973.

§Palmer 1972; Reagan et al. 1968; Lampert and Davis 1964; Atkins and Tretter 1966; Malamud et al. 1954; Boden 1948; Eyster and Wilson 1970; Fogelholm et al. 1974; Dynes and Smedal 1960; Pallis et al. 1961; Henry et al. 1969; Jellinger and Sturm 1970; Wara et al. 1973; Abbatucci 1978.

(1978) of 11 myelopathies and 212 controls, the entire series of 143 cervical and thoracic myelopathies with 508 controls, the 88 thoracic myelopathies with 100 controls, or the 55 cervical myelopathies with 408 controls. A glance at the ED model gives one the impression that the exponents of $N^{0.377}$ and $T^{0.058}$ give, in general, a higher percentage correlation than the NSD model ($N^{0.24}T^{0.11}$) or the BIR model (exponents variable). One should, however, be cautious to conclude that the coefficients in the ED model are the best value.

We have shown that within the range of time, dose and fraction number used in clinical radiation therapy, 1–5% of the myelopathies can be attributed to variations in the treatment time, fraction number and total dose. A higher correlation than a maximum of 5% might have been possible if more patients had received spinal cord doses biologically equivalent to or greater than 6,000–8,000 rads in 6–8 weeks at 1,000 rads/week. However, the majority of dose-time strategems are influenced by the limits which were designed to prevent myelopathy (table 21.1).

DISCUSSION

It appears that the correlation of biologic dose precipitating myelopathy at the 1–5% level is real and most important that this correlation apparently occurs at the same dose-fraction-time events that are necessary to cure patients.

If one's goal were to avoid all probability of myelopathy, then probably many more patients than 5% would die of uncontrolled lymphomas and carcinomas of the aerodigestive tract. Scanning tables 21.2 and 21.3 one can easily see that the majority of the dose-time fractionation events causing radiation myelopathy are identical to those needed for cancer cure.

These are, however, some pithy questions that need to be discussed.

(1) Could the doses to the spinal cord in the patients with myelopathy be underestimated because of hot spots from gaps, overlaps, or multiple fields?

(2) Can irradiation vasculomyelopathy be simulated by the remote effects of cancer on the nervous system? Should patients with local recurrence or distant metastasis always be excluded from an analysis of this kind?

(3) Differences of 10% between institutions in the calibration of radiation apparatus is not unusual. Errors in setup, dosimetry, or treatment planning may combine to allow for further error in the calculation of the dose to the spinal cord. Presumably sufficient numbers of patients nullify these problems, but do they?

(4) Is the definition of the anatomic placement of the spinal cord the same among institutions?

And finally, what information is needed as a minimum base for the intercomparison of clinically equivalent doses and procedures? Will it ever be possible to truly resolve differences between centers by providing better information?

CONCLUSIONS

A review of the literature yielded 143 patients with either thoracic or cervical vasculomyelopathy secondary to radiation. These patients were compared to 508 controls.

A review of the biologic doses using three different models indicated that only 1–5% of the injuries could be attributed to dose-time and fractionation.

It appears that in order to completely avoid myelopathy, many more patients would have to be deprived of a sufficient tumor dose to ensure a high probability of cure.

It is suggested by analogy that the conclusions and principles of this review may be applied to the brain. One hopes there will not be enough patients with cerebral necrosis to prove or disprove this suggestion.

REFERENCES

Abbatucci, J. S. Radiation myelopathy of the cervical spinal cord: time, dose and volume factors. *Int. J. Radiat. Oncol. Biol. Physics* 4:239–248, 1978.

Atkins, H. L., and Tretter, P. Time-dose considerations in radiation myelopathy. *Acta Radiol.* [*Ther.*] (*Stockh.*) 5:79–94, 1966.

Bahn, A. K. *Basic medical statistics.* New York: Grune and Stratton, 1972.

Bhavilai, D. Inadvertent destruction of the spinal cord by radiation therapy. *Surg. Neurol.* 2:333–335, 1974.

Boden, G. Radiation myelitis of the cervical spinal cord. *Br. J. Radiol.* 21:464–469, 1948.

Brown, W. J., and Kagan, A. R. An examination of the pathology of radiation myelopathy following megavoltage irradiation. *Neurol. Soc. Bull.* 43:12–19, 1978.

Bruning, J. L., and Klintz, B. L. *Computational handbook of statistics.* Glenview, Ill.: Scott, Foresman and Co., 1968.

Byfield, J. E. Ionizing radiation and vincristine: possible neurotoxic synergism. *Radiol. Clin. Biol.* 41:129–138, 1972.

Coy, P.; Baker, S.; and Dolman, C. L. Progressive myelopathy due to radiation. *Can. Med. Assoc. J.* 100:1129–1133, 1969.

Den Hoed-Sijtsema, S.; Kaalen, J. G. A. H.; and Crezee, P. The influence of the dose per fraction on radiation damage to the myelum. *Radiol. Clin. Biol.* 40:89–99, 1971.

Dynes, J. B., and Smedal, M. I. Radiation myelitis. *Am. J. Roentgenol.* 83:78–87, 1960.

Ellis, F. Fractionation in radiotherapy. In *Modern Trends in Radiotherapy*, eds. T. J. Deeley and C. A. P. Wood. London: Butterworths, 1967.

Eyster, E. F., and Wilson, C. B. Radiation myelopathy. *J. Neurosurg.* 32:414–420, 1970.

Fogelholm, R.; Haltia, M.; and Andersson, L. C. Radiation myelopathy of cervical spinal cord simulating intramedullary neoplasm. *J. Neurol. Neurosurg. Psychiat.* 27:1177–1180, 1974.

Henry, P. et al. Myelopathie post-radiotherapique tardive. Livrets Med. 1:255–259, 1969.

Jellinger, K., and Sturm, K. W. Delayed radiation lesions of the human spinal cord. *Proceedings of the 6th International Congress of Neuropathology*, pp. 255–264, 1970.

Kagan, A. R.; Bruce, D. W.; and Di Chiro, G. Fatal foam cell arteritis of the brain after irradiation for Hodgkin's disease: angiography and pathology. *Stroke* 2:232–238, 1971.

Kagan, A. R. et al. An examination of some dose-time relationships in therapeutic radiology. *Br. J. Radiol.* 46:354–359, 1973.

Lambert, P. M. Radiation myelopathy of the thoracic spinal cord in long term survivors treated with radical radiotherapy using conventional fractionation. *Cancer* 41:1751–1760, 1978.

Lampert, P. W., and Davis, R. L. Delayed effects of radiation on the human central nervous system. *Neurology* 14:912–917, 1964.

Lindgren, M. On tolerance of brain tissue and sensitivity of brain tumors to irradiation. *Acta Radiol.* [*Suppl.*] (*Stockh.*) 170:1–180, 1958.

Locksmith, J. P., and Powers, W. E. Permanent radiation myelopathy. *Am. J. Roentgenol.* 102:916–926, 1968.

Maier, J. G. et al. Radiation myelitis of the dorsolumbar spinal cord. *Radiology* 93:160–164, 1969.

Malamud, N. et al. Necrosis of brain and spinal cord following x-ray therapy. *J. Neurosurg.* 11:353–362, 1954.

Pallis, C. A.; Louis, S.; and Morgan, R. L. Radiation myelopathy. *Brain* 84:460–479, 1961.

Palmer, J. J. Radiation myelopathy. *Brain* 95:109–122, 1972.

Reagan, T. J.; Thomas, J. E.; and Colby, M. Y. Chronic progressive radiation myelopathy. *J. A. M. A.* 203:128–132, 1968.

Reinhold, H. S.; Haalen, J. B. A. H.; and Unger-Gils, K. Radiation myelopathy of the thoracic spinal cord. *Int. J. Radiat. Oncol. Biol. Physics* 1:651–657, 1976.

Rottenberg, D. A. et al. Cerebral necrosis following radiotherapy of intracranial membranes. *Ann. Neurol.* 1:339–357, 1977.

Rubenstein, L. J. *Tumors of the central nervous system.* Washington, D. C.: Armed Forces Institute of Pathology, 1970.

Wollin, M., and Kagan, A. R. Modification of the biologic dose to normal tissue tolerance. *Acta Radiol.* [*Ther.*] (*Stockh.*) 15:481–492, 1976.

Wara, W. M. et al. Radiation pneumonitis: a new approach to the derivation of time-dose factors. *Cancer* 32:547–552, 1973.

22

Chemotherapy of Metastatic Central Nervous System Carcinoma

William R. Shapiro

The effectiveness of chemotherapy in treating metastatic brain tumors depends both on the nature of the tumor and on the pharmacologic properties of the drugs. The cells of a given tumor may be sensitive to a chemotherapeutic agent yet that agent fails to destroy the tumor because it cannot reach it in sufficient concentration. Thus, while drug sensitivity still depends on the tumor, the optimum drug pharmacology depends on the tumor's location, and for brain tumors, the blood-brain barrier may complicate drug entry.

There is no blood-brain barrier in the center of fully developed brain tumors (Vick et al. 1977), but there may be a barrier along the growing edge of the tumor (Levin et al. 1975) and there is certainly one in the surrounding brain. The blood-brain barrier prevents certain chemotherapeutic agents (notably those that are greater than 200 daltons, water-soluble, and ionized at physiologic pH) from entering the brain at usual doses and routes of administration (Rall and Zubrod 1962). Because a metastatic brain tumor begins as a nidus of single cells or a small cluster within intact brain, it is nourished by normal brain blood vessels bearing an intact blood-brain barrier. These small clusters of malignant cells are sequestered out of reach of the therapist treating systemic cancer because the drugs cannot cross an intact barrier.

Another major problem in the chemotherapy of brain tumors is the existence of cerebral edema. Because steroid hormones represent the best available therapy for cerebral edema, they have been used in conjunction with chemotherapeutic agents in treating such patients. In clinical evaluations involving both steroids and chemotherapeutic agents, proper controls are necessary to differentiate the effects of both agents. Indeed, evaluating the results of chemotherapy occupies much of the effort of treating such patients.

It is harder to evaluate the effects of therapy on brain metastases than on primary brain tumors. Survival time is a relatively good measure of results in primary brain tumor therapy, especially for phase III studies in which patients are treated early, but it is of almost no value in evaluating chemotherapy in metastatic brain tumors. In this circumstance the physician must rely on the combination of CT scans and clinical neurologic evaluation. Such a system works well for recurrent primary gliomas: tumor growth can be visualized on the CT scan, and deterioration in the clinical examination usually indicates progressive encroachment on normal neurologic structures. Unfortunately, the scheme has limitations when applied to metastatic brain tumors because of the systemic nature of the cancer.

Brain metastases frequently present late in the patient's clinical course when widespread systemic disease makes the patient so ill that neurologic signs and symptoms are obscured. In fact, with some important exceptions, most patients with metastatic brain tumors do not die of their brain disease but rather die of the complications of their systemic metastases. Only in the case of certain tumors, (for example, melanoma) is the patient highly likely to die directly from the brain tumor and this tumor is often resistant to both radiation therapy and chemotherapy.

Even when clinical neurologic deterioration can be identified, it may not imply drug failure. Recurrent central nervous system symptoms may not represent recurrent tumor but may mean (1) metabolic encephalopathy, a common problem in cancer patients; (2) subacute radiation toxicity that often clears spontaneously; (3) steroid withdrawal symptoms, such as headache, malaise and lethargy, which simulate recurrent tumor; or (4) vascular disease of the brain (nonbacterial thrombotic endocarditis or disseminated intravascular coagulopathy) or central nervous system infection (meningitis, fungal or viral disease, or opportunistic bacterial infections). Finally, such patients may develop meningeal carcinomatosis with its constellation of new and distant neurologic signs.

Metastatic brain tumor may intrude into efforts of the systemic chemotherapist who uses drugs as prophylaxis against future disease. There are now prophylactic adjuvant chemotherapy protocols for breast cancer, lung cancer, the several kinds of germinoma as well as the better known leukemia and lymphoma protocols. All of these tumors may metastasize to the nervous system. Recent experience suggests that such occurrences may recapitulate the acute lymphoblastic leukemia model in which meningeal leukemia impeded progress against the disease until effective central nervous system prophylaxis was established.

Most effective prophylaxis schemes designed to prevent central nervous system metastasis from solid tumors have relied almost exclusively on radiation therapy to the whole brain (Williams et al. 1977; Jackson et al. 1977); drugs, even the nitrosoureas, have been largely ineffective (Alexander et al. 1977). One major problem in chemoprophylaxis may be the blood-brain barrier. As noted above, there is probably no significant impediment to the entry of most drugs into the bulk of an established brain tumor, but a metastasis implants into normal brain where blood-brain barrier function is preserved. As noted in the discussion of the metastatic rat

Table 22.1

BCNU CHEMOTHERAPY OF BRONCHOGENIC CARCINOMA
METASTATIC TO THE BRAIN

Patient Age/Sex	Interval From Primary Diagnosis to Metastatic Brain Tumor	CNS Treatment Prior to BCNU (Response)
52/M	14 months	Radiation (improved)
60/M	Simultaneous	Radiation, cyclophosphamide vincristine (poor)
65/M	Simultaneous	Radiation (poor)
61/M	15 months	Radiation (fair)
43/F	Simultaneous	Radiation (fair)
47/M	12 months	Radiation (poor)
65/M	7 months	Radiation (fair)

brain tumor model, it is probably just this relatively preserved barrier that permits the development of such brain tumors. Finally, metastatic neurologic disease may present as a solid brain tumor, meningeal carcinomatosis or both. Prophylaxis regimens that rely on whole-brain radiation therapy without drugs are sure to lead to an increased incidence of meningeal metastases.

Our experience with chemotherapy of metastatic central nervous system disease includes chemotherapy of solid brain tumors presenting with recurrent symptoms after radiation therapy as well as attempts at chemotherapy in meningeal carcinomatosis. Our results are summarized here.

Results of Chemotheraphy (CNS)	Survival	
	From Diagnosis of Brain Tumor (Mos.)	From Beginning of Chemotherapy (Mos.)
Improved for 5 months	9	7
Progressive disease, no response	10	3
Progressive disease, no response	4	3
Progressive disease, no response	7	1
Progressive disease, no response	4	<1
Progressive disease, no response	2	2
Progressive disease, no response	8	<1

CHEMOTHERAPY OF METASTATIC BRAIN TUMOR

Table 22.1 shows the results of treatment of 7 patients with bronchogenic carcinoma metastatic to the brain. Using chemotherapy with 1,3-bis(2-chloroethyl)-1-nitrosourea (BCNU), patient 1 improved and remained stable for 5 months before deteriorating and dying of a combination of his brain tumor and systemic disease. The other 6 patients all showed progressive disease without central nervous system response. Patient 4 also developed meningeal carcinomatosis. Table 22.2 shows the results of therapy of 7 patients with malignant melanoma treated with BCNU. Not all of these patients received radiation therapy, and those who

Table 22.2

BCNU CHEMOTHERAPY OF MALIGNANT MELANOMA
METASTATIC TO THE BRAIN

Patient Age/Sex	Interval From Primary Diagnosis to Metastatic Brain Tumor	CNS Treatment Prior to BCNU (Response)
54/M	20 months	Radiation (poor)
53/F	8 years	Radiation (poor)
50/M	6 years	None
28/F	15 months	None
27/F	6 years	Radiation (spinal)
45/M	16 months	None (radiation later)
55/F	8 years	Radiation (poor)

did responded poorly. Patient 2 improved after chemotherapy and remained stable for almost 9 months before dying from her brain tumor. Patient 6 stabilized for 4 months and was then changed to CCNU. The other patients showed no evidence of improvement or stability in their neurologic signs. Patient 5 developed meningeal carcinomatosis.

As can be seen from the two tables, patients with bronchogenic carcinoma not infrequently developed symptoms from brain tumor simultaneously with their presentation of the lung cancer. This combination tends to occur in about 5–10% of all lung cancers (Rubin and Green 1968)

Results of Chemotherapy (CNS)	Survival	
	From Diagnosis of Brain Tumor (Mos.)	From Beginning of Chemotherapy (Mos.)
Progressive disease, no response, meningeal cancer	4	3
Improved to normal neurologically	11	9
Slowly progressive, no definite response	11	7
Slowly progressive, no definite response	11	3
Slowly progressive, no definite response, meningeal cancer	8	8
Stabilized 4 months, CNS improved (changed to CCNU)	9	9
Rapidly progressive, no response	1	1

and may be as frequent as 22% in oat-cell carcinomas (Kato et al. 1969). Patients with melanoma may show no signs of neurologic disease for many years after their initial diagnosis. The results of chemotherapy did not appear to be related to the interval between the primary diagnosis and subsequent development of brain tumor. In both diseases metastatic brain tumor was a late complication of cancer, and most patients died within a year after presentation of neurologic disease. The chemotherapy in most cases added little to the overall survival of the patients.

Table 22.3 depicts the results of therapy for 14 patients with different

Table 22.3

CCNU CHEMOTHERAPY OF METASTATIC BRAIN TUMORS

Patient Age/Sex	Primary Tumor	CNS Treatment Prior to CCNU (Response)	Results of Chemotherapy (CNS)	Survival of From Beginning Chemotherapy (Mos.)
45/M	Melanoma	Radiation, BCNU (Improved 4 months)	Slowly progressive, no improvement	3
47/M	Melanoma	None	Slowly progressive, no improvement	4.5
46/F	Melanoma	None	Slowly progressive, no improvement	5
45/M	Melanoma	None	Rapidly progressive (also MTX, ara-C via Ommaya)	2
42/M	Melanoma	Radiation (poor)	Slowly progressive, no improvement	7
42/F	Melanoma	None	Improved, normal CNS for 8 months	8
55/M	Bronchogenic	Radiation (good)	Systemic progressive, CNS stabilized	5
63/F	Bronchogenic	Radiation (fair)	Slowly progressive, no improvement	5
47/M	Bronchogenic	Radiation (fair)	Slowly progressive, no improvement	4
60/M	Bronchogenic	Radiation (simultaneous)	Slowly progressive, no improvement	3
37/M	Bronchogenic (adeno-cancer)	Radiation (fair)	CNS stabilized for 3 months, died of CNS disease	4

Table 22.3 (Continued)

Patient Age/Sex	Primary Tumor	CNS Treatment Prior to CCNU (Response)	Results of Chemotherapy (CNS)	Survival of From Beginning Chemotherapy (Mos.)
55/F	Breast	Radiation (good)	Slowly progressive, no improvement	5.5
40/F	Breast (meningeal cancer)	Radiation (poor)	Progressive no improvement	3
42/F	Breast	Radiation (fair)	Rapidly progressive, no improvement	2

metastatic tumors using the chemotherapeutic agent 1-(2-chloroethyl)-3-cyclo-hexyl-1-nitrosourea (CCNU). This drug was used at a dose of 130 mg/m^2 every 6 weeks although in subsequent studies with primary tumors we have been using 2-week intervals and a reduced dosage (Shapiro and Young 1976). Six patients with melanoma received CCNU. Patient 6 showed improvement with a normal neurologic examination for 8 months, then died suddenly of a cerebellar hemorrhage, presumably at the site of a previous melanoma. Patient 4 developed meningeal carcinomatosis and was treated with methotrexate and cytosine arabinoside via an Ommaya reservoir.[1] The patient showed slowly progressive disease without evidence of central nervous system improvement. Five patients with bronchogenic carcinoma were treated with CCNU. Most had received prior radiation therapy with good to fair results. The CCNU stabilized patient 7 for 5 months until he died of systemic complications of his lung cancer, and patient 11 stabilized for 3 months before he died of recurrent neurologic disease. Finally, 3 patients with breast cancer were treated with CCNU. Patient 13 developed meningeal carcinomatosis and did poorly despite a combination of oral CCNU and methotrexate delivered by Ommaya reservoir.

This overall experience with metastatic brain tumors is generally consistent with the literature on results with single agent nitrosoureas in metastatic brain tumors (Wilson et al. 1976) and indicates an approximately 20% overall response rate. Even under the best of circumstances, however, the responders were neurologically stable for only a short period of

---

[1] An Ommaya reservoir is a hollow silastic device surgically inserted beneath the scalp and connected with the lateral ventricle by a catheter. The device may be entered percutaneously via a small needle to sample CSF or to administer drugs.

time. Whether nitrosoureas added to radiation therapy might be of benefit, especially with combination chemotherapy, is reviewed by Dr. Chan in Chapter 24.

TREATMENT OF MENINGEAL CARCINOMATOSIS

Meningeal carcinomatosis may involve diffuse or widespread multifocal invasion of the leptomeninges by metastatic carcinoma or lymphoma with or without mass lesions in the central nervous system. Our experience with the presentation and pathology of this disease has been previously presented (Olson et al. 1974). In general, the best way to treat meningeal carcinomatosis is to irradiate the entire neuraxis. Unfortunately, such radiation kills a large volume of bone marrow contained within the spine, marrow needed by the patient for his systemic chemotherapy. For this reason we have elected to focus the radiation to the area of clinical disease—usually the head or the lumbar spine—and have attempted to treat the remaining disease by chemotherapy.

Following the lead in the treatment of meningeal leukemia, we chose to use intrathecal chemotherapy (Shapiro et al. 1977). Early in the course of these studies, we determined the distribution and time course of methotrexate administered by lumbar puncture and by Ommaya reservoir (Shapiro et al. 1975). We found that in about 10% of the instances methotrexate administered by lumbar puncture leaks out of the subarachnoid space into the paravertebral tissues. When the drug was injected into the subarachnoid space, therapeutic concentrations (defined as those greater than 1×10^{-6} molar) were achieved in only about half of the patients and only for about 24 hours. On the other hand, if methotrexate was given directly into the Ommaya reservoir, the drug was completely distributed into all the ventricles and the concentration in the ventricles and the lumbar space equalized within 4 hours, falling exponentially with therapeutic levels of 1×10^{-6} molar maintained for about 48 hours. Low but toxic blood levels similarly persist but may be treated by systemic administration of the folate substitute citrovorum factor (CF). Citrovorum factor is rapidly converted to the natural circulating folate 5-methyl tetrahydrofolate whose level in the CSF after oral or intravenous administration remains low (Mehta et al. 1977). Cytosine arabinoside (ara-C), given by Ommaya reservoir, has similar pharmacokinetics to methotrexate.

We have previously reported the results of a preliminary trial in the therapy of meningeal carcinomatosis by combinations of radiation therapy, methotrexate and ara-C (Young et al. 1975). Recently, we reviewed the results of therapy of an additional 47 patients with meningeal carcinomatosis (Glass et al. 1978). Radiation therapy was administered focally to the area of involved neuraxis determined either clinically or radiographically in 40 of the 47 patients. In 7 patients there was no area that required radiation, and these patients were treated only with chemotherapy. Methotrexate and ara-C were used in combination in 37 patients; methotrexate was used alone in 7.

The results were as follows: 45 of 47 cases had sufficient data to assess clinical outcome. Eight patients showed clinical progression until death with a median survival of 1.5 months. Of the remaining 37 patients, 12 had improved neurologic deficits and 25 remained neurologically stable. The periods of improvement and stabilization ranged from 1 week to 2.5 years with a median of 3 months. Five patients survived for 1 year or longer, and 3 were alive at 16 months, 1.5 years and 2.5 years after the diagnosis of leptomeningeal involvement. Thus, the 1-year survival of the entire group was 10%. Of the 45 patients with clinical followup, 15 eventually died of their meningeal disease, 7 of their systemic disease, and 11 from unknown cause. Infections and miscellaneous causes accounted for death in 9 other patients and 3 patients are still living. Thus, of all the patients in whom a cause of death could be defined, half were related to leptomeningeal involvement. There were six autopsies. Five of them revealed evidence of persistent leptomeningeal infiltration which was either focal or widespread.

Table 22.4 shows the therapeutic responses measured by combining the CSF and clinical data in 31 of 45 patients for whom such information was available. Because such patients are usually deteriorating when first treated, both better and stabilized can be considered improvement. CSF opening pressure, protein, glucose, cell count and cytology at the beginning of the treatment were graded and compared to those after treatment. A decrease in the grade was defined as *better*, no change as *stable*, and an increase as *worse*. The clinical course was likewise defined as *better*, *stabilized*, or *worse*. Under these circumstances, marked improvement (both CSF and clinical course were better) occurred in 5 patients; moderate improvement in 14; and minimal improvement in 8. Only 4 patients showed no response, implying worsening in CSF, clinical course or both.

Table 22.4

THERAPEUTIC RESPONSE IN MENINGEAL METASTASIS
31 OF 45 CASES WITH COMPLETE CSF DATA AND CLINICAL FOLLOWUP

		Clinical Course		
		Better	**Stabilized**	**Worse**
CSF Profile	**Better**	5 Marked	11 Moderate	2 Minimal
	Stabilized	3 Moderate	5 Minimal	2 No Response
	Worse	0 Minimal	2 No Response	0 No Response

Table 22.5

TREATMENT RESULTS IN MENINGEAL METASTASIS
31 OF 45 CASES WITH COMPLETE CSF DATA AND CLINICAL FOLLOWUP

		Improvement				No Improvement
		Total	Marked	Moderate	Minimal	
Solid Tumors	26	22 (85%)	4	11	7	4
Breast	16	13 (81%)	3	5	5	3
Lung	4	4	0	3	1	0
Melanoma	2	2	0	2	0	0
Other	4	3	1	1	1	1
Lymphomas	5	5 (100%)	1	3	1	0

The results of treatment in individual tumors are shown in table 22.5. All lymphoma patients improved, including 2 who received chemotherapy without radiation. Of the solid tumors 85% of the patients improved; breast cancer performed the best with 13 of 16 patients responding. Even some of the lung cancer patients responded for a short period of time.

Of some interest was a separate group of 9 patients whose only manifestation of metastatic cancer was meningeal carcinomatosis. Six of these patients responded with a median survival of 10 months while 3 got worse with a median survival of 1.5 months. The median survival of meningeal carcinoma patients with systemic metastases who respond is only 3 months, suggesting that as in solid metastases to the brain, usually such patients die of their systemic disease not of their central nervous system disease.

CONCLUSIONS

The problems of the overall therapy of metastatic central nervous system cancer are many and are only now being approached. Nevertheless, these early results suggest that vigorous therapy of solid metastatic brain tumors, primarily with radiation therapy and perhaps also with chemotherapy, and of meningeal carcinomatosis with combined radiation and chemotherapy is often rewarding, yielding improved neurologic symptoms and modestly prolonged survival.

REFERENCES

Alexander, M. et al. Combined modality treatment for oat cell carcinoma of the lung: a randomized trial. *Cancer Treat. Rep.* 61:1–6, 1977.

Glass, J. P.; Shapiro, W. R.; and Posner, J. B. Treatment of leptomeningeal metastases. *Neurology* 28:351, 1978.

Jackson, D. V. et al. Prophylactic cranial irradiation in small cell carcinoma of the lung, a randomized study. *J. A. M. A.* 237:2730–2733, 1977.

Kato, Y. et al. Oat cell carcinoma of the lung, a review of 138 cases. *Cancer* 23:517–524, 1969.

Levin, V. A.; Freeman-Dove, M.; and Landahl, H. D. Permeability characteristics of brain adjacent to tumors in rats. *Arch. Neurol.* 32:785–791, 1975.

Mehta, B. M.; Shapiro, W. R.; and Hutchison, D. J. Distribution of 5-methyl tetrahydrofolate (5-CH$_3$-THFA) following IV administration of citrovorum factor (CF) with intra-Ommaya methotrexate (MTX). *Proc. Am. Assoc. Cancer Res.* 18:227, 1977.

Olson, M. E.; Chernik, N. L.; and Posner, J. B. Infiltration of the leptomeninges by systemic cancer, a clinical and pathological study. *Arch. Neurol.* 30:122–137, 1974.

Rall, D. P., and Zubrod, C. C. Mechanism of drug absorption and excretion. Passage of drugs in and out of the central nervous system. *Ann. Rev. Pharmacol.* 2:109–128, 1962.

Rubin, P., and Green, J. *Solitary metastases*. Springfield, Ill.: Charles C Thomas, 1968.

Shapiro, W. R.; Young, D. F.; and Mehta, B. M. Methotrexate distribution in cerebrospinal fluid intravenous, ventricular and lumbar injections. *N. Engl. J. Med.* 293:161–166, 1975.

Shapiro, W. R., and Young, D. F. Chemotherapy of malignant glioma with CCNU alone and CCNU combined with vincristine sulfate and procarbazine hydrochloride. *Trans. Am. Neurol. Assoc.* 101:217–220, 1976.

Shapiro, W. R. et al. Treatment of meningeal neoplasms. *Cancer Treat. Rep.* 61:733–743, 1977.

Vick, N. A.; Khandekar, J. D.; and Bigner, D. D. Chemotherapy of brain tumors: the "blood-brain barrier" is not a factor. *Arch. Neurol.* 34:523–526, 1977.

Williams, C. et al. Role of radiation therapy in combination with chemotherapy in extensive oat cell cancer of the lung: a randomized study. *Cancer Treat. Rep.* 61:1427–1431, 1977.

Wilson, C. B. et al. Single-agent chemotherapy of brain tumors, a five-year review. *Arch. Neurol.* 33:739–744, 1976.

Young, D. F.; Shapiro, W. R.; and Posner, J. B. Treatment of leptomeningeal cancer. *Neurology* 25:370, 1975.

23

Adrenocorticosteroid Hormones

Joel R. L. Ehrenkranz
Jerome B. Posner

The single most dramatic advance in the treatment of brain metastasis has been the introduction of adrenal glucocorticoids. These drugs, first used to treat brain metastasis by Kofman and his colleagues (1957), have revolutionized the initial treatment of metastatic brain tumor and have at times restored moribund patients to full neurologic function, often within hours. Although glucocorticoids are now used to treat several brain disorders, in no other illness is the response so consistent and so dramatic as in treating brain metastases (Fishman 1975; Reulen 1976). This chapter reviews the effects of glucocorticoids, both salutary and untoward, on patients with brain metastases and discusses the mechanism(s) by which these agents exert their beneficial effect.

Adrenal corticosteroids are classified as glucocorticoids, mineralocorticoids or androgens, depending upon their predominant clinical effect. Cortisol is the primary endogenous human glucocorticoid; it exhibits some mineralocorticoid activity that can be diminished by the addition of a fluorine atom to the glucocorticoid molecule. The synthetic congeners of cortisol that result from chemical modification (prednisone, prednisolone, methylprednisolone and dexamethasone), besides having less mineralocorticoid activity, are also more potent than cortisol. Although dexamethasone is the most frequently used, equivalent doses of any synthetic glucocorticoid have similar effects on metastatic brain tumors. These agents are, accordingly, grouped together and referred to in clinical neurology and neurosurgery simply as *steroids*; in this chapter the terms *glucocorticoid* and *steroid* are used interchangeably.

HISTORY

It has been known since Ehrlich (1885) that certain dyes injected intravenously stain virtually all tissues of the body except the brain. Goldmann in 1909 injected trypan blue (an agent now widely used today to assess blood-brain barrier function in experimental animals) intravenously into rabbits and confirmed Ehrlich's earlier findings that such dyestuffs did not penetrate the central nervous system. These experiments led to the concept of a blood-brain barrier excluding from the central nervous system substances that gained easy access to most tissues of the body (see also Rapoport 1976). When the brain is injured, as by a metastasis, the blood-brain barrier at the site of injury is lost, allowing previously excluded molecules to enter. Changes in osmotic and oncotic pressure gradients result in extravasation of fluid and brain swelling (Fishman 1975; Reulen 1976). The brain swelling, or edema, surrounding metastatic tumors appears to be responsible for some of the symptoms produced by these lesions, and the dramatic amelioration of neurologic function produced by glucocorticoids is believed to result from resolution of brain edema.

The salutary effects of steroids on brain edema were first demonstrated by Prados, and his colleagues in 1945. These investigators noted that when the brain was exposed to air the blood-brain barrier failed and brain edema developed. If the brain was sprayed with adrenal extract, however, the blood-brain barrier remained intact and the brain did not swell. Several years later, Ingraham and co-workers (1952) recognized the usefulness of cortisone and ACTH in smoothing the postoperative course of patients after surgery for craniopharyngioma. The beneficial effects of cortisone appeared independent of adrenal insufficiency resulting from pituitary damage. Rasmussen and Gulati (1962) later demonstrated that the transient hemiparesis that followed temporal lobectomy for focal cortical seizures was diminished or prevented by cortisone administration.

In 1957 Kofman and his colleagues gave prednisolone to 20 patients with brain metastases. Steroid treatment was undertaken because the investigators had noted striking relief of neurologic symptoms in a patient with breast carcinoma and a brain metastasis who had been given the drug to suppress adrenal function. They noted amelioration of the neurologic state in other patients and concluded this was an effect of steroids on inflammation and edema. Galicich and French (1961) reported dramatic responses to steroid hormones in patients suffering from brain tumors, both primary and metastatic, and attributed the improvement of neurologic symptoms to regression of brain edema. Since that time, the salutary effects of glucocorticoids on the edema surrounding brain tumors have been demonstrated both microscopically (Long et al. 1966) and by direct measurement of water content (Meinig et al. 1976; Shapiro and Posner 1974).

EFFECT OF STEROIDS ON PATIENTS WITH BRAIN METASTASES

Neurologic Signs and Symptoms

The clinical symptoms of brain metastases can be divided into 2 broad groups: focal and generalized (table 23.1). Focal symptoms, which include hemiparesis or hemiplegia, hemianopia and specific abnormalities of cognitive function (such as aphasia and apraxia), are at times a result of destruction of brain tissue by the metastasis. Usually, however, focal symptoms result from a combined direct effect of the metastasis and of its

Table 23.1

EFFECT OF STEROIDS ON PATIENTS WITH BRAIN METASTASES

A. Clinical improvement
   1. Focal signs
   2. Generalized signs

B. Decrease in intracranial pressure
   1. Plateau waves
   2. Baseline pressure

C. Electroencephalographic improvement

D. Improvement in radionuclide brain scans and CT scans
   1. Less edema
   2. Less isotope or contrast accumulation

E. Increase in cerebral blood flow

F. Decrease in peritumoral water content

surrounding edema. Generalized symptoms, which include headache, nausea and vomiting, lethargy, and confusion, are usually not a direct effect of the metastasis but rather a consequence of shifting cerebral structures and increased intracranial pressure from the edema. Both focal and generalized symptoms respond to glucocorticoids, but the symptoms of generalized brain disease usually resolve more rapidly and completely.

Steroid therapy resolves clinical symptoms in 60–80% of patients with brain metastases. Kofman and his colleagues (1957) noted definite improvement in 9 of 15 patients, Ruderman and Hall (1965) in 11 of 17 patients, and Sligar and Posner (Posner 1974) in 21 of 30 patients. In the last study the symptom which responded best was headache with striking improvement in 16 of 19 patients (85%). Focal weakness (hemiparesis) improved in 19 of 26 patients, or only 73%. In this series and others, symptoms of focal dysfunction, especially visual field and sensory abnormalities, were less responsive than symptoms of more generalized brain dysfunction (headache, confusion, lethargy).

French (1966) described the responses of 249 patients with brain tumors (203 primary, 46 metastatic) to dexamethasone; 81% improved. Headache, confusion and lethargy improved in 91%, hemiplegia in 73%, aphasia in 86%, but visual field defects in only 41% and sensory loss in 55%. The response of local signs to steroid therapy suggests that some focal abnormalities such as aphasia and hemiparesis are not a direct result of the tumors but rather of surrounding edema (Perret and Kernohan 1943). Most of the symptoms of cerebellar metastasis also respond well to glucocorticoids, particularly if those symptoms are caused by edema obstructing the cerebral ventricular system; however, it has been our experience that vertigo usually responds poorly to steroids.

Clinical Pharmacology

The clinical response to glucocorticoids is usually evident within 24–48 hours. In some patients improvement is noticed 4–5 hours after an intravenous injection of glucocorticoid (Gutin 1977; Ransohoff 1972). Maximum clinical improvement usually occurs within 3–7 days (Gutin 1975) and may be sustained for several weeks. If additional treatment is not given, however, patients usually relapse within weeks. Hazra and colleagues (1972), studying patients with brain metastases from carcinoma of the lung, reported significant improvement in 4 of 6 patients treated with steroids alone but a median survival of less than 3 months. With radiotherapy, there was initial improvement in 19 of 25 patients and a somewhat longer median survival of 3–6 months. Horton and coworkers (1971) found no advantage of radiation therapy and steroids over steroids alone in the treatment of brain metastases, but the number of patients treated was small. Gottlieb, Frei and Luce (1972) described 4 patients with malignant melanoma who survived over a year with steroid treatment alone. Bernard-Weil and coworkers (1963, 1972) reported long remissions in patients with malignant glioma treated with both corticosteroids and vasopressin.

Dexamethasone is the most widely used glucocorticoid for the treatment of brain metastasis. There is, however, no evidence that one glucocorticoid is superior to another in the treatment of cerebral edema. Dexamethasone was originally used by Galicich and his colleagues (1961) because it lacks mineralocorticoid effect. Mineralocorticoids are usually associated with fluid retention and peripheral edema and thus are avoided when treating cerebral edema. Paradoxically, aldosterone, a naturally occurring mineralocorticoid, has been reported to prevent cerebral edema after intracranial surgery (Schmiedek et al. 1976). Dexamethasone is usually given orally in a dose of 4 mg every 6 hours or 4 times/day. Patients who do not respond to 16 mg/day may respond to higher doses (Renaudin et al. 1973; Lieberman et al. 1977).

Dose-response curves of steroid effect on cerebral edema have not been constructed. Consequently the optimal dose, frequency of administration and best agent are not known. If a patient fails to respond to 16 mg daily, we double the dose every 48–72 hours up to 96 mg/day. No additional untoward side effects are caused by higher doses when given for a short time (Marshall et al. 1977). For acutely ill patients, higher doses may be given initially. We have given up to 100 mg of dexamethasone intravenously without significant untoward effects.

Recent evidence places the plasma half-life of dexamethasone at 4.7 hours, but the biologic half-life as measured by plasma corticosteroid suppression is 7.0 hours (Meikle and Tyler 1977). We have found no substantial difference in clinical response when steroids are given at longer intervals (twice a day or even once daily), but every-other-day prednisone has not been effective.

After intravenous injection of radioactive corticosteroids, no significant amount of radioactivity is detectable in brain after 60 minutes, and a significant drop in CSF concentration is observed after 90 minutes (Gutin 1977). The therapeutic effects of steroids do not appear to be linearly related to drug concentrations in brain. Certain brain structures, especially the septum, hippocampus and choroid plexus, are able to concentrate cortisol up to 27 times the concentration of blood (McEwen et al. 1968), and experimental ependymoblastoma in mice has also been shown to accumulate radioactive dexamethasone (Schwartz et al. 1972).

Dexamethasone can be administered orally, intramuscularly or intravenously. Glucocorticoids cross the blood-brain barrier easily, but much of the drug is protein-bound, and the entry of steroid into the normal central nervous system varies inversely with protein binding (Marynick et al. 1977). A bolus injection of a large dose of glucocorticoid to saturate protein binding should promote the entry of more drug into the central nervous system.

Between 15% and 40% of patients with brain metastases suffer seizures (see Chapter 11). The drug of choice for treatment of these seizures is phenytoin. Phenytoin induces microsomal enzymes and has striking effects on the metabolism of dexamethasone. In one study, phenytoin decreased the plasma halflife of dexamethasone by 51% and increased the clearance rate by 140% (Werk et al. 1969). Investigators have observed that previously effective doses of dexamethasone are no longer effective if the patient is given phenytoin, phenobarbital or diazepam (Haque et al. 1972; Stjernholm and Katz 1975; Brooks et al. 1972; Werk et al. 1969; McLelland and Jack 1978). The presumed mechanism of action of these drugs is to increase hepatic clearance of dexamethasone. This untoward interaction can be solved either by increasing the dose of dexamethasone or switching to another corticosteroid (such as methylprednisolone), the plasma levels of which are said to be less affected by the addition of phenytoin (Vincent 1978). We also have the clinical impression that patients on phenytoin and dexamethasone maintain less stable levels of phenytoin. When dexamethasone is being tapered, the blood levels of phenytoin rise and previously therapeutic doses of phenytoin become toxic.

The therapy of cerebral edema requires pharmacologic, not physiologic, doses of steroid hormones. The 16 mg/day dose of dexamethasone is much greater than the usual steroid output of the adrenal glands (37.5 mg of cortisol daily, equivalent to 1.5 mg dexamethasone). The maximally stimulated adrenal glands can produce 375 mg of cortisol a day (equivalent to 15 mg of dexamethasone) (Capon et al. 1976). Brain tumors per se do not elevate either serum or CSF cortisol (Murphy et al. 1967). Thus, the effects of steroids on the pathology of cerebral edema represent pharmacologic effects and may have little to do with normal brain–adrenal gland relationships.

Effects of Glucocorticoids on Neurologic Diagnostic Procedures

Procedures sometimes employed in evaluating patients for metastatic brain tumor (see Chapter 11) include lumbar puncture, electroencephalography, radionuclide brain scanning, CT scanning, and arteriography. Glucocorticoids have specific effects on abnormalities detected by these tests (table 23.1).

Lumbar Puncture. In 70% of patients with brain tumor, the CSF pressure and protein are increased (Fishman 1977). The increased protein concentration probably results from leakage across the blood-brain barrier; the degree of protein elevation reflects the tumor's distance from the ventricular system or subarachnoid space. With glucocorticoid therapy, the concentration of protein may return to normal, presumably secondary to a decrease in blood-brain barrier permeability (Weinstein et al. 1973).

Glucocorticoids decrease CSF pressure elevations in patients with metastatic and primary brain tumors but there is no direct relationship between the improvement of clinical symptoms and the decrease in CSF pressure. Kullberg and West (1965) demonstrated that in patients with brain tumors, symptoms often improve before CSF pressure begins to decrease, and in at least one of their patients, clinical improvement occurred in the absence of any change in CSF pressure. Two alterations of the CSF pressure occur after steroid treatment of brain tumors. The plateau waves or sudden increases in intracranial pressure (possibly due to episodic vasoparalysis and sometimes characterized by increasing neurologic dysfunction) disappear within minutes of corticosteroid injection (Lundberg 1960). The baseline intracranial pressure also falls in most patients whose CSF pressure is elevated prior to treatment, but this change may not occur for 24–48 hours and does not correlate with clinical response. At times, plateau waves may disappear without a substantial change in base-line intracranial pressure (Alberti et al. 1978).

Electroencephalography (EEG). Abnormal EEGs are strikingly improved in patients with brain metastases after steroid therapy, and the degree of improvement generally parallels the patient's clinical response (Matsuoka et al. 1978). Figure 23.1 illustrates EEG improvement in a patient with a brain metastasis from carcinoma of the lung. Matsuoka and colleagues (1978) followed the EEG changes in 5 patients with metastatic brain tumors, mapping the distribution and degree of delta activity by topographic display. Diminution of the delta distribution was observed within 20 minutes of intravenous dexamethasone.

Matsuoka and coworkers (1978) have attributed the changes in the EEG to a reduction in peritumoral edema. Support for their concept comes from the experimental work of Schaul and colleagues (1976), who produced cerebral edema in cats by coagulation lesions. Some of the animals then received a wide craniotomy. When the lesion caused only moderate brain edema, the EEG was unaltered. If massive edema occurred, slow wave activity was present only in the unoperated animals. The wide

Figure 23.1.

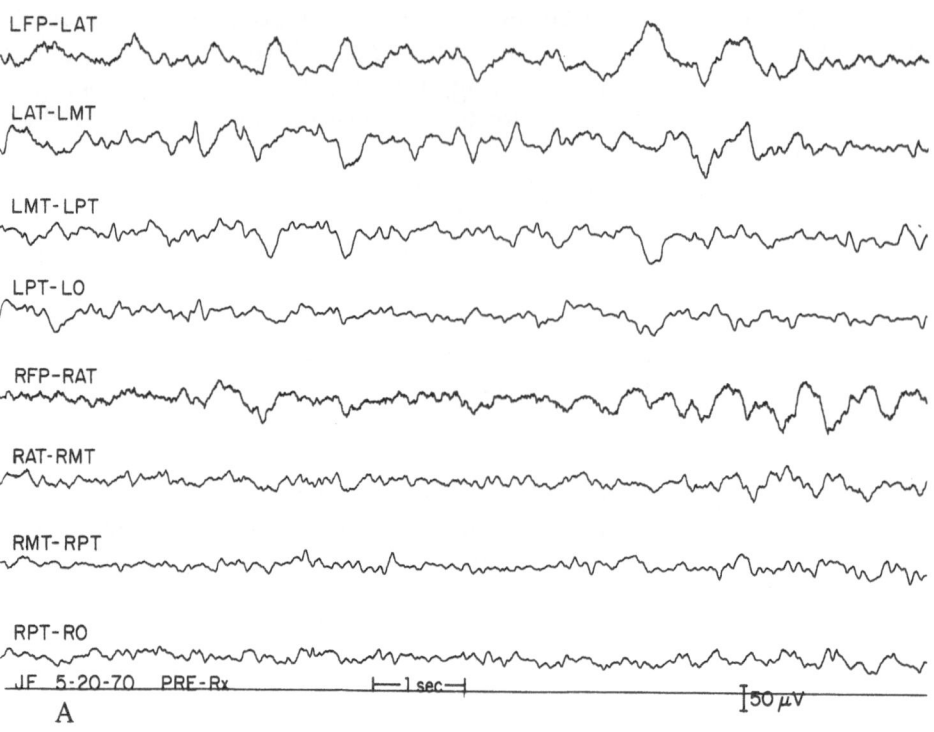

Electroencephalographic (EEG) response to steroids. This patient suffered from carcinoma of the lung metastatic to the left frontal lobe. A. The first EEG was taken when the patient was lethargic and aphasic and had a right hemiparesis. The first 4 leads are along the left temporal area from front to back; the second 4 leads are along the right temporal area from front to back. Note the large slow waves in the left frontopolar (FP) and anterotemporal (AT) areas, which are reflected by smaller voltage slow waves on the homologous right side. There is virtually no normal 8–13/second alpha activity in the posterior leads. B. Six days after treatment with 60 mg of prednisone daily. The patient was awake and alert with normal language and very mild weakness of the right side. There is still slow activity at the site of the tumor in the left FP and AT areas, but normal background activity now appears in the posterior leads in the left and the right-sided leads are close to normal.

craniotomy appeared to prevent the EEG abnormalities associated with cerebral edema. Thus, the delta activity in the EEG does not result from cerebral edema directly but is mediated by structural shifts associated with edema. Corticosteroids were not used in these studies. Steudel and co-workers (1976) reported a correlation between the size of peritumoral edema as identified by CT scan and the degree of focal EEG changes. As in other experiments, delta activity was absent with small amounts of edema but present when the edema became prominent (Schaul).

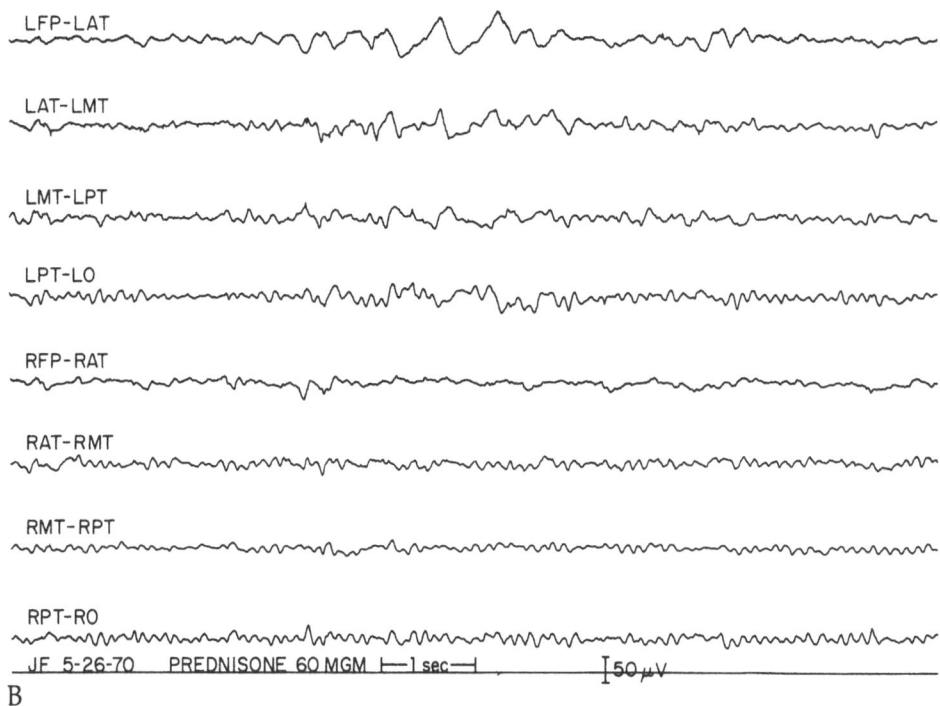

LFP-LAT

LAT-LMT

LMT-LPT

LPT-LO

RFP-RAT

RAT-RMT

RMT-RPT

RPT-RO

JF 5-26-70   PREDNISONE 60 MGM ⊢—1 sec—⊣   ⊥50 μV

B

Radionuclide Brain Scan. Glucocorticoids alter the radionuclide brain scans of patients with brain metastases. Marty and Cain (1973) studied the effects of steroid administration on the technetium brain scan of 12 patients with brain tumors. Ten of the patients showed a reduction in the brain lesion activity after dexamethasone therapy. They attributed the decreased uptake of technetium to decreased peritumoral edema. Fletcher and colleagues (1975) report similar results. Waxman and coworkers (1978) studied the effects of steroids on the technetium glucoheptonate and gallium brain scans of patients with brain tumors (mostly metastases). Gallium uptake was less in patients on steroid therapy. They observed no such effect on the technetium glucoheptonate scan. In no instance did the brain scan revert to normal after steroid therapy.

Computed Tomography (CT, CAT). Steroids also have a marked effect on the CT scan. After injection of contrast, the CT scan usually delineates a brain metastasis from surrounding edema. The tumor appears radiodense and the edema radiolucent (see Chapter 12). Steroids produce amelioration of the surrounding edema in many patients with brain metastases (Steudel et al. 1976; Lanksch et al. 1976). Lanksch and coworkers (1976) measured the water content of tissue surrounding brain tumors and compared it with the CT scan. They found that the low density areas on CT represented areas of increased water content (edema). Crocker and colleagues (1976) found that dexamethasone decreased the accumulation of both ^{99m}Tc-pertechnetate (for radionuclide brain scans) and iothalamate (for CT scans) in the tumor but did not alter the apparent size of the lesion.

Arteriography and Cerebral Blood Flow. Glucocorticoids alter the blood flow and metabolism of the brain surrounding metastases. Weinstein and coworkers (1973) studied 8 patients with metastatic brain tumors treated with dexamethasone: 5 of the 8 patients had complete clearing of their neurologic signs, and 2 others improved. In 3 patients, regional blood flow was measured before and after steroid treatment. In all 3 patients mean hemispheric blood flow was decreased before treatment. During glucocorticoid therapy, total hemispheric blood flow returned to normal levels in 2 patients but did not change significantly in the third. Blood flow was lowest in the regions immediately surrounding the tumor. Blood flow to those areas increased after steroid treatment in all 3 patients. Interestingly, in the one area in which peritumoral blood flow was above normal prior to treatment, there was a decrease after steroid therapy. Two patients in whom mean cerebral blood flow returned to normal had complete amelioration of their clinical symptoms at the time the cerebral blood flow studies were repeated. The third patient had had only a moderate improvement. Similar results were obtained in a study by Hadjidimos and colleagues (1973). Capon and coworkers (1976) demonstrated that the increase in cerebral blood flow occurs before there is a demonstrable change in the size of the tumor and its surrounding edema, as evidenced by blood vessel shifts on arteriography.

Brain Water Content. It is possible to quantify brain edema by measuring the brain water content. In a study of patients with primary brain tumors (gliomas and meningiomas) and metastatic tumors, steroids have been shown to have no effect on the water content of the cerebral cortex (gray matter). In the white matter, however, the water content was 79.9% in untreated patients and 77.3% in patients treated with dexamethasone, an 8% decrease in brain volume. If patients were treated with both dexamethasone and furosemide, the water content was 75.5%, a further 5% decrease in brain volume (Lanksch et al. 1976). These data demonstrate a direct effect of steroids on brain edema and suggest that combinations of agents are more effective than single agents (Meinig et al. 1976; Long et al. 1976).

Untoward Effects of Steroids on the Brain

Glucocorticoids have marked effects on the physiology and metabolism of normal brain. These effects bear no clear relationship to the salutary clinical effects of steroids on the brain metastasis and its surrounding edema. Some of these changes are undesirable (table 23.2).

Glucocorticoids increase excitability of the brain and decrease the threshold both to electroshock and pentylenetetrazol-induced seizures. The lowered seizure threshold apparently results from intracerebral electrolyte alterations, particularly in intracellular sodium (Woodbury 1972). High doses of glucocorticoids given intraperitoneally to normal mice occa-

Table 23.2

SOME EFFECTS OF GLUCOCORTICOIDS ON BRAIN

A. Neurophysiology and behavior
    1. Increases excitability (seizures)
    2. Slows EEG and increases voltage
    3. Alters behavior (psychosis)

B. Brain metabolism
    1. No effect on electrolytes of normal brain
    2. No effect on cerebral blood flow or metabolism
    3. Increases brain glycogen
    4. Decreases protein synthesis
    5. Reduces carbohydrate use
    6. Decreases GABA concentration

C. Other effects
    1. Decreases CSF formation
    2. Inhibits glial growth
    3. Induces enzymes

sionally produce seizures, but there is no definite evidence that the doses of steroids used in humans produce seizures (Czerwinski et al. 1972; Novak et al. 1970). We have had the clinical impression, however, that some patients with brain metastases develop focal or generalized convulsions shortly after being started on steroids.

Glucocorticoids often alter behavior. Changes in mood are common in patients taking steroids, and both euphoria and depression have been reported (Axelrod 1976; Boston Collaborative Study 1972). Initially glucocorticoids produce a sense of well-being which may in part be related to the amelioration of clinical symptoms. Patients' appetites improve, and they feel generally stronger. Associated with this sense of well-being, however, there may be insomnia, agitation, and an increase in physiologic tremor. At times steroids may produce frank psychosis characterized by alterations in mood, illusions, hallucinations and paranoid ideation. Steroid psychosis may be a dose-related side effect. Fortunately, steroid psychosis is rare, and the incidents we have observed in patients on high-dose steroids were usually transient.

Some of the systemic side effects associated with glucocorticoid therapy are summarized in table 23.3. Several recent reviews have been devoted to side effects of steroids (Axelrod 1976; Bond 1977). Glucocorticoids decrease the resistance to infection, particularly to opportunistic infecting agents (Bond 1977). Steroids enhance the likelihood of metastasis from experimental tumors (Fidler and Lieber 1972). Steroids promote muscle catabolism and produce myopathy. Most patients with brain

Table 23.3

SOME SYSTEMIC EFFECTS OF GLUCOCORTICOIDS OF RELEVANCE
TO BRAIN METASTASIS

A. May promote metastatic spread

B. Decreases muscle strength (steroid myopathy)

C. Gastrointestinal bleeding and perforation

D. Steroid withdrawal syndromes

E. Decreases resistance to infections

F. Decreases carbohydrate tolerance

metastases who have been on steroids for more than 3–4 weeks have some degree of proximal muscle weakness. The weakness is clinically characterized by difficulty rising from the toilet seat or getting out of a low chair. The weakness is usually a nuisance rather than a true disability.

Changes in fatty distribution are well known and usually of no major consequence. Gastrointestinal bleeding, ulceration and perforation have been reported as a complication of steroid therapy (Jack and Porter 1978). Retrospective statistical analysis does not support a relationship between gastrointestinal bleeding and corticosteroid therapy, but the added risk of intracranial pathology, which by itself may produce gastrointestinal ulceration in the setting of glucocorticoid therapy, may produce bleeding (Silen 1977).

Preliminary evidence suggests that prophylactic administration of the gastric H_2 receptor antagonist, cimetidine, prevents the development of gastrointestinal ulceration (Gudmand-Hoyer et al. 1978). Gastrointestinal perforation, when it does occur, tends to be clinically silent because the anti-inflammatory effects of corticosteroids mask the peritoneal inflammatory response.

A peculiar side effect of high-dose intravenous dexamethasone is an anogenital burning sensation during rapid injection of the drug. The sensation subsides within a few minutes and can be minimized by slow injection (Czerwinski et al. 1972). No such symptoms appear to follow intravenous methylprednisolone injection.

Withdrawal from Steroids

At Memorial Sloan-Kettering Cancer Center we treat brain metastasis with glucocorticoids throughout the period of radiation therapy and then gradually taper to the lowest dose which permits maximum neurologic function. Approximately 50% of patients can be completely withdrawn from the drug, but there is often difficulty during the withdrawal from steroids: (1) When steroids have been clinically effective but other treatment does not substantially alter the tumor, the withdrawal of steroids leads to recurrence of symptoms. Reinstitution of the drug often relieves the symptoms again. (2) The so-called steroid withdrawal syndrome often mimics the signs and symptoms of recurrent brain metastasis but occurs even in patients without brain tumor. Amatruda and colleagues (1965) treated patients with tuberculosis with corticosteroids for 3 weeks. When the drugs were withdrawn, the patients complained of headache and postural dizziness. They became lethargic and anorexic, and some developed nausea and vomiting. The syndrome was reversed by reinstitution of steroids but was not related to laboratory evidence of adrenal insufficiency. Such symptoms in patients with brain metastases would likely be attributed to recurrence of the tumor.

In some patients, withdrawal of steroids after prolonged usage leads to increased intracranial pressure and papilledema (Byyny 1976). Pseudotumor cerebri also occurs in Addison's disease and may be a result of increased brain sodium (Woodbury 1972). A peculiar symptom that suggests a steroid withdrawal syndrome is called *pseudorheumatism* (Rotstein and Good 1957). As steroids are withdrawn, many patients develop muscle and joint pains, often so severe that they are unable to walk. The steroid withdrawal syndrome can usually be circumvented by slowing the reduction in steroid dosage.

MECHANISMS OF GLUCOCORTICOID ACTION IN BRAIN METASTASES

Glucocorticoid hormones may exert their salutary effects on patients with symptomatic brain metastases in one of several ways:

(1) Glucocorticoids may directly affect the tumor by decreasing its size or rate of growth.

(2) Glucocorticoids may directly improve neurologic function even without changing the metastasis or its surrounding edema.

(3) Glucocorticoids may decrease cerebral edema by reducing its production or increasing its reabsorption.

(4) Independent of effects on edema, glucocorticoids may lower intracranial pressure, allowing for improvement of blood flow to potentially hypoxic areas of brain.

(5) Systemic effects of glucocorticoids may also contribute to their effects on brain metastases.

These potential effects of steroids on brain metastases are not mutually exclusive, and there is some evidence that each of them plays a role.

Oncolysis

There is no clinical evidence that solid tumors metastatic to brain are responsive to steroid therapy. In fact, in the first study of steroids and brain metastases, Kofman and coworkers (1957) noted dramatic improvement in patients with brain metastases from breast cancer even when the peripheral tumor did not respond. A metastatic lesion's sensitivity to steroids should parallel that of the primary (but see Slack and Bross 1975). Experimental evidence, both in vivo and in vitro, suggests that steroids have effects on certain types of primary and metastatic brain tumors: Kotsilimbas and colleagues (1967) implanted melanomas into the brains of mice and then treated the animals with steroids. They noted that the tumor size was smaller and survival longer in those animals treated with steroids, and suggested that the decreased water content of the surrounding tissues was a result of the smaller tumor size rather than a direct effect of the steroids. Gurcay and coworkers (1971) demonstrated inhibition of tumor growth in a rat glioma transplanted in the brain.

In tissue-cultured human glioblastoma and in subcutaneously implanted rat glioma and mouse ependymoblastoma, very high concentrations of dexamethasone and prednisolone inhibit growth (Grasso 1976; Guner et al. 1977; Mealey et al. 1971; Wright et al. 1969). This effect appears to be related to nonspecific cytotoxic damage.

In vitro growth inhibition by corticosteroids is dose-dependent (Grasso and Johnson 1977) and is associated with selective effects on enzyme and cyclic adenosine monophosphate (AMP) metabolism; the cell cycle of treated tumor cells appears lengthened, and oxygen utilization and anaerobic glycolysis are reduced (Wright et al. 1969). In a series of studies on both experimental primary and metastatic brain tumors, Shapiro and Posner (1974) demonstrated some effects of steroids: although incorporation of thymidine into DNA was inhibited by the glucocorticoid and the tumors so treated were smaller, effects on survival were minimal or absent. Thus, it is doubtful that in humans with brain metastases glucocorticoids bring about their dramatic responses by affecting the tumor itself.

Brain Excitability

Independent of pathologic states, corticosteroids directly affect cerebral function. Effects on developmental enzyme induction (Asmitia and McEwen 1974), stabilization of the resting membrane potential (Gruener and Stern 1972), single cell firing (Foote et al. 1972), and EEG activity (Feldman and Dafny 1970) have been described. The absence of endogenous steroids, whether experimental or clinical, is associated with CNS abnormalities which include changes in sensory threshold (for example, a patient with Addison's disease can detect odors at 1/10,000 of the normal threshold concentration) (Henkin 1975), in sodium (Baethmann and Van Harreveld 1972), and in calcium metabolism (Woodbury 1972).

Such widespread effects on neuronal function raise the possibility that in patients with brain metastases improvement may be related to these changes. In areas where cerebral function is depressed, glucocorticoids may facilitate neural activity independent of effects on underlying pathology. Support for this hypothesis comes from observations which suggest improvement in symptoms before changes in cerebral edema, tumor growth, or CSF pressure occur (Kullberg and West 1965). Pappius and McCann (1969) demonstrated in experimental animals that after a freeze injury which produced cerebral edema and slowing of the EEG, administration of adrenal corticosteroids normalized the EEG and thus electrical activity of the brain independent of alterations of water or electrolyte content of the surrounding edema. Matsuoka and coworkers (1978) noted improvement in the EEG within 20 minutes after injection of steroids in patients with brain metastases before significant changes in tumor or edema could occur.

Corticosteroids produce numerous specific effects both acutely and chronically on the healthy brain. They also correct disrupted brain function in patients with metastatic brain tumors. Whether glucocorticoid effects on normal brain are therapeutic to diseased brain requires further evaluation.

Cerebral Edema

Why brain edema produces symptoms is not known. Two possible mechanisms include ischemic dysfunction and toxic inhibition of neural activity. Edema, by increasing the volume of one compartment of brain at the expense of another, alters local tissue pressure and shifts cerebral structures within the closed cranial cavity. These cerebral herniations interfere with the blood supply to specific areas of brain. If these pathological shifts can be reversed, neurologic symptoms resolve. Another effect of cerebral edema might be direct toxic inhibition of local neural activity, particularly axonal transmission. The chemical composition of cerebral edema differs from normal brain extracellular fluid. Neurons and glia bathed in a transudate of plasma may not function normally. Perhaps the clearance of edema removes toxic components, resulting in improvement of symptoms.

Glucocorticoids have profound effects on cerebral edema surrounding brain metastases, and most clinicians and investigators believe that this effect accounts for the striking clinical improvement. Both clinical and experimental evidence support this hypothesis. Patients with brain metastases and little surrounding edema (as evidenced by CT scan) are less improved by steroid therapy than those patients with tumor surrounded by large amounts of edema.

Glucocorticoids may decrease peritumoral edema either by reducing edema production or by increasing clearance of edema (table 23.4). Each of these general mechanisms may be the result of several specific mechanisms (figs. 23.2 and 23.3).

Table 23.4

SOME POSTULATED EFFECTS OF STEROIDS ON CEREBRAL EDEMA

A. Decreased edema formation (decreased vascular permeability)
1. Reduce inflammation
2. Stabilize vascular membrane
3. Scavenge free radicals

B. Increased edema reabsorption
1. Bulk flow
   a. Decreased CSF formation
   b. Decreased CSF pressure
   c. Increased CBF (serotoninergic inhibition)

2. Transport
   a. Increased sodium transport ($Na^+ - K^+$ ATPase)
   b. Pinocytosis?

Edema Production

Vascular Permeability. Glucocorticoids decrease the permeability of injured blood vessels, limiting extravasation of edema (Ransohoff 1972). In patients with brain metastases, the amount of protein which enters the tumor from the plasma decreases after dexamethasone treatment (Reulen et al. 1972). Experimental evidence indicates that disruption of normal capillary permeability in the brain by radiofrequency or cold lesions, by tryethyltin, amphetamines and hypertension, or by prolonged seizures is prevented by pretreatment with glucocorticoids (Rovit and Hagan 1968; Long et al. 1976; Studer et al. 1973; Johannson 1978; Eisenberg et al. 1970). Steroid adjuvants, antioxidants, and alpha and beta sympathetic antagonists are without effect in these models (Long et al. 1976). No reported histologic changes in vessel morphology correlate with the therapeutic effects of glucocorticoids.

Local increases in serotonin concentration may contribute to increased vascular permeability in cerebral edema (Klatzo 1972). The additional serotonin presumably results from platelet release, as brain serotonin is concentrated in small and rather discrete areas of the central nervous system and this effect is thought to be a general one. Corticosteroids increase tryptophan hydroxylase activity in brain and increase tryptophan pyrolase activity in both brain and liver. The former enzyme helps synthesize; the latter degrades serotonin. The clinical significance of corticosteroid alterations in serotonin metabolism and their relationship to cerebral edema requires additional study.

Sodium Metabolism. Sodium and water concentrations are uniformly elevated in vasogenic edema associated with brain tumors. The

Figure 23.2.

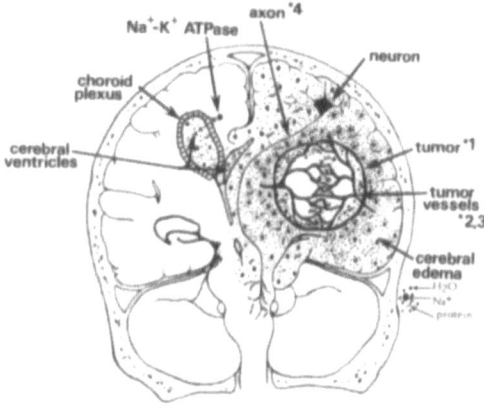

Effect of steroid therapy on production of cerebral edema in patients with brain metastases. Cerebral edema is produced by leakage of protein- and sodium-rich fluid through capillaries within the metastasis. Steroids may act by: (1) decreasing the size of the tumor itself, (2) decreasing the permeability of tumor vessels to large molecular substances, (3) restoring vasomotor stability, and (4) facilitating neuronal or axonal transmission. Mechanisms 1 and 2 would decrease the actual amount of cerebral edema present. Mechanism 3 might increase cerebral metabolism in the area surrounding the tumor, and mechanism 4 might improve neuronal functioning without altering the actual amount of edema.

Figure 23.3.

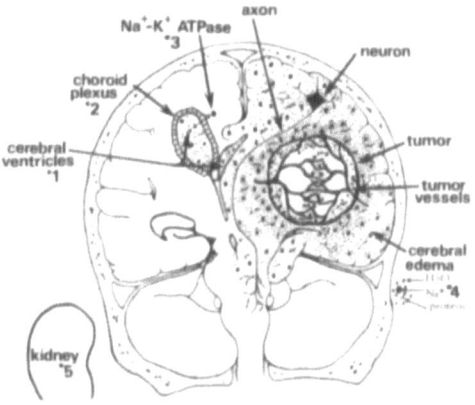

Effects of steroids on clearance of cerebral edema. Steroids may promote clearance of cerebral edema by: (1) decreasing CSF pressure, allowing more edema fluid to flow into the ventricular system, (2) decreasing CSF production, (3) enhancing Na⁺-K⁺ ATPase, (4) decreasing brain sodium, and (5) promoting systemic diuresis (high-dose steroids). All of these mechanisms are discussed in the text.

primary insult is probably an increased sodium concentration; water follows passively along the osmotic gradient so produced. Other pathologic states associated with increased brain sodium are also associated with increased intracranial pressure and cerebral edema. Examples of this include Addison's disease (Baethmann and Van Harreveld 1972) and steroid withdrawal or pseudotumor cerebri; both are corrected by the administration of corticosteroids.

One possible mechanism of glucocorticoid effect on sodium metabolism is via sodium-potassium adenosine triphosphatase (Na^+-K^+ ATPase). Renal, adrenal (Hendley et al. 1972) and intestinal (Charney et al. 1975) ATPase activity increase with corticosteroid administration. This has not been demonstrated in brain (Stastny 1971; Gallagher and Glaser 1968). Brain tumors are reported to increase Na^+-K^+ ATPase activity in surrounding neural tissue (Laws and O'Connor 1970). Brain areas resistant to cerebral edema, the arcuate nucleus and corpus callosum, are also resistant to the tumor-associated increase in Na^+-K^+ ATPase (Ransohoff 1972). The choroid plexus, which couples sodium transport to CSF formation, concentrates corticosteroids (McEwen et al. 1968) and in some species contains an Na^+-K^+ ATPase that is suppressed by these hormones (Miller et al. 1977; Weiss and Nulsen 1970). Corticosteroids appear to decrease sodium extravasation, enhance sodium clearance, and by action on the choroid plexus, decrease CSF production (Schwartz et al. 1972). These effects may be mediated by Na^+-K^+ ATPase.

Anti-inflammatory Effect.   Corticosteroids are known to have potent anti-inflammatory properties. This activity, at one time attributed to stabilization of lysosomal membranes, may bear on cerebral edema. Oxygen-free radicals have been proposed as the toxic molecules which produce leaks in cerebral vessels by disrupting membrane activity. They may likewise disrupt neural integrity and produce neurologic dysfunction in areas of peritumoral edema. Corticosteroids, because of their hydrophobic properties and lipid solubility, are thought to be able to intercollate into cell membranes and stabilize them against peroxidation (Ortega et al. 1972). Stabilization of both blood vessel and neuronal membranes would lead to decreased edema production and improved neurologic function. Ortega and colleagues (1972) have proposed free radical scavenging as the mechanism of corticosteroid improvement in cerebral edema. Corticosteroids do have nonspecific antioxidant effects (Long et al. 1972), but there is no clear evidence to support the theory of oxygen-free radical toxicity in brain edema.

Edema Clearance

Glucocorticoids promote clearance of cerebral edema by increasing the bulk flow of edema fluid into the lateral ventricles where it can be reabsorbed via normal CSF pathways (fig. 23.3) (Pappius 1975). Corticosteroids are reported to decrease CSF production by about 50%, probably by inhibiting Na^+-K^+ ATPase in the choroid plexus (Schwartz et al. 1972). Decreased CSF production leads to increased clearance of edema provided CSF absorption remains the same. Furosemide and acetazolamide, also reported to be effective agents in treating cerebral edema, appear to work in this fashion (Pappius 1972). Steroids, perhaps via this mechanism, decrease CSF pressure and increase brain compliance (Miller et al. 1977).

A further result of decreased CSF production is a fall in CSF pressure. When CSF pressure falls, the tissue–ventricle pressure gradient increases, resulting in increased bulk flow of edema into the ventricle. Steroid hormones also increase cerebral blood flow in the area of peritumoral edema. Why cerebral blood flow increases is not clear. It may be because there is less edema to compress small blood vessels. Its effect is to increase local tissue pressure, however, augmenting the gradient between the brain and ventricles and promoting increased bulk flow.

Systemic Effects

Adrenal corticosteroids, including cortisol, prednisone and dexamethasone, produce a systemic diuresis decreasing the peripheral edema associated with the nephrotic syndrome and heart failure (Heidorn and Schermm 1955), with cirrhosis and ascites (Stormont et al. 1959), and also with reduced sodium and water retention following craniotomy (Bouzarth et al. 1972). This diuretic effect appears independent of changes in aldosterone levels (Thomas and El-Shaboury 1971). It contributes to the resolution of cerebral edema.

CONCLUSIONS

Adrenocorticosteroids are the drugs of choice for the initial treatment of brain metastases. These drugs ameliorate clinical symptoms in 70–80% of patients and often stabilize their course for weeks to months. Steroids appear to have their primary effect on cerebral edema and probably act by both decreasing capillary permeability and by increasing the clearance of edema fluid. The mechanism(s) of action are not known but appear to be multiple. Until the mechanism(s) is established and a reproducible measure of response (such as a biochemical test) developed, it will be difficult to construct response curves to compare the various synthetic glucocorticoids with respect to efficacy.

REFERENCES

Alberti, E. et al. The effect of large doses of dexamethasone on the cerebrospinal fluid pressure in patients with supratentorial tumors. *J. Neurol.* 217:173–181, 1978.

Amatruda, T. T.; Hurst, M. M.; and D'Esopo, N. D. Certain endocrine and metabolic facets of the steroid withdrawal syndrome. *J. Clin. Endocr.* 25:1207–1217, 1965.

Axelrod, L. Glucocorticoid therapy. *Medicine* 55:39–65, 1976.

Azmitia, E. C., and McEwen, B. S. Adrenal cortical influence on rat brain tryptophan hydroxylase activity. *Brain Res.* 78:291–302, 1974.

Baethmann, A.; and Van Harreveld, A.: Physiological and biochemical findings in the central nervous system of adrenalectomized rats and mice. In *Steroids and brain edema*, eds. H. J. Reulen and K. Schurmann. Berlin: Springer-Verlag, 1972.

Bernard-Weil, E., and David, M. Preoperative hormonal treatment in cases of cerebral tumor. *Neurochirurgia* 4:127–134, 1963.

Bernard-Weil, E. et al. Clinical effects of combined vasopressin corticosteroid therapy in patients with recurrent grade III astrocytomas. *Neurochirurgia* 4:127–134, 1972.

Bond, W. Toxic reactions and side effects of glucocorticoids in man. *Am. J. Hosp. Pharm.* 34:479–485, 1977.

Boston Collaborative Drug Surveillance Program. Acute adverse reactions to prednisone in relation to dosage. *Clin. Pharm. Therap.* 13:694–698, 1972.

Bouzarth, W. E.; Shenkin, H. A.; and Gutterman, P. Adrenal cortical response to neurosurgical problems, noting the effects of exogenous steroids. In *Steroids and brain edema*, eds. H. J. Reulen and K. Schurmann. Berlin: Springer-Verlag, 1972.

Brooks, S. M. et al. Adverse effects of phenobarbital on corticosteroid metabolism in patients with bronchial asthma. *N. Engl. J. Med.* 286:1125–1128, 1972.

Byyny, R. L. Withdrawal from glucocorticoid therapy. *N. Engl. J. Med.* 295:30–32, 1976.

Capon, A. et al. Changes in regional cerebral blood flows produced by dexamethasone in patients with brain metastases. *Acta Neurol. Belg.* 76:325–330, 1976.

Charney, A. N. et al. Na^+-K^+ activated adenosine triphosphate and intestinal electrolyte transport. *J. Clin. Invest.* 56:653–660, 1975.

Crocker, E. F. et al. The effect of steroids on the extravascular distribution of radiographic contrast material and technetium pertechnetate in brain tumors as determined by computed tomography. *Radiology* 119:471–474, 1976.

Cruess, R. L. Steroid-induced avascular necrosis of the head of the humerus. *J. Bone Joint Surg.* 58:313–317, 1976.

Czerwinski, A. W. et al. Effects of a single, large, intravenous injection of dexamethasone. *Clin. Pharm. Therap.* 13:638–642, 1972.

Diez, J. A.; Sze, P. Y.; and Ginsburg, B. E. Effects of hydrocortisone and electric foot shock on mouse brain tyrosine hydroxylase activity and tyrosine levels. *Neurochem. Res.* 2:161–170, 1977.

Ehrlich, P. Das Sauerstoffbedurfnis des Organismus. In *Eine Far-benanalytische Studie*. Berlin: 1885, Hirschwald.

Eisenberg, H.; Barlow, C.; and Lorenzo, A. Effect of dexamethasone on altered brain vascular permeability. *Arch. Neurol.* 23:18–22, 1970.

Feldman, S., and Dafny, N. Effects of adrenocortical hormones on the electrical activity of the brain. In *Progress in brain research*, vol. 32, ed. D. Deweid, and *J.A.M.A.* Weijnen. Amsterdam: Elsevier Publ. Co., 1970.

Fidler, I. J., and Lieber, S. Quantitative analysis of the mechanism of glucocorticoid enhancement of experimental metastasis. *Res. Comm. Chem. Path. Pharm.* 4:607–613, 1972.

Fishman, R. A. Brain edema. *New Engl. J. Med.* 293:706–711, 1975.

Fishman, R. A. Cerebrospinal fluid. In *Clinical neurology*, Hagerstown, Maryland: Harper & Row, 1977.

Fletcher, J. W. et al. Brain scans, dexamethasone therapy, and brain tumors. *J.A.M.A.* 232:1261–1263, 1975.

Foote, W. E. et al. Effect of hydrocortisone on single unit activity in midbrain raphe. *Brain Res.* 41:242–244, 1972.

French, L. A. The use of steroids in the treatment of cerebral edema. *Bull. N.Y. Acad. Med.* 42:301–311, 1966.

Galicich, J. H., and French, L. A. Use of dexamethasone in the treatment of cerebral edema resulting from brain tumors and brain surgery. *AP-DT* 12:169–174, 1961.

Gallagher, B. B., and Glaser, G. H. Seizure threshold, adrenalectomy, and Na-K stimulated ATPase in rat brain. *J. Neurochem.* 15:525–528, 1968.

Goldmann, E. E. Die aussere und innere Sekretion des gesunden und kranken Organismus im Lichte der "vitalen farbung." *Beitr. Z. Klin. Chir.* 64:192–265, 1909.

Gottlieb, J. A.; Frei, E.; and Luce, J. K. An evaluation of the management of patients with cerebral metastases from malignant melanoma. *Cancer* 29:701–705, 1972.

Graber, A. L. et al. Natural history of pituitary adrenal recovery following long-term suppression with corticosteroids. *J. Clin. Endocr. Metab.* 25:11–16, 1965.

Grasso, R. J. Transient inhibition of cell proliferation in rat glioma monolayer cultures by cortisol. *Cancer Res.* 36:2408–2414, 1976.

Grasso, R. J., and Johnson, C. E. Dose-response relationships between glucocorticoids and growth inhibitors. *Proc. Soc. Exp. Med. Biol.* 154:238–241, 1977.

Gruener, R., and Stern, L. Corticosteroids: effects on muscle membrane excitability. *Arch. Neurol.* 26:181–185, 1972.

Gudmand-Hoyer, E. et al. Prophylactic effect of Cimetidine in duodenal ulcer disease. *Br. Med. J.* 1:1095–1096, 1978.

Guner, M. et al. Effects of dexamethasone and betamethasone on *in vitro* cultures from human astrocytoma. *Br. J. Cancer* 35:439–447, 1977.

Gurcay, O. et al. Corticosteroid effect on transplantable rat glioma. *Arch. Neurol.* 24:266–269, 1971.

Gutin, P. H. Corticosteroid therapy in patients with cerebral tumors: benefits, mechanisms, problems, practicalities. *Sem. Oncol.* 2:49–56, 1975.

Gutin, P. H. Corticosteroid therapy in patients with brain tumors. In *National Cancer Institute Monograph #46*, 1977.

Hadjidimos, A. et al. The effects of dexamethasone on RCBF and cerebral vasomotor response in brain tumors. *Europ. Neurol.* 10:25–30, 1973.

Haque, N. et al. Studies on dexamethasone metabolism in man: effect of diphenylhydantoin. *J. Clin. Endocr.* 34:44–50, 1972.

Hazra, T.; Mullins, G. M.; and Lott, S. Management of cerebral metastasis from bronchogenic carcinoma. *Hopkins Med. J.* 130:377–383, 1972.

Heidorn, G. H., and Schermm, F. R. The clinical use of corticotropin (ACTH) and adrenal corticosteroids. *Am. J. Med. Sci.* 229:621–631, 1955.

Hendley, E. D. et al. Effects of adrenalectomy and hormone replacement on Na$^+$-K$^+$ ATPase in renal tissue. *Am. J. Physiol.* 222:754–760, 1972.

Henkin, R. I. Effects of ACTH, adrenocorticosteroids, and thyroid hormone on sensory function. In *Anatomical neuroendocrinology*, eds. E. Stumpf and L. D. Grant. Basel: S. Karger, 1975.

Horton, J. et al. The management of metastases to the brain by irradiation and corticosteroids. *Am. J. Roent.* 3:334–336, 1971.

Ingraham, F. D.; Matson, D. D.; and McLaurin, R. L. Cortisone and ACTH as an adjunct to the surgery of craniopharyngiomas. *N. Engl. J. Med.* 246:568–571, 1952.

Jick, H., and Porter, J. Drug-induced gastrointestinal bleeding. *Lancet* 1:87–89, 1978.

Johannson, B. Effect of dexamethasone on protein extravasation in the brain in acute hypertension induced by amphetamine. *Acta Neurol. Scand.* 57:180–185, 1978.

Johnson, I.; Gilday, D. L.; and Hendrick, E. B. Experimental effects of steroids and steroid withdrawal on cerebrospinal fluid absorption. *J. Neurosurg.* 42:690–695, 1975.

Klatzo, I. Pathophysiologic aspects of brain edema. In *Steroids and brain edema*, ed. H. J. Reulen and K. Schurmann. Berlin: Springer-Verlag, 1972.

Kofman, S. et al. Treatment of cerebral metastases from breast carcinoma with prednisolone. *J.A.M.A.* 163:1473–1476, 1957.

Kotsilimbas, D. G. et al. Corticosteroid effect on intracerebral melanomata and associated cerebral edema. *Neurology* 17:223–226, 1967.

Kullberg, G., and West, K. A. Influence of corticosteroids on the ventricular fluid pressure. *Acta Neurol. Scand.* (suppl.) 13:445–452, 1965.

Lanksch, W. et al. CT findings in brain edema compared with direct chemical analysis of tissue samples. In *Dynamics of brain edema*, eds. H. M. Pappias and W. Feindel. Berlin: Springer-Verlag, 1976.

Laws, E. R., and O'Connor, J. S. ATPase in human brain tumors. *J. Neurosurg.* 33:167–171, 1970.

Lieberman, A. et al. Use of high-dose corticosteroids in patients with inoperable brain tumors. *J. Neurol. Neurosurg. Psychiat.* 40:678–682, 1977.

Long, D. M.; Hartmann, J. F.; and French, L. A. The response of human cerebral edema to glucosteroid administration. An electron microscopic study. *Neurology* 16:521–528, 1966.

Long, D. M.; Maxwell, R. E.; and French, L. A. The effects of glucosteroids upon experimental brain edema. In *Steroids and brain edema*, ed. H. J. Reulen and R. Schurmann. Berlin: Springer-Verlag, 1972.

Long, D. M.; Maxwell, R.; and Choi, K. S. A new therapy regimen for brain edema. In *Dynamics of brain edema*, ed. H. M. Pappius and W. Feindel. Berlin: Springer-Verlag, 1976.

Lundberg, N. Continuous recording and control of ventricular fluid pressure in neurosurgical practice. *Acta Psychiat. Neurol. Scand. Suppl.* 149:1–193, 1960.

Marshall, L. F.; King, J.; and Langfitt, T. W. The complications of high-dose corticosteroid therapy in neurosurgical patients: a prospective study. *Ann. Neurol.* 1:201–203, 1977.

Marty, R., and Cain, M. L. Effects of corticosteroid (dexamethasone) administration on the brain scan. *Radiology* 107:117–121, 1973.

Marynick, S. P., et al. Studies on the transfer of steroid hormones across the blood-cerebrospinal barrier in the rhesus monkey. II. *Endocrinology* 101:562–567, 1977.

Matsuoka, S. et al. The effect of dexamethasone on electroencephalograms in patients with brain tumors. With specific reference to topographic computer display of delta activity. *J. Neurosurg.* 48:601–608, 1978.

Mayman, C. I., and Tijerina, M. L. Inhibitory effect of steroids on Na^+-K^+ ATPase of human choroid plexus. *Neurology* 28:368, 178.

McEwen, B.; Weiss, J.; and Schwartz, L. Selective retention of corticosterone by limbic structures in rat brain. *Nature* 220:911–912, 1968.

McLelland, J., and Jack, W. Phenytoin/dexamethasone interaction: a clinical problem. *Lancet* 1096–1097, 1978.

Mealey, J.; Chen T. T.; and Schanz G. P. Effects of dexamethasone and methylprednisolone on cell cultures of human glioblastomas. *J. Neurosurg.* 34:324–334, 1971.

Meikle, A. W., and Tyler, F. H. Potency and duration of action of glucocorticoids; effects of hydrocortisone, prednisone and dexamethasone on human pituitary-adrenal function. *Am. J. Med.* 63:200–207, 1977.

Menig, G.; Aulich, A.; Wende, S.; and Reulen, H. J. The effect of dexamethasone and diuretics on peritumor brain edema: comparative study of tissue water content and CT. In *Dynamics of brain edema*, ed. H. M. Pappius, W. Feindel. Berlin: Springer-Verlag, 1976.

Miller, J. D.; Sakalas, R.; Ward, J. D. et al. Methylprednisolone treatment in patients with brain tumors. *Neurosurgery* 1:114–117, 1977.

Murphy, B. E. P.; et al. Adrenal corticoid levels in human cerebrospinal fluid. *Canad. Med. Assoc. J.* 97:13–17, 1967.

Novak, E.; Stubbs, S. S.; Seckman, C. E. et al. Effects of a single large intravenous dose of methylprednisolone sodium succinate. *Clin. Pharm. Therap.* 11:711–717, 1970.

Ortega, B. O.; Demopoulos, H. B.; Ransohoff, J. Effects of antioxidants on experimental cold-induced cerebral edema. P. 167. In *Steroids and brain edema*, eds. H. J. Reulen, K. Schurmann. Berlin: Springer-Verlag, 1972.

Pappius, H. M. Effects of steroids on cold injury edema. In *Steroids and brain edema*, eds. H. J. Reulen, R. Schurmann. Berlin: Springer-Verlag, 1972.

Pappius, H. M. Normal and pathological distribution of water in brain. P. 194. In *Fluid environment of the brain*, eds. H. F. Cserr, J. D. Fenstermacher, V. French. New York: Academic Press, 1975.

Pappius, H. M., and McCann, W. P. Effects of steroids on cerebral edema in cats. *Arch. Neurol.* 20:207–216, 1969.

Perret, G. E., and Kernohan, J. W. Histopathologic changes of the brain caused by intracranial tumors. *J. Neuropath. Exp. Neurol.* 2:341–352, 1943.

Posner, J. B. Diagnosis and treatment of metastases to the brain. *Clin. Bull.* 4:47–57, 1974.

Prados, M.; Strowger, B.; and Feindel, W. H. Studies on cerebral edema. II. Reaction of the brain to exposure to air; physiologic changes. *Arch. Neurol. Psychiat.* 54:290–300, 1945.

Ransohoff, J. The effects of steroids on brain edema in man. Pp. 211–217. In *Steroids and brain edema*, ed. H. J. Reulen and K. Schurmann. Berlin: Springer-Verlag, 1972.

Rapoport, S. I. *Blood-Brain barrier in physiology and medicine*. New York: Raven Press, 1976.

Rasmussen, T., and Gulati, D. R. Cortisone in the treatment of postoperative cerebral edema. *J. Neurosurg.* 19:535–544, 1962.

Renaudin, J.; Fewer, D.; Wilson, C. B. et al. Dose dependency of Decadron in patients with partially excised brain tumors. *J. Neurosurg.* 39:302–305, 1973.

Reulen, H. J. Vasogenic brain edema. *Br. J. Anaesth.* 48:741–752, 1976.

Reulen, H. J.; Hadjidimos, A. M.; Schurmann, K. The effect of dexamethasone on water and electrolyte content and on CBF in perifocal brain edema in man. In *Steroids and brain edema*, eds. H. J. Reulen, K. Schurmann. Berlin: Springer-Verlag, 1972, p. 239.

Rotstein, J., and Good, R. A. Steroid pseudorheumatism. *Arch. Int. Med.* 99:545-555, 1957.

Rovit, R., and Hagan, R. Steroids and cerebral edema: the effects of glucocorticoids in abnormal capillary permeability following cerebral injury in cats. *J. Neuropath. Exp. Neurol.* 27:277–299, 1968.

Ruderman, N. B., and Hall, T. C. Use of glucocorticoids in the palliative treatment of metastatic brain tumors. *Cancer* 18:298–306, 1965.

Sadasivudu, B.; Rao, T. I.; and Murthy, C. R. K. Metabolic effects of hydrocortisone in mouse brain. *Neurochem. Res.* 2:521–532, 1977.

Schaul, N.; Ball, G.; Gloor, P.; and Pappius, H. M. The EEG in cerebral edema. Pp. 144–149 in *Dynamics of brain edema*, ed. H. M. Pappius, W. Feindel. Berlin: Springer-Verlag, 1976.

Schwartz, M. L.; Tator, C. H.; and Hoffman, H. J. The uptake of hydrocortisone in mouse brain and ependymoblastoma. *J. Neurosurg.* 36:178–183, 1972.

Shapiro, W. R., and Posner, J. B. Corticosteroid hormones. *Arch. Neurol.* 30:217–221, 1974.

Silen, W. Peptic ulcer. P. 1494 in *Harrison's Textbook of Medicine*. New York: McGraw-Hill, 1977.

Slack, N. H., and Bross, I. D. J. The influence of site of metastasis on tumour growth and response to chemotherapy. *Br. J. Cancer* 32:78–86, 1975.

Stastny, F. Hydrocortisone as a possible inductor of Na^+-K^+ ATPase in the chick cerebral hemispheres. *Brain Res.* 25:397–410, 1971.

Steudel, W. I.; Beck, U.; and Becker, H. Perifocal edema in computerized tomography and EEG changes in patients with tumors of cerebral hemispheres. P. 188–191 in *Cranial computerized tomography*, ed. W. Lanksch, and E. Kazner. Berlin: Springer-Verlag, 1976.

Stjernholm, M. R., and Katz, F. H. Effects of diphenylhydantoin, phenobarbital, and diazepam on the metabolism of methylprednisolone and its sodium succinate. *J. Clin. Endocrinol. Metab.* 41:887–893, 1975.

Stormon, J. M. et al. The effect of prednisone and amphenone on fluid and electrolyte balance and on aldosterone secretion of patients with cirrhosis and ascites. *J. Lab. Clin. Med.* 53:396–416, 1959.

Studer, R. K.; Siegle, B. A.; Norgan, J.; and Potchen, E. J. Dexamethasone therapy of triethyltin induced cerebral edema. *Exp. Neurol.* 38:429–437, 1973.

Thomas, J. P., and El-Shaboury, A. H. Aldosterone secretion in steroid-treated patients with adrenal suppression. *Lancet* 1:623–625, 1971.

Vincent, F. M. Phenytoin/dexamethasone interaction. *Lancet* 1:1360, 1978.

Waxman, A. D.; Beldon, J. R.; Richli, W. et al. Steroid-induced suppression of gallium uptake in tumors of the central nervous system: concise communication. *J. Nucl. Med.* 19:480–482, 1978.

Weinstein, J. D.; Toy, F. J.; Jaffe, M. E. et al. The effect of dexamethasone on brain edema in patients with metastatic brain tumors. *Neurology* 23:121–129, 1973.

Weiss, M. H., and Nulsen, F. E. The effects of glucocorticoids on CSF flow in dogs. *J. Neurosurg.* 32:452–458, 1970.

Werk, E. E.; Choi, Y.; Sholiton, L. et al. Interference in the effect of dexamethasone by diphenylhydantoin. *N. Engl. J. Med.* 281:32–34, 1969.

Woodbury, D. M. Biochemical effects of adreno-cortical steroids on the central nervous system. Pp. 255–287 in *Handbook of neurochemistry*, vol. VII. New York: Plenum Press, 1972.

Wright, R. L.; Shaumba, B.; and Keller, J. The effect of glucocorticosteroids on growth and metabolism of experimental glial tumors. *J. Neurosurg.* 30:140–145, 1969.

24

Combined Chemotherapy and Irradiation in the Treatment of Brain Metastases from Lung Cancer

Paul Y. M. Chan
John E. Byfield
Thomas Campbell
Leonard Sadoff
Aroor R. Rao

As noted elsewhere in this volume, treatment of brain metastases by either radiotherapy or chemotherapy, with or without steroids, has been disappointing: although radiation therapy has been shown to improve the quality of life (Hendrickson 1975; Order et al. 1968), the average duration of survival is only 3–6 months. Among patients with lung cancer and brain metastases, the response is very poor particularly with non-oat cell carcinoma. This chapter reports our experience with concomitant doxorubicin hydrochloride (Adriamycin), CCNU and radiation therapy in the treatment of brain metastases from lung cancer exclusively.

PATIENTS AND METHODS

Patients with brain metastases from primary carcinoma of the lung were entered into this study between June 1975 and October 1977. Diagnosis of brain metastases was established by a positive radionuclide brain scan. Each patient's performance status was classified according to the RTOG neurologic function levels (Hendrickson 1975; Order et al. 1968). Four levels were designated: (1) Able to work, neurologic findings minor or absent; (2) able to be at home although nursing care might be required, neurologic findings present but not serious; (3) requires hospitalization and medical care with major neurologic findings; (4) requires hospitalization and in serious physical or neurologic state including coma. Complete

364

blood count, hemoglobin, hematocrit, urinalysis, electrocardiogram, liver profile and occasionally bone marrow studies were obtained for all the patients prior to entry.

The treatment program consisted of concomitant administration of doxorubicin hydrochloride, CCNU, and external radiotherapy. Cyclophosphamide (Cytoxan) was also given to patients with oat-cell carcinoma. Doxorubicin hydrochloride (40–50 mg/m²) was administered intravenously every 3 weeks whereas CCNU (50–60 mg/m²) was given simultaneously by mouth with doxorubicin hydrochloride on day 1 and every 6 weeks. For patients with oat-cell carcinoma, cyclophosphamide (300 mg/m²) was added on day 1 and every 3 weeks.

Four MV X-irradiation to the whole brain was carried out concomitantly with chemotherapy. The tumor dose to the brain was 2,000 rads given in 5 consecutive days and repeated after a 3-week rest. Thus a total of 4,000 rads was delivered in the first 5 weeks. Dexamethasone (4 mg) was given immediately on the diagnosis of brain metastasis and was repeated every 6–8 hours. Complete blood count, urinalysis, and EKG were done prior to each cycle of chemotherapy. No chemotherapy was given when the white blood count was below 2,500/mm³, the hemoglobin was below 10gm%, the platelet count was below 100,000 mm³, or the EKG tracing was abnormal.

EVALUATION OF PATIENTS

On the eighth week, when the patients returned for the third course of doxorubicin hydrochloride, their neurologic function was assessed as complete, partial, or absent. The response was evaluated every 3 weeks until death. Three months after the inception of treatment, a radionuclide brain scan was obtained and graded as normal, 50% improvement, no change, or worse. It was mandatory that patients were taken off steroid therapy before doing the brain scan. When the patient died, attempts were made to obtain an autopsy; failing this, the cause of death was determined on the basis of clinical findings. Special attention was paid to whether the cause of death was the result of brain metastasis.

RESULTS

Over 28 months, 24 patients with brain metastases from primary lung cancer were entered into the study. The average age was 53 years (range 44–65); there were 17 male and 7 female patients (table 24.1).

According to histopathologic diagnosis of the primary lesions, 3 patients had oat-cell carcinoma; of the others, 15 had epidermoid carcinoma, 4 had adenocarcinoma, and 2 had large anaplastic-cell carcinoma.

In an analysis of clinical signs and symptoms, 62% or 15 patients had headaches; 70%, motor deficits; 21%, sensory deficits; 50%, aphasia and

Table 24.1

24 PATIENTS WITH BRAIN METASTASIS OF PRIMARY LUNG CANCER
(JUNE 1975–OCTOBER 1977)

Age	Average	53 years
	range	44–65
Sex	Male/	17
	female	7
	ratio	2.4:1
Cell type	Oat cell carcinoma	3
	Non-oat cell carcinoma	21

Signs and Symptoms	**Number of Patients**	**%**
Headaches	15	62
Motor deficit	17	70
Sensory deficit	5	21
Aphasia and intellectual impairment	12	50
Changes of awareness	8	33
Seizures	4	16
Papilledema	6	25
Cerebellar signs	5	21
Multiple symptoms and signs	16	66

intellectual impairment; 33%, changes of awareness; 15%, seizures; 25%, papilledema; and 21%, cerebellar signs. Sixteen patients (66%) showed multiple symptoms and signs of brain metastases (table 24.1). Two of the 24 patients (patients F.W. and G.B. in table 24.2), had simultaneous presentation of cerebral metastases and primary lung cancer at diagnosis.

Of the 24 patients, 22 patients were evaluated (table 24.3) with two exclusions (1 patient committed suicide, and the other refused further treatment after the first course of radiation). The mean total dosage of doxorubicin hydrochloride was 160 mg/m²; CCNU, 200 mg/m²; and cyclophosphamide, 3,295 mg/m². Alopecia occurred in all patients. Over

50% of the patients experienced nausea and anorexia, but otherwise treatment was well tolerated. No hematopoietic toxicity or cardiotoxicity was apparent. Among the 22 evaluable patients, the neurologic function response was complete in 82% and partial in 18% (table 24.4). The median duration of response has been 8 months (table 24.2).

Three months after completion of treatment, 15 patients had normal radionuclide brain scans (fig. 24.1), 5 patients showed 50% improvement (fig. 24.2), and only 2 patients showed no changes (table 24.4).

In analyzing the causes of death, two of the 14 deaths were directly due to brain lesions; the others died of intrathoracic spread or wider dissemination of disease. One patient died of acute myocardial infarction which was not related to doxorubicin hydrochloride toxicity. Autopsies were performed for 3 of the 14 deaths. The postmortem findings on 1 patient (S.F.) provided no evidence of brain metastases, thus confirming both the clinical assessment and brain scan which indicated a complete response.

At present, 8 patients are still alive after 10–18 months. Among these 8 survivors, 2 patients show no evidence of disease and have lived 12 and 18 months, respectively (fig. 24.3). The median survival time of 22 evaluable patients has been 8 months.

DISCUSSION

Since Chao and others (1954) reported their Roentgen-ray therapy experience for the treatment of cerebral metastasis, external irradiation has become a standard palliative procedure. In general, radiation therapy with or without steroids at a tumor dose of 3,000–4,000 rads given in 2–4 weeks has been reported to yield a 60–70% neurologic improvement, a remission duration of 3–5 months, and a survival of 3–6 months (Chao et al. 1954; Deeley and Edwards 1968; Newman and Hansen 1974; Nisce et al. 1971; Order et al. 1968). In a series of 81 patients receiving a single dose of 1,000 rads and steroids, Shehata and others (1974) reported an excellent response in 35%, a fair response in 40%, and no response in 25%; a mean survival of 5 months was recorded.

Whole-brain irradiation certainly improves the quality of survival in patients with brain metastases. Adrenocorticosteroids are a very valuable adjunct in the management of brain metastasis and often cause a dramatic, but short-lived response (see Chapter 23). According to RTOG studies reported by Hendrickson (1975), steroids improved neurologic function more quickly in the first 3 weeks; by the fourth week, there was no difference in improvement between patients who received steroids and those who did not receive steroids. Thus the value of the antineoplastic effect of steroids was questioned, and it was concluded that steroids offer no survival advantage.

One of the main uses of steroid therapy emphasized in the literature is to provide a reliable indication of response to future treatment. A good

Table 24.2

CONCOMITANT DOXORUBICIN HYDROCHLORIDE, CCNU, AND RADIATION THERAPY IN 24 PATIENTS WITH BRAIN METASTASIS OF PRIMARY LUNG CANCER

Name	Sex	Age	Cell Type	Status of Primary Lesion	Functional Level	Other Sites of Metastasis	Brain Metastasis		
							XRT† 4,000 Rads	DH‡ mg/m²	CCNU mg/m²
B. M.	F	44	Epidermal	Post-lobectomy 6 mos.	IV	—	x	280	400
A. C.	M	52	Adeno-carcinoma	PR 4 mos. RA	III	Liver?	x	140	180
R. C.	M	53	Epidermal	Lobectomy 8 mos.	II	Lung	x	120	160
S. F.	F	49	Adeno-carcinoma	Lobectomy 2 wks.	II	—	x	160	180
F. W.	M	50	Epidermal	CR at 3 mos. on RA	III	Brain and lung lesions at diagnosis	x	240	620
R. G.	F	54	Large anaplastic	CR 6 mos. post-RA	IV	—	x	180	300
M. M.	M	61	Adeno-carcinoma	Post-lobectomy 3 yrs.	III	—	2,000 rads	80	100
H. G.	F	63	Epidermal	CR 10 mos. post-RA	II	—	x	160	300
R. B.	M	64	Epidermal	PR 4 mos. on RA	III	—	x	120	180
F. H.	M	61	Oat cell	CR 4 mos. on RB	IV	—	x	140	160

Therapy Cyclophosphamide mg/m²	Response and Duration in Mos.	Survival in Mos.	Brain Scan at 3 Mos.	Final Functional Level	Cause of Death Brain	Cause of Death Other	Remarks
—	CR 13	14	Negative	II	Yes 2 wks.	Post craniotomy	Relapse at 13 mos. and CT scan positive
—	PR 6	6	↓50%	I	No	Lung and liver	
—	CR 7	7	↓50%	I		Lung	
—	CR 8	8	Negative	I		Lung	Brain negative at autopsy
—	CR 18	18	Negative	I		Alive	
—	CR 12	12	Negative	I	No	MI	
—	— —	—	—	I	—	—	
—	CR 8	8	Negative	I	No	Liver and bones	
—	PR 7	8	↓50%	III	Yes	Metastases to bone, liver, adrenal glands	Seen at autopsy
4,600	PR 6	6	↓50%	I	No	Dissemination	

Table 24.2 (Continued)

Name	Sex	Age	Cell Type	Status of Primary Lesion	Functional Level	Other Sites of Metastasis	Brain Metastasis		
							XRT † 4,000 Rads	DH ‡ mg/m²	CCNU mg/m²
P. B.	M	62	Oat cell	CR 3 mos. post-RB	II	—	x	220	360
L. T.	M	53	Epidermal	CR 2 mos. on RA	III	—	x	180	200
G. B.	F	52	Epidermal	PR 3 mos. on RA	II	Brain and lung lesions at diagnosis	x	180	240
R. S.	M	46	Epidermal	PR 6 mos. on RA	II	Bone and liver	x	120	160
J. S.	M	51	Epidermal	CR 4 mos. post-RA ′	III	—	x	180	300
M. S.	M	64	Oat cell	CR 1 mo. post-RB	III	Liver	x	140	200
C. L.	M	57	Adeno-carcinoma	Lobectomy 2 yrs.	II	Bone?	x	180	200
S. V.	F	57	Epidermal	CR 14 mos. post-RA	III	—	x	140	200
S. B.	M	61	Epidermal	Post-lobectomy 13 mos.	II	Intrathoractic recurrence	x	180	300
R. S.	F	46	Epidermal	CR 16 mos. post-RA	II	—	x	180	400
J. I.	M	54	Epidermal	PR 10 mos. on RA	III	—	x	140	120

Table 24.2 (Continued)

Therapy Cyclophos- phamide mg/m²	Response and Duration in Mos.	Survival in Mos.	Brain Scan at 3 Mos.	Final Functional Level	Cause of Death Brain	Other	Remarks
9,800	CR 15	15	Negative	I		Alive	Liver metastasis
—	CR 5	5	Negative	I	No	Lung	
5,200	CR 12	12	Negative	I		Alive	CT scan also negative
—	CR 5	5	NC	I	No	Dissemination	
—	CR 12	12	Negative	I		Alive	NED
2,400	CR 2	3	Negative	II	No	Hepatic coma	
—	CR 11	11	Negative	I		Alive	Bone metastasis?
—	CR 6	7	Negative	II	No	Lung, adrenal glands	CT scan and autopsy, Brain positive
—	CR 11	11	↓50%	I		Alive	Lung recurrence
—	CR 10	10	Negative	I		Alive	Relapse in lung?
—	CR 4	10	—	I	No	Dissemination	

Table 24.2 (Continued)

Name	Sex	Age	Cell Type	Status of Primary Lesion	Functional Level	Other Sites of Metastasis	Brain Metastasis		
							XRT† 4,000 Rads	DH‡ mg/m²	CCNU mg/m²
W. L.	M	61	Epidermal	Pneumonectomy 20 mos.	II	—	x	170	160
M. L.	M	62	Large anaplastic	No therapy	IV	—	2,000	50	100
K. W.	M	63	Epidermal	Lobectomy 26 mos.	III	Bone	x	160	200

*CR = complete response; PR = partial response; NR = no response; NC = no change.
RA = Regimen consists of doxorubicin, bleomycin, and radiation therapy.
RB = Regimen consists of doxorubicin, cyclophosphamide, and radiation therapy.
†XRT = External radiation therapy.
‡DH = Doxorubicin hydrochloride (Adriamycin).

Therapy Cyclophosphamide mg/m²	Response and Duration in Mos.	Survival in Mos.	Brain Scan at 3 Mos.	Final Functional Level	Cause of Death Brain	Other	Remarks
—	PR 2	3	NC	I	No	Dissemination	
—	— —	—	—	—	—	—	Refused further treatment
—	CR 10	10	Negative	I		Alive	Bone metastasis

Table 24.3

24 PATIENTS WITH CEREBRAL METASTASIS (OF PRIMARY LUNG CANCER) TREATED WITH DOXORUBICIN, CCNU AND RADIOTHERAPY

Pretreatment RTOG Functional Stage	I	II	III	IV	Total
Number of patients	0	10	10	4	24
Evaluated	0	10	9	3	22
Not evaluated 1 suicide 1 refusal of further treatment	0	0	1	1	2

Table 24.4

RESULTS OF TREATMENT

	I	II	III	IV	Total	(%)
Posttreatment RTOG Functional Stage						
Complete response	0	9	7	2	18	(82)
Partial response	0	1	2	1	4	(18)
No response	0	0	0	0	0	
Brain scan 3 mos. after treatment (off steroid)						
Normal	0	7	5	2	14	(66)
50% improvement	0	2	2	1	5	(24)
No change	0	1	1	0	2	(10)
No follow-up brain scan	0	0	1	0	1	
Worsened	0	0	0	0	0	

Causes of death in 14 patients	Number of Patients	%
Brain death	2	(14)
Intrathoracic disease	5	(36)
Liver, bone, or generalized metastases	6	(43)
Other	1	(7)
Median survival time 8 mos.*		

*8 patients still alive at 10, 10, 11, 11, 11, 12, 15, and 18 mos; 2 patients, no evidence of disease at 12 and 18 mos.

Figure 24.1.

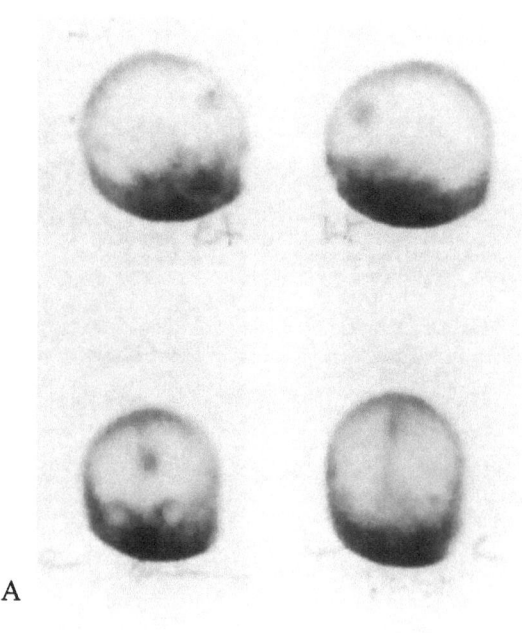

A

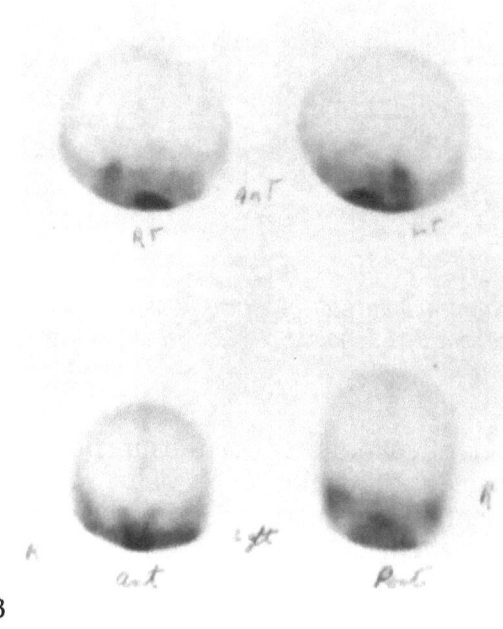

B

A. *Pretreatment radionuclide brain scan of patient B. M. on 8-19-75. (Details in table 24.2). B. Posttreatment radionuclide brain scan of patient B. M. showed normal uptake on 11-18-75.*

Figure 24.2.

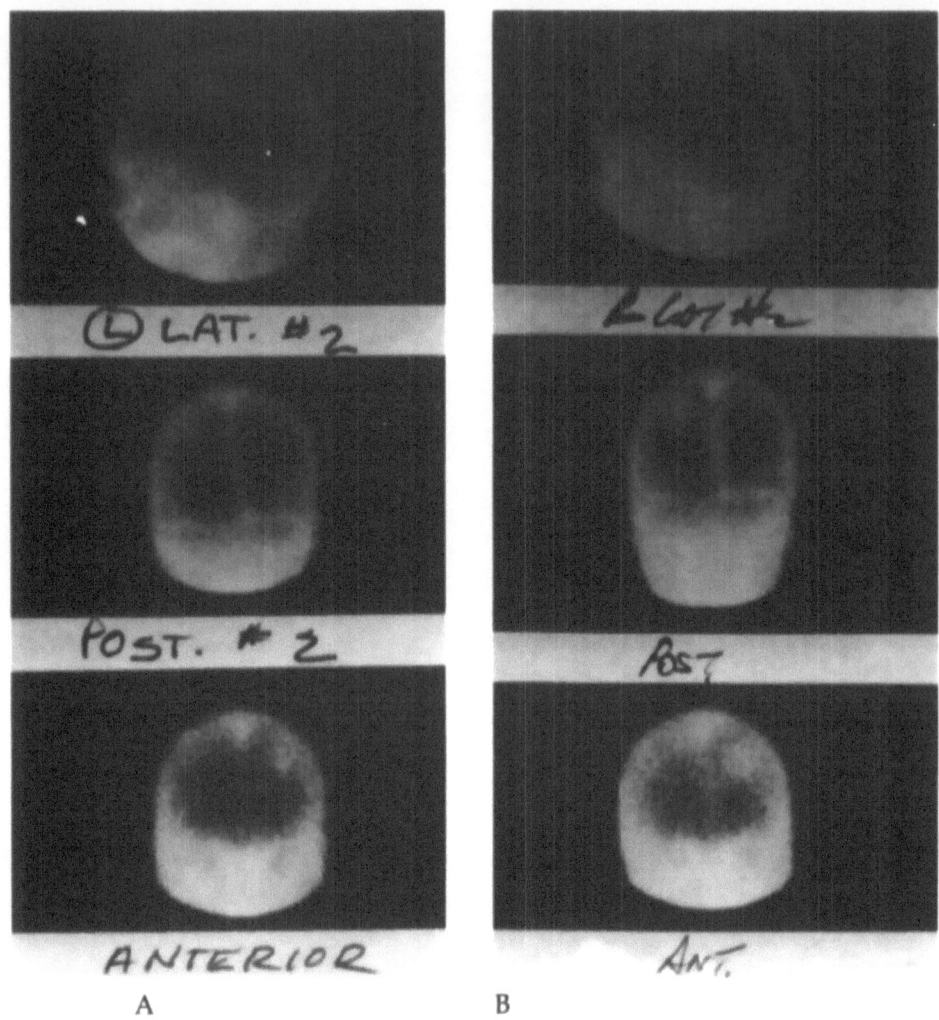

A

B

A. *Pretreatment brain scan of patient R. B. on 2-3-77. B. Posttreatment brain scan of patient R. B. showed 50% decrease in uptake on 5-27-77.*

response to steroids often indicates that the functional impairment is temporary and reversible and that the degree of brain damage is minimal. By and large, treatment after a good steroid response may bring complete temporary remission. On the other hand, failure to respond to steroid therapy often indicates irreversible brain damage. It is therapeutically sound to initiate aggressive treatment as soon as the diagnosis of brain metastasis is established and before functional impairment and brain damage become permanent and irreversible.

A parallel relationship was observed between clinical response and

Figure 24.3.

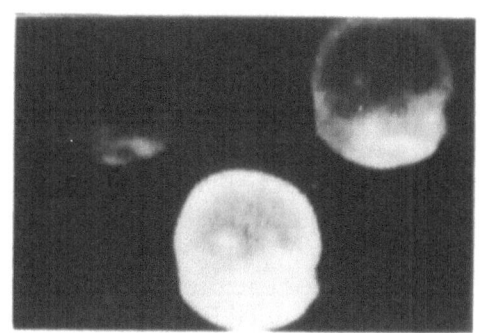

A

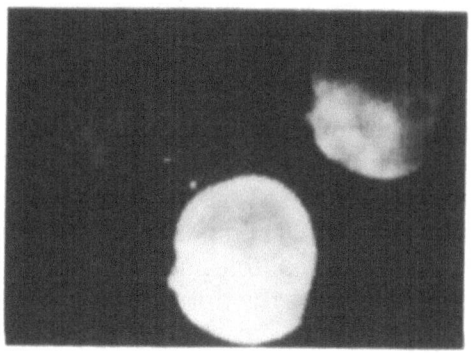

B

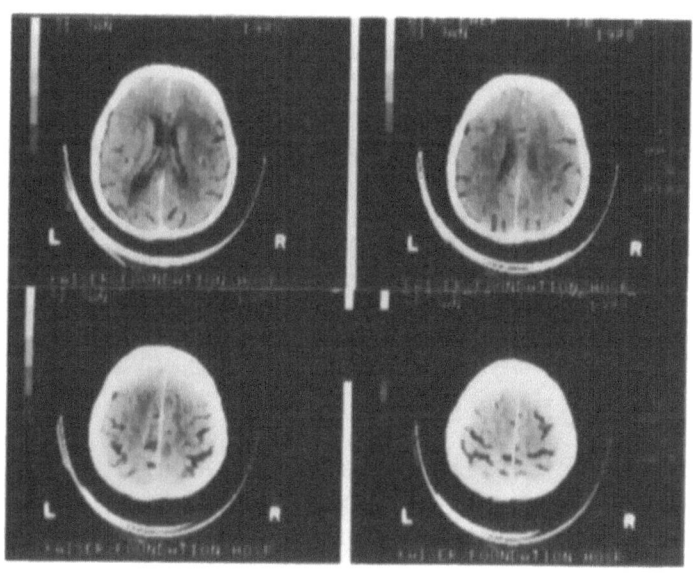

C

A. *Pretreatment brain scan of patient G. B. on 7-6-77. B. Posttreatment brain scan of patient G. B. showed normal uptake on 10-14-77. C. CT scan of patient G. B. on 1-31-78.*

the radionuclide brain scan (table 24.4), and the conversion of a positive to negative brain scan was always associated with a good clinical response. Clinical improvement in neurologic function may not be reflected in a brain scan for at least 3 months, however. Computed tomography (CT) scans became available to us 10 months after this study began. We have therefore only performed three CT scans for brain metastasis (table 24.2). One patient (G.B.) had a negative brain scan and also a negative CT scan (figs. 24.5, 24.6, and 24.7); another patient (S.V.) had a negative brain scan but a positive CT scan. There is no doubt that CT is more accurate than radionuclide scanning, not only in identifying metastases but also in establishing differential diagnoses (see Chapter 12). In future studies, CT scans will be done after negative radionuclide brain scans.

The objective of concomitant administration of chemotherapy and radiotherapy is to simultaneously enhance local cell-kill in the irradiated volume and to control metastases. Doxorubicin hydrochloride has been shown to have radioenhancement properties in vitro (Byfield et al. 1977), and Cortes and others (1974) have reported one patient with brain metastasis from a primary lung cancer who showed complete tumor regression on the radionuclide scan after receiving doxorubicin. Doxorubicin cannot prevent brain metastases, however. Table 24.2 shows that several patients developed brain metastasis while being treated with doxorubicin for lung cancer. Doxorubicin is not lipid soluble and is a relatively large molecule. It is therefore not expected to cross the normal blood-brain barrier (Chapter 6). Once the blood-brain barrier is no longer intact (see Chapter 7), then doxorubicin hydrochloride is able to reach metastatic lesions in the brain.

CCNU is potentially one of the more promising nitrosoureas for the treatment of brain metastases because of its lipid solubility. Fewer and others (1972) used CCNU to treat 4 patients with brain metastases from primary lung cancer but reported a favorable response in only one. In the present pilot study, we have observed a promising improvement in responses and survival rates in patients receiving doxorubicin hydrochloride, CCNU and radiotherapy compared with our experiences with radiotherapy alone for similar patients. These encouraging results warrant further laboratory investigation and a phase III randomized study.

REFERENCES

Byfield, J. E. et al. Cellular effects of combined Adriamycin and X-irradiation in human tumor cells. *Int. J. Cancer* 19:194–204, 1977.

Chao, J. H.; Phillips, R.; and Nickson, J. J. Roentgen-ray therapy of cerebral metastases. *Cancer* 7:682–689, 1954.

Chu, F. C. H., and Hilaris, B. B. Value of radiation therapy in the management of intracranial metastases. *Cancer* 14:577–581, 1961.

Cortes, E. P.; Takita, H.; and Holland, J. F. Adriamycin in advanced bronchogenic carcinoma. *Cancer* 34:518–525, 1974.

Deeley, T. J., and Edwards, J. M. R. Radiotherapy in the management of cerebral secondaries from bronchial carcinoma. *Lancet* 1:1209–1212, 1968.

Fewer, D. et al. Phase II study of 1-(2-chloroethyl)-3-cyclohexyl-1-nitrosourea (CCNU; NSC-79037) in the treatment of brain tumors. *Cancer Chemother. Rep.* 56:421–427, 1972.

Hendrickson, F. R. Radiation therapy of metastatic tumors. *Semin. Oncol.* 2:43–46, 1975.

Newman, S. J., and Hansen, H. H. Frequency, diagnosis and treatment of brain metastases in 247 consecutive patients with bronchogenic carcinoma. *Cancer* 33:492–496, 1974.

Nisce, L. Z.; Hilaris, B. S.; and Chu, F. C. H. A review of experience with irradiation of brain metastases. *Am. J. Roentgenol.* 111:329–333, 1971.

Order, S. E. et al. Improvement in quality of survival following whole-brain irradiation for brain metastasis. *Radiology* 91:149–153, 1968.

Shehata, W. M.; Hendrickson, F. R.; and Hindo, W. Rapid fraction technique and retreatment of cerebral metastases by irradiation. *Cancer* 34:257–261, 1974.

25
Surgical Therapy of Brain Metastases

Joseph Ransohoff

Metastatic brain disease is probably the most common central nervous system complication of systemic cancer and is not a problem which lends itself to easy or simplistic answers. The treatment modalities available include surgical excision, radiation therapy, and chemotherapy as well as combinations of all three methods. With very rare exceptions, surgery is restricted to those patients with single intracranial metastases whereas radiation therapy and chemotherapy are applicable to patients with multiple intracranial tumors.

The treatment of patients with metastatic brain disease requires input from several disciplines including neurology, neuroradiology, neurosurgery, internal medicine, oncology, and radiation therapy if maximal results are to be obtained. The advent of computed transaxial tomography (CT) scanning and the use of high-dose corticosteroids with surgical and nonsurgical treatment have significantly improved our capacity to care for these patients. In carefully selected patients, total excision of solitary intracranial metastases can prolong meaningful life by many months.

In a review of the problem of metastatic brain disease, it is important to differentiate between immunology of the central nervous system and the remainder of the body. The anatomy and physiology of the immune response in the central nervous system differs from that in other tissues. The brain has no lymphatic system. In addition, the blood-brain barrier, which in large part results from so-called tight junctions between capillary endothelial cells, shields the brain to a large extent from systemic humoral and cellular immunity. As a result, immunoglobulins are not able to permeate freely into the central nervous system under normal conditions. The lymphocyte is also generally barred from the central nervous system. Indeed, the only cell normally found in the central nervous system which may be classified as lymphoreticular is the controversial microglial cell. Thus, because of the presence of the blood-brain barrier and the absence of lymphatics, the immune response is markedly reduced in the central nervous system as compared with the rest of the body. Indeed, the central nervous system is often considered an immunologically privileged site. The anterior chamber of the eye, the thyroid and the testicle are other tissues to which this designation has been sometimes applied.

CLINICAL PRESENTATION

Patients with a single intracranial metastatic tumor, the prime candidates for excision followed by radiation therapy and chemotherapy, may present in quite different stages of the disease process and carry quite different prognoses. Patients may present with the classic signs of brain tumor, including increased intracranial pressure, seizures, or focal neurological deficits. The diagnostic workup may demonstrate a primary cancer, or the metastatic nature of the tumor may not be recognized until pathologic examination. By and large, these patients have the best prognosis in the entire group: their systemic immunologic defense mechanisms presumably are controlling their primary disease, but the immunologically privileged characteristics of the central nervous system have enabled the tumor to grow to symptomatic size within the brain.

At the other end of the prognostic scale are the patients in whom brain metastases are found while undergoing workup for symptomatic systemic cancer. These patients are much more common now that CT scanning is employed during the diagnostic workup. The outlook of these patients is as dependent upon the prognosis of the primary tumor as on that of the metastatic brain disease.

A third intermediate, and possibly the most interesting, group of patients with metastatic brain disease are those whose primary cancer is under good control with various modalities of treatment before the metastatic brain tumor makes itself known. Melanoma is the prime example of this situation: if a single intracranial melanoma nodule can be totally excised and followed by radiation therapy, the prognosis reverts to the status prior to the development of the brain tumor and is dependent on continued response to chemotherapy.

In summary, one sees patients with brain tumors that are metastatic, patients with widespread metastatic disease including brain tumors, and patients with central nervous system metastases developed late in the course of their systemic disease. The selection of appropriate therapy must be based on each patient's general health and immunologic competency, on the central nervous system's inadequate defense mechanisms as compared to the organism as a whole, and the stage in the overall course of the disease at which a particular patient presents with metastatic brain tumor.

In an excellent review of the diagnosis and treatment of metastasis to the brain at Memorial Sloan-Kettering Cancer Center, Posner (1974) described 171 patients with intracerebral metastases discovered in 1,905 autopsies during the 3 years between 1970 and 1973. Even at autopsy in this cancer center, over one-third (65) of these metastatic lesions were single.

In a series of patients undergoing intracranial surgery for metastatic brain tumors, Lang and Slater (1964), Stortebecker (1954), Vieth and Odom (1965), Richards and McKissock (1963), and Raskind and others (1971) reported a consistent distribution of primary malignancies, and a review of 100 consecutive cases from our medical center revealed a similar distribution (table 25.1). Carcinoma of the lung far outstrips all other tumors as a source of intracranial metastases (accounting for up to 65% in some

Table 25.1

PRIMARY SITE OF 100 SURGICALLY EXCISED METASTATIC
BRAIN TUMORS

Site	Number of Patients
Lung	28
Unknown	22
Breast	15
Melanoma	14
Genitourinary	10
Others	11

series). In decreasing frequency thereafter, the primary sites include breast, kidney, gastrointestinal tract, melanoma, and a host of rarer tumors. Those patients in whom the primary site cannot be determined often carry an excellent prognosis.

The neurologic signs and symptoms in patients with metastatic brain disease have no pathognomonic characteristics but are similar to those seen with most intracranial mass lesions including the gliomas. A high percentage of patients with intracranial metastases have headaches associated with personality change, memory loss, and mild confusion. These symptoms, along with nausea and vomiting, are evidence of increased intracranial pressure and diffuse cerebral dysfunction and are usually due to the extensive brain edema often associated with metastatic brain tumors. The other more specific signs include seizures (either focal or generalized), hemiparesis, and aphasia and visual field defects. Cerebellar metastases are fairly common and present with ataxia and pressure signs. In contrast to patients harboring primary tumors of the central nervous system, patients with metastatic brain disease may give a history of significant weight loss and malaise.

THE DIAGNOSTIC WORKUP

Systemic Evaluation

Similar diagnostic measures are used in the systemic evaluation of a patient with intracranial tumor irrespective of its nature. The minimal general workup should include posteroanterior and lateral chest films and conventional tomography, if indicated, routine blood and urine determinations, and sedimentation rate. Of 158 patients with metastatic brain tumors described by Stortebecker (1954), only 25% had a sedimentation rate below 10 mm/hour; another 25% had a sedimentation rate of 10–20 mm; and the remaining 50% were over 20 mm.

Except in those with a history of malignant disease, intracranial metastases are usually suspected on the basis of specialized neurologic studies. The application of corticosteroids in the management of increased intracranial pressure has reduced the urgency of most diagnostic workups and has allowed time for a carefully planned program of evaluation. If neurologic studies suggest metastatic brain tumors, a search usually can be conducted for the primary or for other metastases at least to the extent of chest tomography, intravenous pyelography, mammography, radionuclide liver and bone scans, and total body CT scanning, if available. In view of the low incidence of gastrointestinal tract metastases to the central nervous system, preoperative studies of this system are rarely indicated. Patients may also be subjected to nonspecific immunologic challenge with mumps vaccine and streptokinase-streptodornase (Varidase). Nonresponders are probably in a state of anergy from carcinomatous disease and are poor candidates for operation.

Neurologic Evaluation

Neurologic evaluation of a patient with signs and symptoms suggestive of an intracranial mass usually requires specific studies in a routine sequence, starting with skull radiography, electroencephalography and radionuclide brain scanning. (See also Chapters 11 and 12.) Skull films may show thinning and erosion of the dorsum sellae and posterior clinoids and thus suggest increased intracranial pressure of long standing. Occasionally, shifting of a calcified pineal gland and local hypervascularity of the skull may indicate the site of a tumor, either a metastatic lesion or a meningioma, particularly if it is receiving a significant blood supply from the dura mater. Electroencephalography has only lateralizing value although diffuse slowing can be associated with intracranial pressure.

The radionuclide brain scan (^{99m}Tc) can have considerable value, and operative treatment is excluded when there is clearcut evidence of multiple lesions. It must be remembered, however, that brain scanning does not demonstrate all metastatic tumors. The lower limit of tumor size demonstrated is approximately 0.5–1 cm, and one tumor may show uptake on the brain scan and a second may not be visible at all or may show only as a faintly suspicious shadow. This phenomenon probably is due to differences in the quantity of edema in the white matter surrounding the tumor: in a single patient one tumor may produce little or no edema while another tumor in the opposite hemisphere produces a great deal. Tumors with little or no edema are less visible on the radionuclide scan.

During the initial phase of evaluation, patients should be placed on anticonvulsant therapy (diphenylhydantoin, 0.1 gm three times daily) even if they have not had seizures before admission, and corticosteroids should be added if there are signs of increased pressure or a focal neurologic deficit. We prefer methylprednisolone, which generally is started at 120 mg/day and is maintained at this level throughout the diagnostic evaluation until a decision is made concerning surgery, radiation therapy, chemotherapy, or combinations of these. Recent experience with massive doses of corticosteroids (1–1.5 gm of methylprednisolone/day) have shown dramatic reversal of severe obtundation and marked neurologic deficit in patients with massive brain edema (Renaudin et al. 1973; Lieberman et al. 1977).

When available, computed transaxial tomography (CT) has great value in the diagnostic workup of patients with intracranial tumors. Ventricular size and position are clearly visible. Patients with a posterior fossa lesion (even those without signs of papilledema) will almost always show enlarged ventricles and a shift of the fourth ventricle. Intravenous injection of 200 cm³ sodium diatrizoate (Hypaque) greatly enhances the definition of metastatic tumors and meningiomas, but primary gliomas are not opacified as dramatically. Finally, bilateral cerebral angiography via a femoral catheter provides a definitive diagnosis except in patients with a posterior fossa tumor for whom vertebral angiography and ventriculography may also be required (the latter on rare occasions). Lumbar puncture rarely is necessary in the workup of a brain tumor patient unless one suspects intracranial infection or is searching for malignant cells in the cerebrospinal fluid.

SURGICAL MANAGEMENT

Surgical excision of intracranial metastases should be limited to those patients in whom a thorough workup demonstrates a single intracranial lesion. Deeply placed lesions, either primary or metastatic, in the midportion of the dominant hemisphere are not surgically accessible. Most metastatic tumors arise from the cortical gray–white junction, however, and are accessible to the surgeon. Except when there is a strong possibility of brain abscess, needle biopsy may have considerable academic interest, but because of the risk, it should be done only to gain information that will influence therapy significantly (for example, the choice of a chemotherapeutic agent).

When operation is chosen, based on the location of the lesion, the patient's age, the general medical status, the host-tumor relationship, and the surrounding social factors, the surgeon's goals are to achieve a total excision, to see the patient through safely, and to secure the best result possible. The operation must be planned carefully with a wide exposure of the brain, preferably including one polar aspect, either frontal, temporal, or occipital. This will permit complete or nearly complete excision, and if needed, a lobectomy should be performed to provide adequate internal decompression. Fortunately, metastatic tumors commonly develop a pseudocapsule, and often the gross lesion can be excised intact. The bone flap is reinserted firmly at the completion of the procedure. Rarely is there any justification for discarding the bone and leaving the dura open to provide external decompression. This procedure, which generally indicates inadequate planning and poor execution, results in futher herniation of viable brain and development of a bulging skin flap; the patient may linger in a terminal state. The planned approach has little place for intraoperative frozen section to determine the nature of the lesion. In most instances, the surgeon is committed to a definitive procedure before submitting the patient to surgery and rapid section techniques are often misleading.

Objective evaluation of the results of surgical extirpation of single metastatic disease is difficult. As Posner (1974) has pointed out, no random study has compared the effects of surgical extirpation and radiation therapy to those of radiation therapy alone. This type of study could be done only in patients in whom systemic tumor has been demonstrated. Advances in chemotherapy and immunotherapy probably will make such research more difficult to conduct in view of the varying responses of the central nervous system to these therapies.

We believe all patients who have undergone successful removal of an intracranial metastatic tumor should be given postoperative radiation therapy. The Radiology Therapy Oncology Group has been investigating various treatment regimens in a random study of the palliation of metastatic brain disease. After having cooperated in the study, Drs. J. Newell and R. J. Carella of the Department of Radiation Therapy at New York University have recommended 4,000 rads in 10 treatments or 5,000 rads in 15 treatments. The same dosage is recommended for patients with multiple intracranial metastases as the primary treatment modality.

The Radiation Therapy Oncology Group is currently initiating a study of the use of misonidazole and radiation in the treatment of brain metastases (RTOG 78-12) (Dische et al. 1977; Urtasun et al. 1976). This agent, which enhances the effect of ionizing radiation on hypoxic cells, has evoked considerable interest and is currently under evaluation by the Brain Tumor Study Group for the treatment of malignant gliomas.

The effect of adding chemotherapy and immunotherapy to this regimen has not been evaluated adequately. When specific and well established therapeutic regimens for the primary tumor are available (such as in melanoma), the patient should continue therapy until death. The effects of some drugs such as lipid-soluble nitrosoureas and other promising agents are currently under investigation for treatment of primary brain tumors (glioblastomas) and can be considered for administration in conjunction with radiation therapy. These drugs may be valuable for treatment of metastatic brain disease, but once again, no authoritative random study has been conducted to determine their usefulness.

SURGICAL EXTIRPATION AND SURVIVAL

The literature contains many reports of surgical removal of metastatic brain tumor. Lang and Slater (1964) reported a median survival time of 4 months and an average survival time of 12 months in 208 patients undergoing intracranial surgery for metastatic brain tumor. Richards and McKissock (1963) described 108 patients in whom apparent total excision of the tumor was achieved; 22 of them survived for 1 year or more. In a series from Memorial Hospital (Posner 1974), those patients who received surgery and radiation therapy had a median survival of 4 months and 21% survived for 1 year or more. Raskind and others (1971) reported 100 patients who underwent surgery for what appeared to be a single metastatic tumor; 15 of them survived for more than 1 year. Table 25.2 shows our results in the last 100 patients who underwent intracranial surgery for what appeared to be single metastatic tumors; they are similar to Posner's results.

Our experience suggests that selected patients with an apparently single intracranial metastatic tumor in a surgically accessible region have a 25% chance or better of meaningful survival for 1 year or longer after surgical removal and radiation therapy. Two illustrative case reports emphasize this point.

J. L., a 37-year-old female, was misdiagnosed on the basis of radionuclide brain scans and cerebral angiography as having a right frontal glioma in 1969. She was treated with 4,500 rads of radiation therapy and

Table 25.2

RESULTS OF COMBINED SURGERY, RADIATION, AND/OR CHEMOTHERAPY

Tumor Origin	Number of Patients	Survival (Mos.)					
		Primary	1–6	6–12	12–18	18–24	Over 24
Lung	28	5	11	3	4	2	3
Unknown	22	2	3	8	5	2	2
Breast	15	0	5	3	4	0	3
Melanoma	14	2	2	3	1	2	3
Genitourinary	10	1	3	4	2	0	0
Others	11	0	4	3	2	1	1
Totals	100	10	28	24	18	7	13

Figure 25.1.

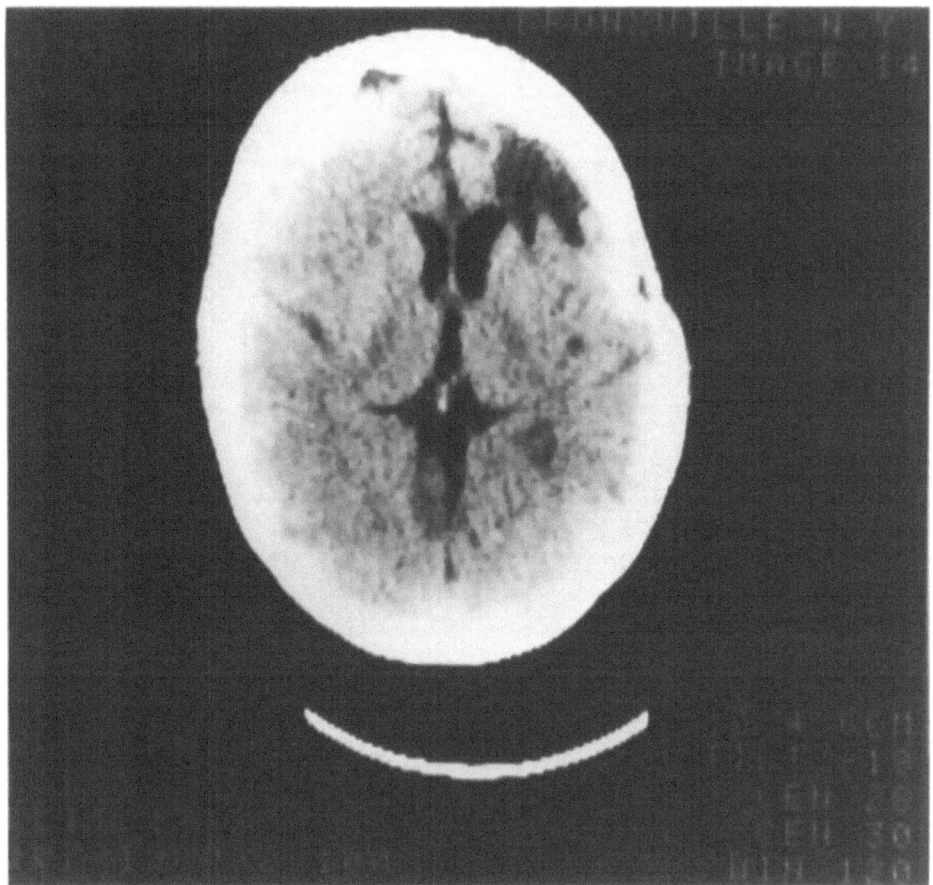

Patient J. L. with single intracranial metastasis and unknown primary. CT scan 8 years after radiation and surgical excision of right frontal metastatic tumor.

maintained on corticosteroids. In 1970, 8 months after radiation therapy, a right frontal undifferentiated metastatic tumor was totally excised. She is presently maintained on phenobarbitol. Repeated workup has failed to reveal a primary tumor. She is asymptomatic. Fig. 25.1 shows postoperative right frontal changes on her CT scan 8 years after surgery.

F. B., a 53-year-old female, underwent radical mastectomy for carcinoma of the breast followed by radiation therapy in 1970. In March of 1976, a juge right parietal, metastic brain tumor (fig. 25.2A) was found. The tumor was totally removed. She received 4,000 rads of whole brain therapy in 3 weeks immediately after operation. She has been maintained on 5-flurouracil, cyclophosphamide, and methotrexate since craniotomy. She remains fully functional (fig. 25.2B) 24 months after craniotomy.

Figure 25.2.

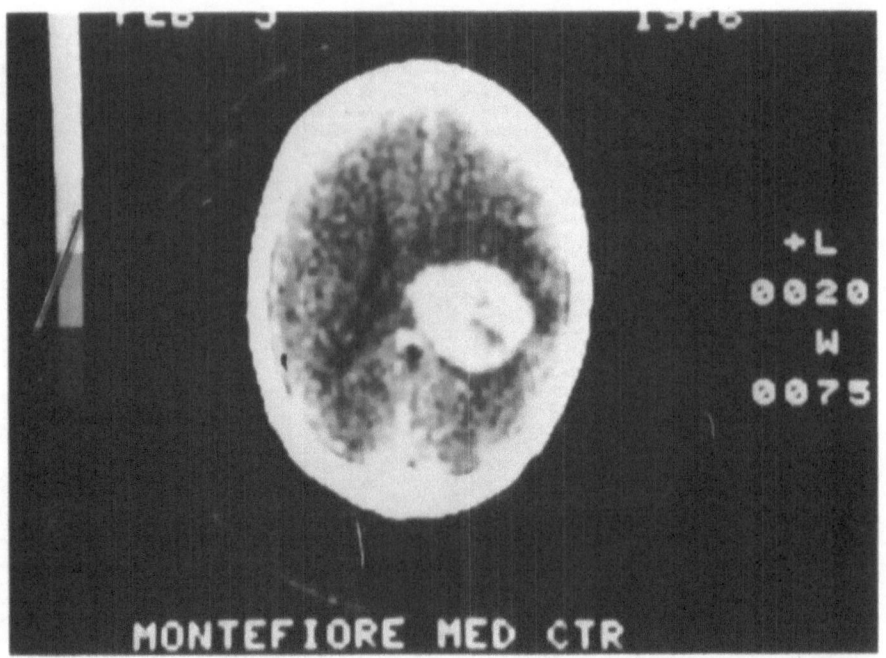

A

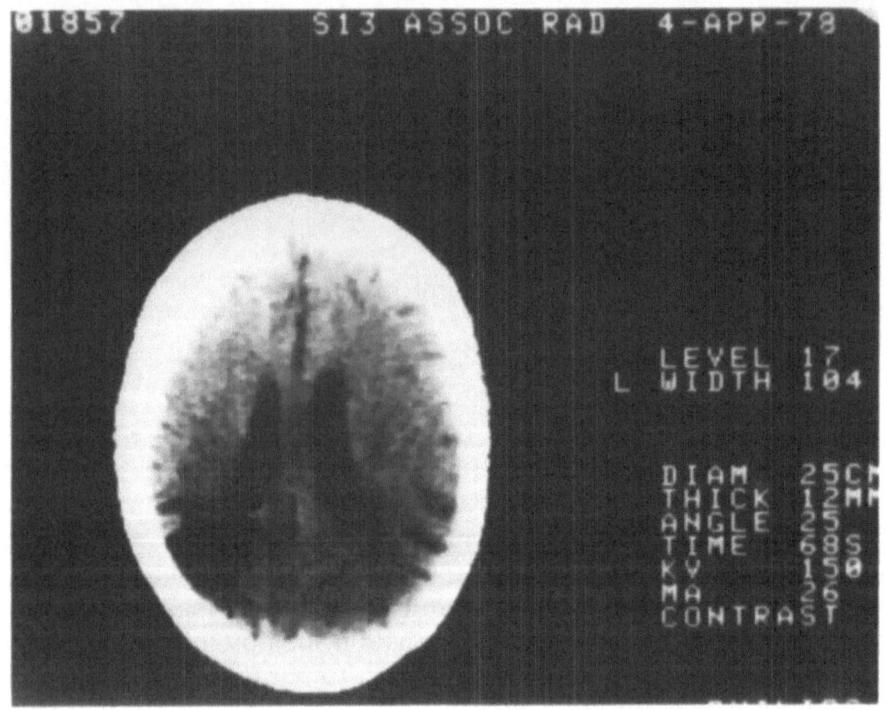

B

*Patient F. B. with breast cancer metastatic to brain. A. Preoperative CT scan.
B. CT scan 2 years after total excision, radiation therapy and chemotherapy.*

When systemic tumor presents itself primarily with central nervous system symptoms or signs, the patient may benefit significantly from intracranial surgery and radiation therapy. In the future, advances in chemotherapy and immunotherapy may further prolong life, particularly as progress is made in systemic and central nervous system tumor therapy. Thoughtful planning, multifactored decision making, and aggressive surgery are essential for success in the treatment of metastatic brain tumor.

REFERENCES

Dische, S. et al. Clinical testing of the radiosensitizer RO-07-0582. Experience with multiple doses. *Br. J. Cancer* 35:567–579, 1977.

Lang, E. J., and Slater, J. Metastatic brain tumors: results of surgical and nonsurgical treatment. *Surg. Clin. North Am.* 44:865–872, 1964.

Lieberman, A. et al. Use of high dose corticosteroids in patients with inoperable brain tumors. *J. Neurol. Neurosurg. Psych.* 40:678–682, 1977.

Posner, J. B. Diagnosis and treatment of metastases to the brain. *Clin. Bull.* 4:47–57, 1974.

Raskind, R. et al. Survival after surgical excision of single metastatic brain tumors. *Am. J. Roentgenol.* 111:323–328, 1971.

Renaudin, J. et al. Dose dependency of Decadron in patients with partially excised brain tumors. *J. Neurosurg.* 39:302–305, 1973.

Richards, P., and McKissock, W. Intracranial metastases. *Br. Med. J.* 1:15–18, 1963.

Stortebecker, T. P. Metastatic tumors of the brain from a neurosurgical point of view: a follow-up study of 158 cases. *J. Neurosurg.* 11:84–111, 1954.

Urtasun, R. C. et al. Metronidazole as a radiosensitizer. *N. Engl. J. Med.* 295:901–902, 1976.

Vieth, R. G., and Odom, G. L. Intracranial metastases and their neurosurgical treatment. *J. Neurosurg.* 23:375–383, 1965.

26

Treatment of Brain Metastases by Surgical Extirpation

Francis W. Gamache, Jr.
Joseph H. Galicich
Jerome B. Posner

The idea of surgically extirpating a single brain metastasis has a compelling logic which makes it attractive to many oncologists and neurosurgeons. The prevailing view that removal of a solitary brain metastasis will cure the patient, whereas radiation therapy and chemotherapy only palliate lends support to those who favor surgical extirpation for apparently solitary brain metastases. Occasional reports in the literature describe longterm survivors after surgical extirpation of single (Modesti and Feldman 1975; Tarnoff et al. 1976) or more rarely, multiple brain metastases (Dayes et al. 1977; Haar and Patterson 1972). The number of such reported cures is small, however, and there are no randomized prospective studies comparing the efficacy of surgical extirpation of brain metastases with that of whole-brain irradiation alone. Retrospective analyses comparing surgical extirpation with radiation therapy have generally shown either a modest advantage for surgical extirpation or no difference between the two treatments (Order et al. 1968; Montana et al. 1972; Posner 1974).

This chapter presents a retrospective analysis of 94 patients with presumptive single metastatic brain lesions treated by surgical extirpation at the Memorial Sloan-Kettering Cancer Center between 1968–1977. Surgical extirpation was followed in most instances by whole-brain irradiation. The study was undertaken to evaluate in detail several aspects of surgical extirpation of brain metastases which might interest oncologists and neurologists considering such therapy for their patients.

Specific attention is paid to the following aspects: (1) factors influencing survival, (2) the quality of survival after surgical extirpation, (3) the complications of the surgical procedure itself, and (4) the cause of death of patients undergoing surgical extirpation of brain metastases.

We have also attempted to define clinical criteria with which to identify individual patients who are good candidates for surgical extirpation.

390

METHODS

The records of all patients undergoing craniotomy for treatment of hematogenously spread brain metastases in the years 1968–1977 at Memorial Hospital were reviewed. Patients who proved at operation to have either primary brain tumors or whose systemic tumor involved the cranial cavity by direct extension from extracranial structures were excluded, but patients in whom the metastasis was not found at operation (negative exploration) were included. There were 94 patients selected for operation from over 1,000 patients with metastatic brain tumors evaluated and treated during this ten year period. All 94 patients were believed to be suffering from a single intracranial metastatic lesion as determined by carotid and vertebral cerebral arteriography and, in the last 4 years, by computed tomography (CT) (see Chapter 12).

Other criteria for selection were not predetermined but involved some of the following considerations: that patients be free of extracranial tumor or have extracranial tumor either under good control or probably controllable by surgery, radiation or chemotherapy. Some patients underwent operation despite advancing systemic disease because the brain tumor was producing intractable neurologic symptoms, such as uncontrollable seizures or increased intracranial pressure. Patients suffering serious neurologic symptoms threatening death from herniation at times underwent surgery as an emergency without full evaluation of the extent of extracranial disease. Patients whose tumors were believed to be slow-growing and not radiosensitive were sometimes selected as well.

Because there were no predetermined criteria, the selection was at times capricious but generally involved patients who were in better condition than those chosen to undergo radiation therapy alone. Of the 94 patients, 76 patients (particularly those considered to have radiosensitive tumors) received whole-brain irradiation postoperatively (table 26.1). There were 58 patients who received postoperative immunotherapy or chemotherapy. Most of these had been receiving such therapy preoperatively.

All patients received adrenocorticosteroids (usually dexamethasone, 16 mg or more daily) prior to surgery and continued on corticosteroid therapy through the duration of postoperative radiation therapy. When radiation therapy was completed, the steroid dose was decreased. If neurologic symptoms recurred, steroids were again employed and maintained at the smallest dose which controlled the symptoms. Patients were followed postoperatively by both the neurosurgical and oncology services. Although 8 different surgeons, both residents and attendings, participated in the operations, the majority were performed by one surgeon (J. H. G.).

RESULTS

The clinical findings in the 94 patients selected for operation are summarized in table 26.1. The most common tumors were lung carcinoma (23

Table 26.1

SURGICAL EXTIRPATION OF BRAIN METASTASIS: PATIENT DATA

Primary Tumor	Number of Patients	Age		Interval*		Headache
		Range (Yrs.)	Median (Yrs.)	Range (Mos.)	Median (Mos.)	
Lung	23	36–74	58	0–75	6	13
Melanoma	18	25–69	39	2–240	31	10
Breast	11	49–58	53	3–192	38	6
Sarcomas	8	9–62	17.5	9–98	16.5	3
Germ-cell tumors	9	22–52	36	1–45	17	3
Undetermined origin	8	43–70	60	0–7	—	5
Kidney	7	44–75	65	0–33	8	3
Uterus	3	33–62	60	33–108	71	2
Colon	4	43–66	65	5–72	27	3
Prostate	1		71	—	60	0
Ovary	1		10	—	11	1
Neuroblastoma	1		13	—	23	1
TOTALS	94	9–75	—	0–240	17.5	50 (54%)

*From diagnosis of primary tumors to diagnosis of brain metastasis
†HIF = higher integrative functions; ICP = signs of increased intracranial pressure

patients), melanoma (18 patients) and breast carcinoma (11 patients). Breast cancer is the most common neoplasm treated at Memorial Sloan-Kettering Cancer Center, but patients with lung cancer and melanoma were more commonly selected for surgery: the lung because of the high incidence of lung lesions with single brain metastases (and without systemic disease), and melanoma because of its radioresistance. The fourth large category, sarcomas (8 patients), included Ewing's sarcoma, osteo-

	Neurologic Findings†				Extracranial Tumor		Additional Therapy RT Chemotherapy and/or	
HIF	Seizures	Hemiparesis	ICP	Visual Field Abn.	Present	Absent	Immunotherapy	
8	5	9	8	3	14	9	23	15
8	4	8	6	2	14	4	11	12
3	1	7	6	0	6	5	10	7
4	5	2	3	1	7	1	5	7
1	6	3	2	8	7	2	8	7
3	2	6	2	0	3	5	5	1
3	2	5	5	0	4	3	5	3
3	0	2	2	1	2	1	3	2
1	2	1	2	0	3	1	4	2
1	0	1	0	0	0	1	1	0
1	0	0	1	0	1	0	1	1
0	0	1	0	1	1	0	1	1
36 (39%)	27 (29%)	45 (48%)	37 (40%)	16 (17%)	62 (66%)	32 (34%)	76 (81%)	58 (62%)

genic sarcoma, leiomyosarcoma, myxoliposarcoma and chondrosarcoma. In 8 patients, the site of origin of the cancer could not be determined.

The patients ranged in age from 9 to 75 years. Age did not appear to affect the outcome of surgery. The median interval between discovery of the primary tumor and discovery of the brain metastasis was 17 months. There was considerable variability in the interval among patients with the same primary tumor and between types of tumors. Thus, although the median interval between diagnosis of carcinoma of the lung and development of a brain metastasis was short (6 months), the range varied from zero (those whose lung cancer was discovered after the brain metastasis) to over 6 years. The brain metastasis was also sometimes the first symptom of cancer in patients with renal carcinoma and cancers whose primary source could not be determined. There were no patients with malignant melanoma, breast carcinoma, sarcoma, carcinoma of the uterus, or colon cancer who first presented with cerebral symptoms. In these patients the duration between the onset of the primary cancer and the brain metastasis was often several years. The significance of the interval between diagnosis of the primary tumor and the brain metastasis is considered later in the chapter.

The signs and symptoms which prompted evaluation for brain metastasis are also listed in table 26.1. They are generally similar to those reported by others (see Chapter 11). Headache was present in approximately half of the patients, and changes in cognitive function in 39%. Mild focal weakness was present in slightly less than half of the patients, and signs of increased intracranial pressure (lethargy, papilledema, vomiting, hiccups) were present in 40%. Focal or generalized convulsions occurred in 29%, and 17% had visual field deficits. Surprisingly, 5 of 6 patients (84%) with germ cell tumors presented with homonymous hemianopia from occipital metastases. This finding was present in only 8 of 72 patients with other kinds of tumor.

Two-thirds of the patients were believed to have systemic disease at the time of surgery and one-third were believed to be free of extracerebral disease. Eighteen patients (19%) were considered surgical emergencies having rapidly developed signs of increased intracranial pressure and incipient herniation. Posterior fossa (cerebellar) tumors were present in 17 patients (18%).

Table 26.2 details the survival after craniotomy. Eight patients died within 30 days of surgery (an operative mortality of 8.5%). Five of the postoperative deaths were in patients whose operation was done as an emergency because of brain herniation. If only elective procedures are considered (76 patients), the operative mortality was 4%. In 4 patients, a tumor was either not located or was too close to the motor cortex to be removed safely. All of these patients had surgery before preoperative localization by CT scan (see Chapter 12) was being used routinely. In a fifth patient, negative exploration was followed several weeks later by successful removal of the tumor after localization by CT. Two of the 4 patients with negative explorations are alive and without evidence of brain metastasis at 32 and 55 months postoperatively; 2 patients are dead at 11 and 25 months postoperatively.

The median survival after surgery depended on the primary tumor and ranged from 2.5 months for neuroblastoma to 8 months for carcinoma of the uterus. Approximately one-quarter of the patients survived one year, and 9% survived 2 years. No patient survived more than 5 years. The percentage of longterm survivors (greater than 2 years) was highest in carcinoma of the breast (38%), but 10% of patients with carcinoma of the lung survived for more than 2 years. One of 15 patients with malignant melanoma survived more than 3 years.

Of the 72 patients who survived more than 30 days, 65 (90%) were improved at 2 months; 44 had marked improvement in neurologic symptoms and signs and had returned to full activity (table 26.3). There were 21 patients who were somewhat improved from their preoperative state but continued to have neurologic problems which prevented them from returning to full activity. Seven patients were either not improved or were worse as a result of the operation. In general, the patients who improved most were those who had suffered preoperatively from raised intracranial pressure or only mild-to-moderate neurologic dysfunction (lethargy, obtundation, hemiparesis). Patients who improved least suffered preoperatively from severe neurologic dysfunction, especially dementia or hemiplegia.

Table 26.4 lists some complications of surgery other than death or negative exploration. Sixteen patients (17%) underwent 21 surgical re-explorations because of neurologic deterioration after initially being alert and awake in the postoperative period. Half of these patients deteriorated in the first 24 hours after surgery and were re-operated at that time; in the other patients, neurologic deterioration began later or developed more slowly so that the operation was deferred for 48 hours or more. Subdural hematomas, often small, were discovered in 7 of 21 re-explorations; intraparenchymal hemorrhage into the tumor bed occurred in 2; and subdural loculation of CSF with associated brain swelling developed in 2 patients. The exploration was either negative or revealed only brain swelling in 6 instances. Two patients developed brain abscesses: one was evacuated on the 18th postoperative day, the other required serial aspirations (three). Thirteen of 16 patients undergoing surgical re-exploration survived more than 30 days. The number of surgical re-explorations has dropped dramatically with the availability of postoperative CT scans.

We attempted to analyze factors which might allow selection of patients who would be longterm survivors. We found several factors. The longer the interval between discovery of the primary tumor and development of brain metastasis, the longer the patients survived after surgical extirpation (table 26.5). Those 52 patients in whom the interval between discovery of the primary tumor and that of brain metastasis was greater than a year had a median survival of 7.2 months, significantly longer ($p <$ 0.05, chi-square analysis) than those 41 patients in whom the interval between primary tumor and cerebral metastasis was less than a year (5 months). The subgroups by tumor type are too small for statistical analysis, but patients with carcinoma of the breast and lung and long intervals between the discovery of the primary tumor and the brain metastasis seemed to do better than those with shorter intervals.

Survival also correlated with neurologic condition at the time of craniotomy (table 26.6). Patients who underwent emergency craniotomy survived only 2.3 months after surgery, whereas those undergoing elec-

Table 26.2

SURVIVAL FROM TIME OF CRANIOTOMY

Primary	Total Number of Patients	30-Day		Median (mos.)	1-Yr.	
		(Number)	(Percentage)		(Number)	(Percentage)
Lung	23	22	95	5	6	26
Melanoma	18	16	88	4.0	4	22
Sarcoma	8	8	100	7.5	3*	43
Breast	11	9	82	5.0	5	45
Choriocarcinoma	9	9	100	7.75	2*	22
Undetermined	8	8	100	5.25	1*	14
Kidney	7	5†	72	5	0	0
Uterus	3	3	100	8	1	33
Colon	4	3	75	4.8	0	0
Prostate	1	1	100	5	0	0
Ovary	1	1	100	6	0	0
Neuroblastoma	1	1	100	2.5	0	0
TOTALS	94	86	91.5	5.5	20	25

*One patient lost to followup.
†Two patients lost to followup.

tive craniotomy survived 7 months. The differences are statistically significant ($p < 0.001$, Gehan-Breslow analysis). When only elective operations are considered, patients with supratentorial lesions survived longer (7 months) than patients with posterior fossa lesions ($p < 0.0001$). Survival statistics for patients undergoing emergency craniotomies for tumors at these sites were not significantly different.

The presence of disease outside the nervous system appeared to have no effect on survival (table 26.7). The median survival of those patients

2 Yrs.		3 Yrs.		4 Yrs.		5 Yrs.		
(Number)	(Percentage)	(Number)	(Percentage)	(Number)	(Percentage)	(Number)	(Percentage)	Autopsy
2	9	2	9	1*	5	0	0	5
1	6	1	6	0	0	0	0	2
1*	17	1	17	0	0	0	0	1
3	27	1	9	1	9	0	0	1
0	0	0	0	0	0	0	0	0
0	0	0	0	0	0	0	0	0
0	0	0	0	0	0	0	0	3
0	0	0	0	0	0	0	0	0
0	0	0	0	0	0	0	0	1
0	0	0	0	0	0	0	0	0
0	0	0	0	0	0	0	0	1
0	0	0	0	0	0	0	0	1
7	9	5	6	2	3	0	0	15

with disease outside the nervous system was exactly the same as those who were believed to be free of extracranial tumor.

By the time this study was completed, 91 of the 94 patients were dead. We attempted to discern the cause of death in 59 patients for whom clinical information concerning the terminal course was available (table 26.8). The major causes of death were disseminated systemic disease (17 patients), acute pulmonary embolus (10 patients), and aspiration pneumonia (7 patients). Only 10 patients (17%) died primarily from their neurologic dis-

Table 26.3

CLINICAL STATE OF 94 PATIENTS AT 2 MONTHS AFTER SURGERY

	Number of Patients	Percentage of Total	Percentage of Survivors
Marked improvement (full activity)	44	47	61
Somewhat improved (home, limited activity)	21	22	29
Essentially unchanged (disabled)	7	8	10
Dead	22	23	—
TOTALS	94	100	100

ease. Two additional patients died of intracranial hemorrhage in the postoperative period.

Only 19 patients were examined at autopsy (table 26.9). The small number of autopsies in part reflects the large number of patients dying at home or in other hospitals. Of the 19 patients who were examined at autopsy, 17 had active systemic cancer. Thirteen of the 19 patients had central nervous system metastatic disease at autopsy. In 6 patients there was local recurrence at the surgical site; 2 had a new single metastasis distant from the original surgical site; and 9 had multiple metastatic lesions in the brain. Six patients had developed meningeal carcinomatosis. Only 2 of the 19 patients were free from cancer. One died of a pulmonary embolus shortly after his craniotomy, and one died of sepsis and a brain abscess at the site of a previous craniotomy.

DISCUSSION

The results of surgical extirpation of brain metastases achieved in this study compare favorably with those previously reported in the literature (table 26.10). The operative mortality of 8.5% is as low as any previously reported and is considerably lower than that reported in the early studies. Perhaps this reflects the salutary effects of steroids in controlling cerebral edema. However, Haar and Patterson (1972) found no difference in mortality when comparing patients treated with steroids with those not.

Our operative mortality would have been lower (4%) if we considered only elective patients because many of the deaths occurred in patients who were desperately ill prior to surgery. In short, careful selection of patients for craniotomy clearly affects survival statistics. The 90% improvement rate in those patients who survived is impressive and compares favorably with those few surgical studies which consider the quality of survival (see table 26.10).

Despite the initial good response, half of the patients were dead by 6 months, and only one-quarter survived a year. None of our patients have survived 5 years. Although several reports in the literature describe prolonged survival after surgical extirpation, very few patients can be expected to survive in good or stable neurologic condition for extended periods.

The 94 patients reported here represent only about 10% of those patients who were seen and evaluated by the neurologic and neurosurgical services for the treatment of brain metastasis during the period covered in this report. This small number of patients who are candidates for surgery explains why most published reports in the literature either include only small numbers or encompass extended periods of time during which there may be changes in the surgical approach. Thus, Harr and Patterson's (1972) study of 167 patients covered 36 years and Stortebecker's (1954) 125 cases 30 years.

One of the reasons for reporting the current series is that the operations were performed by a limited number of surgeons over a short period of time. Thus surgical techniques and pre- and postoperative treatment differed only by small degrees. Even since this series was prepared, however, there have been improvements in preoperative techniques which promise to change the outcome of some surgical procedures. For example, CT localization of metastatic lesions decreases the number of negative explorations (we have had only one negative exploration since we began to localize by CT scanning, a procedure done after this study closed). CT localization also allows the surgeon to identify and remove smaller lesions with less operative trauma than was heretofore possible. Postoperative CT scanning in patients who develop neurologic deterioration allows the surgeon to distinguish hemorrhages which need to be extirpated from brain swelling, which can be treated with hypertonic agents and steroids, thus preventing many of the postoperative re-explorations noted in this series.

How do the results of surgical extirpation compare with whole-brain radiation therapy, a less arduous treatment for patients suffering from systemic cancer? The results of several radiation therapy studies are included elsewhere in this monograph. The 30-day mortality, when reported, is often high because radiation therapy is frequently undertaken when patients are in extremis. The acute complications of radiation therapy are few at the radiation dosages used in these studies (Young et al. 1974), and thus the 30-day mortality reflects the severity of illness. The median survival of 3–6 months is certainly less than that of patients treated surgically, as are

Table 26.4

SURGICAL REEXPLORATIONS IN 16 OF 94 TOTAL PATIENTS
(21 REOPERATIONS)

Primary	Finding at Reexploration	Total Number of Patients
Lung	SDH	4
	NEG	2
Melanoma	SDH	2
	CSF loculation	2
	BrSw	1
Choriocarcinoma	Abscess	4
	BrSw	1
Undetermined	BrSw	1
Kidney	SDH	1
	NEG	1
	IPH	1
Colon	IPH	1
TOTAL		21

*One patient had multiple tumors discovered at craniotomy with small CSF loculation and much brain swelling on reexploration.

Time Elapsed Between Craniotomy and Reexploration and Number of Reexplorations (Hrs.)				Other	30-Day Mortality
12	24	48	72		
	1	1		SDH {1 5th POD 1 6th POD	0
			2		0
2					0
		2†			1
			1		0
				1 18th POD/1 patient 1, 2, 4 mos. postop. (reexplored ×3)	0
				1 6th POD	0
	1				0
1					0
	1				0
	1				1
	1				1
3	5	3	3	7	3

NOTE: SDH = subdural hematoma
NEG = negative exploration and associated brain swelling
BrSw = brain swelling with removal of bone plate
IPH = intraparenchymal hematoma
POD = postoperative day

Table 26.5

DISEASE-FREE INTERVAL VS. MEDIAN SURVIVAL

	Interval ≤ 12 months*			Interval > 12 months		
	Number of Patients	Median Survival (Mos.)	Survival > 1 year	Number of Patients	Median Survival (Mos.)	Survival > 1 year
Lung	16	4.5	3	7	11	3
Melanoma	3	2	0	15	6	4
Sarcoma	2	t	1	6	7.5	2
Breast	3	5	0	8	9	4
Choriocarcinoma	3	3.5	0	6	7.8	1
Undetermined primary	7†	5.5	1	—	—	—
Others	7	6	0	10	3.6	1
TOTAL	41	5	5	52	7.2	15

*Interval (mos.) between diagnosis of primary and diagnosis of cerebral metastasis.
†One patient is 11 months postcraniotomy and still disease-free (primary has not declared itself); this patient has not been included in the table here.

Table 26.6

CONDITION AT THE TIME OF CRANIOTOMY AND SURVIVAL

Elective Craniotomies			
Site	Number of Patients	Median Survival (Mos.)	30-Day Mortality
Supratentorial	67	7	3
Posterior fossa	9	2	2
TOTAL	76	7 overall median	5 (6.5%)

the one-year and longterm survivals. Approximately 60% of patients who undergo radiation therapy are improved by the treatment, and this figure is likewise lower than that reported in our surgical series.

Data comparing radiation therapy alone with surgery followed by radiation therapy are not strictly comparable. Patients undergoing surgical extirpation are likely to be in better physical and neurologic condition than those being radiated because a poor operative risk is frequently denied surgery. Patients undergoing surgical extirpation are less likely to have extensive systemic disease and more likely to have a single brain metastasis. Patients receiving radiation therapy, on the other hand, are more likely to have extensive systemic disease and multiple brain metastases. Thus, one might expect the median and longterm survival statistics to be better in patients treated by surgical extirpation. In our own series, however, approximately 20% of the patients were in extremis (neurologic) when surgery was undertaken, and two-thirds of the operated patients had metastatic disease outside the CNS. Despite these factors tending to make our patients greater operative risks, the results of this study compare favorably with those from either the radiation or surgical literature.

Several other attempts have been made to compare the results of surgical extirpation with radiation therapy. Order and colleagues (1968) compared their patients with carcinoma of the lung who received radiation therapy with the surgically treated patients of Lang and Slater (1964). The differences between the 2 groups were not statistically significant although at each point there appeared to be more survivors in the radiation group. Lang and Slater's series had a high operative mortality, however, because most of the patients were treated before steroids were used for adjunctive therapy. Montana and colleagues (1972) reported the results of 15 craniotomies (in patients with single and multiple metastatic lesions) and compared those figures with the results from 47 patients irradiated (in different fashions) for single, multiple and an undetermined number of

Emergency Craniotomies			
Site	Number of Patients	Median Survival (Mos.)	30-Day Mortality
Supratentorial	9	2	1
Posterior fossa	9	4	2
	18	2.3 overall median	3 (16.6%)

Table 26.7

EXTRACRANIAL DISEASE AT THE TIME OF CRANIOTOMY AND SURVIVAL

| | Extent of Disease (Positive) | | | |
| | | | 1-Year Survival | |
Primary	Number of Patients	Median Survival (Mos.)	Number of Patients	(Percentage)
Lung	14	4.5	2*	15
Melanoma	14	3.8	2†	18
Sarcoma	7‡	4	2*	33
Breast	6	9	3	50
Choriocarcinoma	7	8	2	28.5
Undetermined	3	5	1	33
Others	11	5	1*	10
TOTAL	62	5 overall	13	23

*One patient lost to followup.
†Two patients lost to followup.
‡One patient's status preoperatively was unclear but was probably positive for extracranial disease.
§One patient still living.

metastatic lesions. The results were not statistically different. Essentially the same findings were observed in Berry's study (1974) comparing 22 patients undergoing surgical resection with 102 patients receiving only radiation therapy, although at all points the surgical group had a slightly greater percentage of survivors. In our previously reported series, surgically treated patients appeared to live longer (Posner 1974) but at no point are the data statistically different. Interestingly, in these series in which patients were broken down by functional class before treatment, there appeared no substantial difference between those patients selected for surgery and those selected for radiation therapy.

One argument frequently mustered for surgical extirpation of single brain metastases is the occasional longterm survivor or apparent cure produced by such treatment. We achieved no such prolonged survival in our

	Extent of Disease (Negative)			
			1-Year Survival	
	Number of Patients	Median Survival (Mos.)	Number of Patients	(Percentage)
	9	6	4*	50
	4	8.5	2	50
	1	24§	1	100
	5	5	2	40
	2	6.2	0	0
	5	5.5	0*	0
	6	6.5	0†	0
	32	5.75 overall	9	32

series. Other series summarized in table 26.10 indicate that this occurs although the percentage of prolonged survivors is quite small.

Surgical extirpation of brain metastases at least guarantees that the pretreatment diagnosis is correct. Because histologic verification of brain metastases treated with radiation is not obtained (except at autopsy, if performed), occasional longterm survivors in the radiation therapy series may be the result of errors in diagnosis. When Posner (1974) reviewed the patients who received whole-brain irradiation for presumptive brain metastases prior to 1971 and who were examined at autopsy, he discovered a 50% error rate. If a patient survives for a long period of time after radiation, it is possible that the diagnosis was incorrect rather than radiation therapy effective. Raskind and Weiss (1970) have emphasized in their report that errors in diagnosis are often made.

With careful neurologic evaluation and neurodiagnostic techniques, including computed tomography, the error rate is likely to be much smaller. When strict neurologic criteria including contrast studies were re-

Table 26.8

CAUSE OF DEATH

Cause	Number of Patients
Disseminated disease	17*
Acute pulmonary embolus	10
Pneumonia	7
Sepsis	7
Recurrence/extension of neurologic disease	10†
Other (CP arrest, respiratory failure, GI hemorrhage)	8
TOTAL	59

*Many patients were suffering from effects of widely disseminated disease when last examined, but since details of events surrounding death were not always clear, such patients' causes of death are not included in these figures.
†Includes one from meningeal melanoma and one brain abscess.

quired to make a diagnosis of cerebral metastasis, our error rate fell to less than 2% (Posner 1974).

Evaluation of radiation therapy series in the literature requires a knowledge of the criteria used for establishing the diagnosis, but a report of prolonged survival after irradiation of a brain metastasis should not imply that there was an error in diagnosis. Several case reports describe long survivals after irradiation of seemingly well-documented brain metastases (Deeley and Edwards 1968). We have reported 5 patients in whom autopsy examination suggested complete sterilization of a brain metastasis by radiation therapy (Cairncross et al. 1979).

In the absence of a controlled study, it is impossible to be certain whether surgical extirpation has any advantage over radiation therapy alone for the treatment of brain metastases. The finding that surgically treated patients live a little longer can be explained in part by the fact that good risk patients are likely to be treated with surgery and that poor risks tend to be treated by radiation alone.

All patients who undergo surgical extirpation should receive postoperative whole-brain irradiation, both to treat the bed of the brain metastasis removed and any microscopic lesions which may be present elsewhere in the brain. At the time of autopsy, 68% of our patients had tumor involving the brain, and about one-third had local recurrence at the operative site. Nearly half of those with brain metastases at autopsy had multiple lesions. The role of chemotherapy in the postoperative treatment of patients is unclear.

One of the interesting findings from this study is the frequent stormy postoperative course requiring re-operation. The only previous study which discussed re-operations (Harr and Patterson 1972), reported a postoperative complication rate of 24% and an 8% re-operation rate. Among our patients 17% underwent re-operation.

In most instances, our patients requiring re-exploration developed lethargy, often with accentuation of their preoperative neurologic signs, within 48 hours of surgery. When they were re-explored, subdural hematomas, CSF loculations, or simply brain swelling were encountered. Usually these patients did well postoperatively. One-third of our re-explorations (7 of 21) disclosed subdural hematomas. Many of these hematomas were small (less than 50 cc) and were accompanied by cerebral edema. The latter was probably responsible for the patients' neurologic deterioration. In 8 of the 21 re-explorations, brain swelling alone (of various degrees) was found as the explanation for the postoperative deterioration.

Two patients who developed intracerebral hematoma did well for about 12 hours and then developed sudden rather than subacute decompensation characterized by stupor, respiratory distress, motor dysfunction, and third nerve palsy. Both patients developed brainstem compression and subsequently died despite re-operation. Both were studied at autopsy. There was no residual tumor in one; but in the other, a small tumor nodule (not suspected preoperatively) was found adjacent to the surgical site and was the cause of swelling, herniation and hemorrhage. Ransohoff (1975) has emphasized the importance of small neighboring metastatic nodules which are not diagnosed preoperatively and which later account for postoperative deterioration.

One patient was explored 24 hours after the original operation. Brain swelling was found, and she did well for about 24 hours and then deteriorated again. The second time no operation was carried out, but she was treated with large doses of steroids and intravenous mannitol. She subsequently recovered after about 48 hours and did well thereafter. Indeed we have since had patients who presented in a similar fashion and in whom cerebral arteriography was performed: when the arteriograms were normal, those patients responded to large doses of dexamethasone together with hyperosmolar agents. Thus, the data from the current series suggest that deterioration between 12–72 hours after surgery calls for a CT scan; unless there is clear evidence of a significant hematoma, the patient probably need not be re-explored but instead should be treated with steroids and hyperosmolar agents as necessary to control symptoms.

Unusually high doses of steroids (40–80 mg/day dexamethasone)

Table 26.9

PATHOLOGIC CORRELATIONS FOR 19 PATIENTS
EXAMINED BY AUTOPSY

	Number of Autopsies	Evidence of Systemic Disease Preoperatively		CNS-Free
		Positive	Negative	
Lung	6	5	1	1
Melanoma	2	2	0	0
Breast	1	1	—	0
Sarcoma	1	1	—	0
Kidney	4	1	3	2
Colon	1	1	—	1
Ovary	1	1	—	1
Neuroblastoma	1	1	—	0
Choriocarcinoma	2	1	1	1†
TOTALS	19	14	5	6

*Patient died from acute pulmonary embolus.
†Brain abscess.

might be useful in protecting against or in treating postoperative neurologic deterioration (Renaudin et al. 1973). Using this treatment in several patients, the symptoms usually resolved within 48 hours. The symptoms were believed to be due to cerebral edema with subdural hematoma or loculated spinal fluid collection playing a minor role. Re-exploration and removal of the bone plate, despite adequate (complete) excision of the metastatic tumor, may nevertheless be necessary when medical treatment alone fails to halt neurologic deterioration. Exact guidelines for the clinician in this dilemma remain to be clarified.

The problem of negative explorations, which was significant in the

		Autopsy Findings			
Local Recurrence	New Single Metastasis	Multiple Metastases	Meningeal Carcinomatosis	Systemic Disease	
				Present	Absent
3	1	4	3	6	0
0	0	2	2	2	0
0	1	0	1	1	—
0	0	1	0	1	—
2	0	0	0	3	1*
0	0	0	0	1	—
0	0	0	0	1	—
0	0	1	0	1	—
1	0	1	0	1	1
6	2	9	6	17	2

early part of this study, now appears largely solved by the ability of CT to localize the precise site of the tumor. This allows the surgeon to locate the tumor even when it is not visible on the surface of the brain. Thus, judicious use of the CT scan, both before and after operation, makes management of the surgical patient much easier today than in the past.

The most surprising finding in this study was the lack of correlation between the degree of systemic disease and the length of survival after surgery. There are two reasons for this: first, patients with widespread systemic disease not expected to live more than a few weeks or months are rarely referred for surgery and are not considered in this study. Furthermore, in this study most of the patients with documented systemic disease were believed to have indolent or easily controllable disease. Secondly,

Table 26.10

SURGICAL TREATMENT OF CEREBRAL METASTASIS

Reference	Number of Patients	30-Day Mortality (Percentage)
Stortebecker (1954)	125	25 (20 days)
Richards and McKissock (1963)†	108	32
Lang and Slater (1964)	208	22
Vieth and Odom (1965)	155	15 (2 weeks)
Raskind et al. (1971)	51	12 (2 weeks)
Haar and Patterson (1972)	167	11
Ransohoff (1975)	100	10
Present study (1978)	94	8.5

*Back to work.
†Total excision only.
‡Alive and well at 6 mos. following surgery.

preoperative studies do not always disclose systemic disease: several of our patients whom we thought to be free of systemic tumor developed lethal metastatic complications during the postoperative period. They died much earlier than we had anticipated.

Even though the literature up to the present time, including this study, provides no basis (controlled study) for determining whether surgical therapy is superior to radiation therapy for the treatment of brain metastases, we believe that our data identify the following patients as those likely to benefit most by surgical extirpation: Patients in whom there has been a long interval between the discovery of their primary tumor and the discovery of their brain metastasis. This was suggested by Livingston and colleagues 30 years ago (1948). Patients with single brain metastases in accessible areas (supratentorial compartment) do better than those with multiple metastases or those whose tumor is deep within the hemisphere or in the posterior fossa. Longterm survivors usually have relatively indolent tumors and systemic disease that can be controlled for prolonged periods by radiation or chemotherapy.

Survival			Neurologically Improved (Percentage)
Median (Mos.)	1-Year	Long Term	
3.6	21	3 > 4 years	32*
<5.0	17	8 > 2 years	—
4.0	20	27 > 2 years	40‡
<6.0	13.5	12 > 2 years	52‡
<6.0	30	4 > 3 years	79
6.0	22	7 > 5 years	—
6+	38	13 > 2 years	—
5.5	25	2 > 4 years	90

The guidelines we recommend for selection of patients for surgical extirpation of a brain metastasis are summarized in table 26.11. The indications for surgery include an *uncertain diagnosis*. Patients with Hodgkin's disease, for example, are more likely to suffer from brain abscesses than brain metastases, and if the two cannot be clinically differentiated exploration for diagnostic purposes is indicated. Many patients in general hospitals enter surgery for what is thought to be a primary brain tumor; the systemic cancer is discovered only after the histologic diagnosis of brain metastasis. In our series, these patients appeared to do no better than those known to be harboring systemic cancers.

A second indication is the *failure of conservative therapy* to control symptoms. If whole-brain irradiation has been given and the patient continues to show signs of increased intracranial pressure or does not recover motor function, or if these signs recur after the patient has received maximal radiation and the patient's systemic condition is still good, surgical extirpation may be indicated. Prior irradiation may make the operation more difficult, but surgical removal is still possible.

There are certain *very slowly growing tumors which resist radiotherapy*, such as alveolar soft-part sarcomas which should be removed if the patient's general health permits.

Table 26.11

SURGERY FOR CEREBRAL METASTASES: INDICATIONS AND CONTRAINDICATIONS

Indications

1. Uncertain diagnosis

2. Recurrence or persistence of severe neurologic disability post-radiation therapy (+ chemotherapy)

3. Certain indolent but radioresistant tumors (such as alveolar soft part sarcoma)

4. Certain single cerebral metastasis?
    a. > 1 year after discovery of primary*
    b. lesion easily accessible
    c. elective patients
    d. no or moderate extracranial disease

Contraindications

1. Multiple cerebral metastases

2. Extensive or disseminated extracerebral disease

3. Stupor or coma

4. < 1 year after diagnosis of primary

*Certain lung and renal tumors presenting as cerebral lesions may be exceptions.

Relative contraindications include *multiple brain metastases* and *extensive or disseminated extracerebral disease* although our findings suggest that some extracerebral disease does not significantly change the prognosis. Cure is considerably less likely if extracerebral disease has not been eradicated, however.

Extirpation of tumors in patients who are stuporous, comatose or herniating (emergency states) should be considered only if these patients were in satisfactory medical and neurologic condition immediately prior to their sudden neurologic decompensation. Patients in the present study in good medical and neurologic condition immediately prior to herniation were often returned to a good functional state and survived for 5–20 months. On the other hand, patients in poor neurologic condition prior to sudden decompensation could be expected to live only a few weeks.

A short interval between discovery of the primary cancer and the appearance of brain metastasis also is a relative contraindication to surgery. In our study, this was especially true for patients with malignant melanoma.

Further delineation of the surgical treatment of brain metastases will, of necessity, await a controlled study comparing surgical extirpation with nonsurgical treatment. Our preliminary experience indicates, however, that several problems may make such a study exceedingly difficult: Many patients are willing to join protocol studies comparing two types of drugs or two types of surgery but are unwilling to be randomized to surgery versus nonsurgery, frequently choosing one or the other treatment modality themselves. Many referring physicians also have definite views about treatment and indicate such to their patients. Furthermore, nonrandomized studies have indicated that differences in outcome between surgical and nonsurgical therapy are likely to be small and that large numbers of patients will be required to achieve statistical significance. Because the outcomes may vary with the nature of the primary tumor, a proposed study must stratify patients into the various primary tumors. Consequently the definitive state on the treatment of solitary accessible brain metastases will be a long time in coming.

REFERENCES

Anderson, R. Diodrast studies of the vertebral and cranial venous systems. *J. Neurosurg.* 8:411–422, 1951.

Berry, H. C.; Parkers, R. G.; and Gerdes, A. J. Irradiation of brain metastases. *Acta Radiol. [Ther.] (Stockh.)* 13:535–544, 1974.

Brady, L. et al. Radiation therapy for intracranial metastatic neoplasia. *Radiol. Clin. Biol.* 43:40–47, 1974.

Breslow, N. A generalized Kruskal-Wallis test for comparing K samples subject to unequal patterns of censorship. *Biometrika* 57:579–594, 1970.

Dandy, W. E. *Surgery of the brain.* Hagerstown, Md.: W. F. Prior Co., Inc., 1945.

Dayes, L. A.; Rouhe, S. A.; and Barnes, R. N. Excision of multiple intracranial metastatic hypernephroma. Report of a case with a 7-year survival. *J. Neurosurg.* 46:533–535, 1977.

Deeley, T. J., and Edwards, J. M. Radiotherapy in the management of cerebral secondaries from bronchial carcinoma. *Lancet* 1:1209–1213, 1968.

Deutsch, M.; Parsons, J. A.; and Mercado, R., Jr. Radiotherapy for intracranial metastases. *Cancer* 34:1607–1611, 1974.

Fager, C. S. Neurosurgery in central nervous system metastasis. *Med. Clin. North Am.* 59:487–494, 1975.

Goran, A., and Murthy, K. K. Solitary cerebral metastasis: long-term survival following surgery. *N.Y. State J. Med.* 77:1780–1782, 1977.

Haar, F., and Patterson, R. H. Surgery for metastatic intracranial neoplasm. *Cancer* 30:1241–1245, 1972.

Lang, E. F., and Slater, J. Metastatic brain tumors. Results of surgical and non-surgical treatment. *Surg. Clin. North Am.* 44:865-872, 1964.

Livingston, K. E.; Horrax, G.; and Sachs, E. Metastatic brain tumors. *Surg. Clin. North Am.* 28:805–810, 1948.

Mayer, E. G.; Boone, M. L.; and Aristizabal, S. A. Role of radiation therapy in the management of neoplasms of the central nervous system. *Adv. Neurol.* 15:201–220, 1976.

Modesti, L. M., and Feldman, R. A. Solitary cerebral metastasis from pulmonary cancer. Prolonged survival after surgery. *J.A.M.A.* 231:1064, 1975.

Montana, G. S.; Meacham, W. F.; and Caldwell, W. L. Brain irradiation for metastatic disease of lung origin. *Cancer* 29:1477–1480, 1972.

Newman, S. J., and Hansen, H. H. Frequency, diagnosis and treatment of brain metastases in 247 consecutive patients with bronchogenic carcinoma. *Cancer* 33:492–496, 1974.

Nisce, L. Z.; Hilaris, B. S.; and Chur, F. C. H. A review of experience with irradiation of brain metastasis. *Am. J. Roentgenol.* 111:329–333, 1971.

Order, S. E. et al. Improvement in quality of survival following whole brain irradiation for brain metastasis. *Radiology* 91:149–153, 1968.

Posner, J. B. Diagnosis and treatment of metastases to the brain. *Clin. Bull.* 4:47–57, 1974.

Posner, J. B., and Shapiro, W. R. The management of intracranial metastases. In *Current controversies in neurosurgery*, ed. T. P. Morley. Philadelphia: W. B. Saunders Co., 1976.

Ransohoff, J. Surgical management of metastatic tumors. *Semin. Oncol.* 2:21–27, 1975.

Raskind, R.; and Weiss, S. R. Conditions simulating metastatic lesions of the brain. Report of eight cases. *Int. Surg.* 43:40–43, 1970.

Raskind, R. et al. Survival after surgical excision of single metastatic brain tumors. *Am. J. Roentgenol.* 111:323–328, 1971.

Renaudin, J. et al. Dose dependency of Decadron in patients with partially excised brain tumors. *J. Neurosurg.* 39:302–305, 1973.

Richards, P., and McKissock, W. Intracranial metastases. *Br. Med. J.* 1:15–18, 1963.

Stortebecker, T. P. Metastatic tumors of the brain from a neurosurgical point of view: a follow-up study of 158 cases. *J. Neurosurg.* 11:84–111, 1954.

Tarnoff, J. F.; Calinog, T. A.; and Byla, J. G. Prolonged survival following cerebral metastasis from pulmonary cancer. *J. Thorac. Cardiovasc. Surg.* 72:933–937, 1976.

Vieth, R. G., and Odom, G. L. Intracranial metastases and their neurosurgical treatment. *J. Neurosurg.* 23:375–383, 1965.

Young, D. F. et al. Rapid-course radiation therapy of cerebral metastases: results and complications. *Cancer* 34:1069–1076, 1974.

Appendix

A SCHEME FOR RECORDING AUTOPSY DATA USED IN THE
NEUROPATHOLOGY SECTION, DEPARTMENT OF PATHOLOGY,
MEMORIAL SLOAN-KETTERING CANCER CENTER

WORK BOOK

NEUROPATHOLOGY

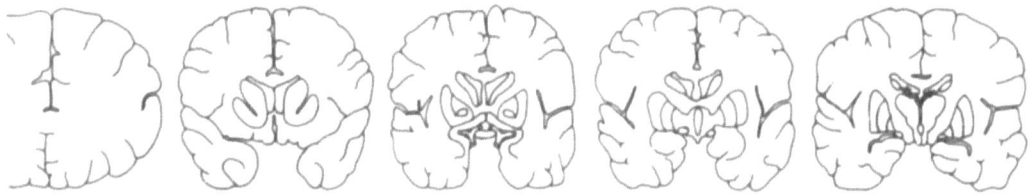

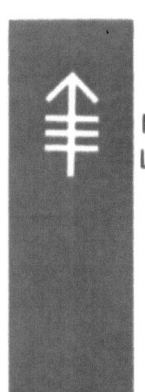

N.L. Chernik, M.D. • Neuropathology Section
L.B. McDowell, M.A. • Department of Medical Illustration

Name _____   Prosector _____

Chart No. _____   Neuropathologist _____

Accession _____   Date _____

Autopsy No. _____

Provisional Neuropathologic Diagnosis:

Microscopic Findings:

Final Neuropathologic Diagnosis:

GROSS APPEARANCE

Cerebral Dura and Calvarium:

Brain   Brain Weight _____
   A. Vessels

   B. Leptomeninges

   C. Size, type and anatomic location(s) of lesion(s):

   D. Mass displacements

   E. Ventricular system

Vertebral Column

Spinal Cord and Nerve Roots

Pituitary Gland / Cavernous Space

Autopsy No. _____

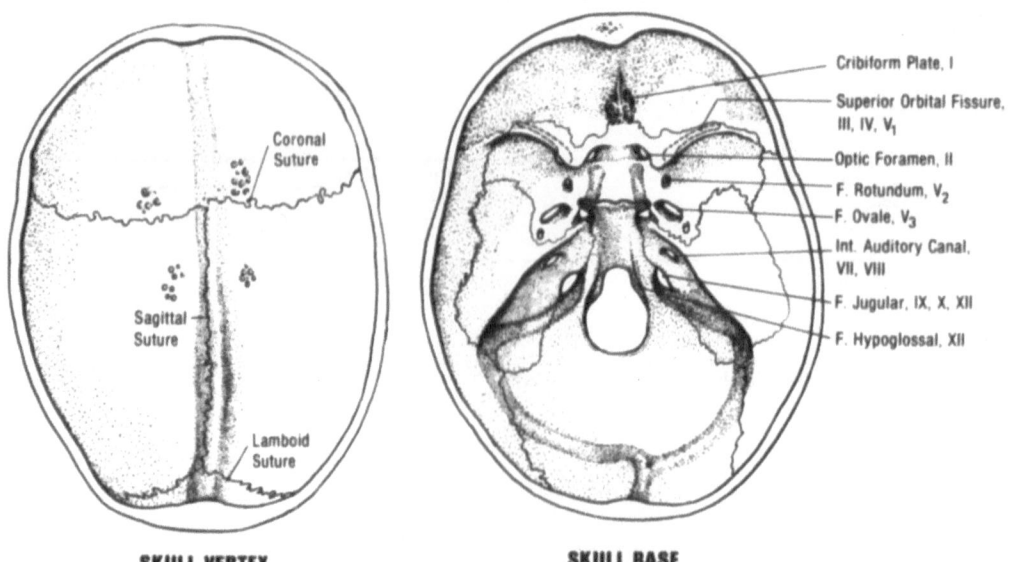

SKULL VERTEX

Coronal Suture

Sagittal Suture

Lamboid Suture

SKULL BASE

Cribiform Plate, I

Superior Orbital Fissure, III, IV, V₁

Optic Foramen, II

F. Rotundum, V₂

F. Ovale, V₃

Int. Auditory Canal, VII, VIII

F. Jugular, IX, X, XII

F. Hypoglossal, XII

1. Internal Carotid
2. Middle Cerebral
3. Anterior Cerebral
4. Vertebral
5. Basilar
6. Posterior Cerebral
7. Post. Inf. Cerebellar
8. Anterior Spinal

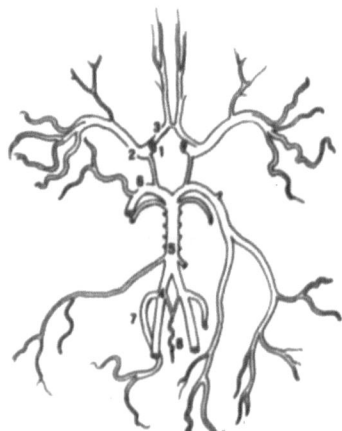

CIRCLE OF WILLIS

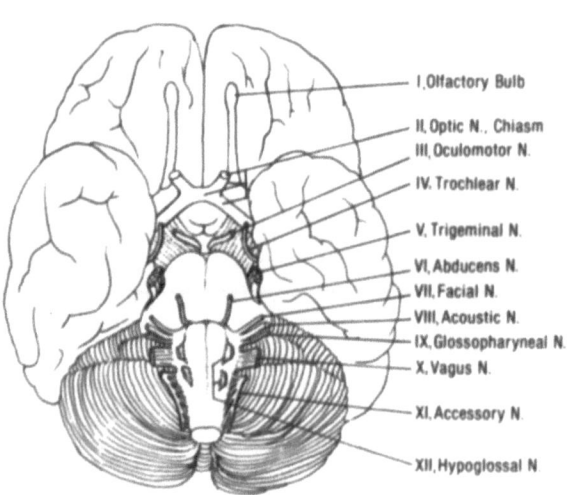

BASE OF BRAIN

I, Olfactory Bulb

II, Optic N., Chiasm

III, Oculomotor N.

IV. Trochlear N.

V, Trigeminal N.

VI, Abducens N.

VII, Facial N.

VIII, Acoustic N.

IX, Glossopharyneal N.

X, Vagus N.

XI, Accessory N.

XII, Hypoglossal N

Autopsy No. _____

☐ Indicate if this page is for final report

A. Frontal Lobes
(poles)

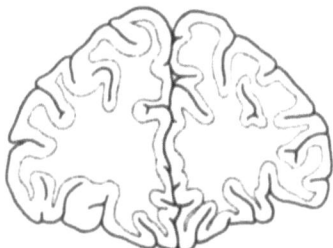

B. Frontal Lobes
(at genu corpus callosum)

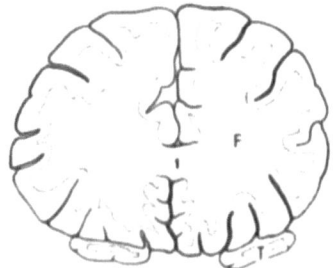

C. Mid Frontal Lobes
(at head of caudate nucleus)

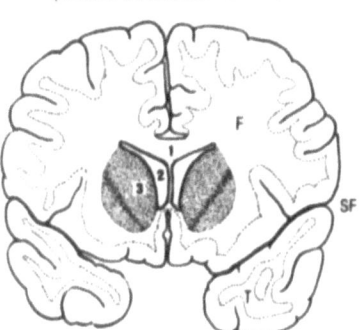

D. Mid Frontal - Temporal Lobes
(at anterior limb internal capsule)

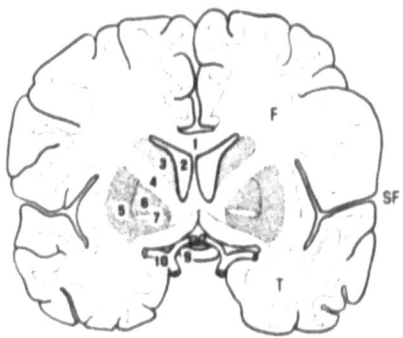

E. Posterior Frontal - Temporal Lobes
(at genu internal capsule)

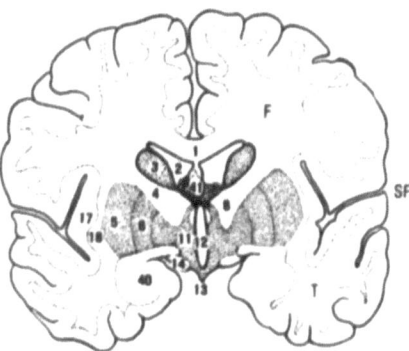

F. Posterior Frontal - Temporal Lobes
(at posterior limb internal capsule)

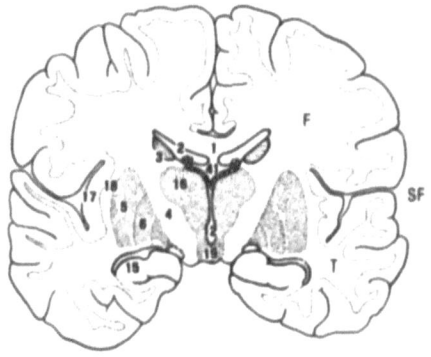

CORONAL BRAIN SECTIONS

Autopsy No. _____

☐ Indicate if this page is for final report

G. Posterior Frontal - Parietal - Temporal Lobes

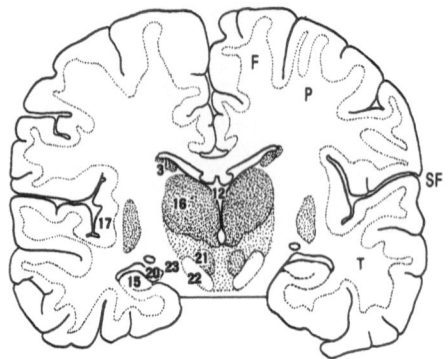

H. Parietal - Temporal Lobes

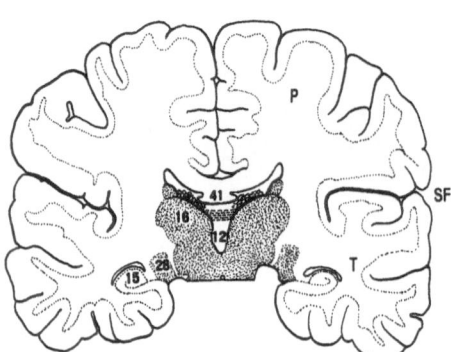

I. Parietal - Temporal Lobes
(at splenium of corpus callosum)

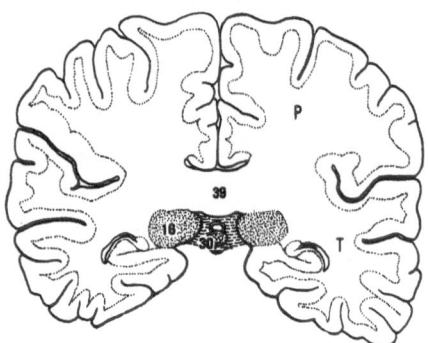

J. Occipital Lobes

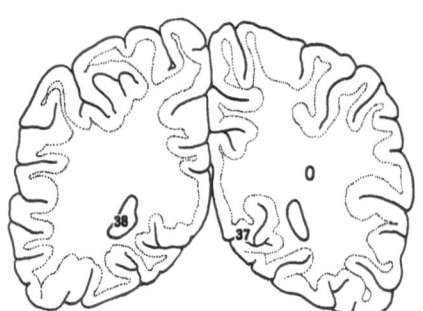

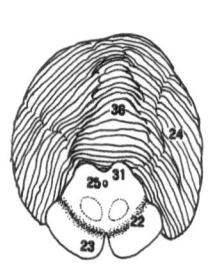

MIDBRAIN

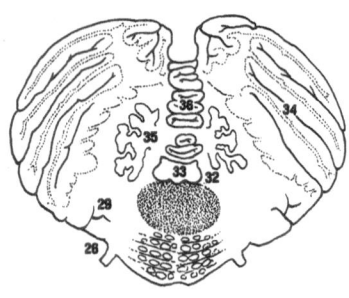

PONS

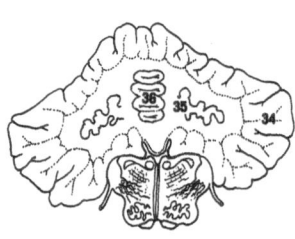

MEDULLA

CORONAL BRAIN SECTIONS

Autopsy No. _____
☐ Indicate if this page is for final report

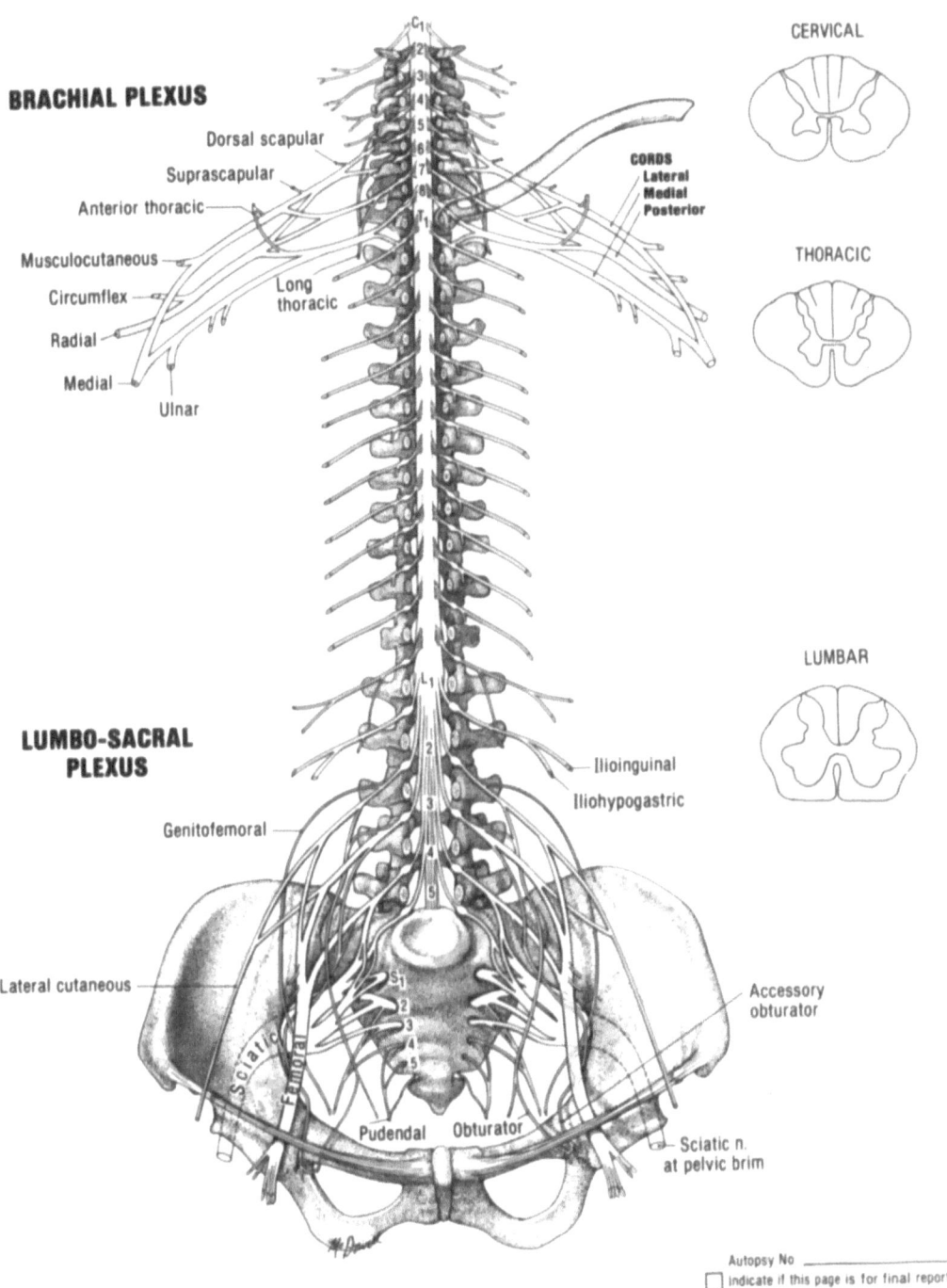

BRACHIAL PLEXUS

CERVICAL

Dorsal scapular

Suprascapular

Anterior thoracic

Musculocutaneous

Circumflex

Radial

Medial

Ulnar

Long thoracic

CORDS
Lateral
Medial
Posterior

THORACIC

**LUMBO-SACRAL
PLEXUS**

LUMBAR

Ilioinguinal

Iliohypogastric

Genitofemoral

Lateral cutaneous

Accessory obturator

Sciatic

Femoral

Pudendal   Obturator

Sciatic n.
at pelvic brim

Autopsy No _____
☐ indicate if this page is for final report

Index

Subject Index

Abscesses
  on CT scan, 220, 223, 233–234
  needle biopsy and, 386
  after surgery, 397
Absorption tests, in immunological studies, 170–176
Acalculia, 194
ACNU, 136–138
Acoustic neurinomas
  on CT scan, 231
  metastases to, 8
Addison's disease, 351
Adenocarcinomas
  cell arrest and, 41
  circulation of, 88
  metastases from, 82, 84
Adrenocorticosteroid hormones, 340–363
  history of use of, 340–341
  surgery and, 393
  See also Steroids
Adriamycin, with radiation therapy, 364–379
Agnosia, 194
Aldosterone, 343
Alexia, 194
α-amino-isobutyric acid (AID), 141–142
α-feto protein, 44
Ammonia, labeled, 250
Amnesia, 194
Angiography, 208
Anticoagulant drugs, 41
Antigens. See Cell-surface antigens
Aphasia, 194, 195, 341
Apraxia, 194, 341
Arabinoside. See Cytosine arabinoside
Arachnoidal membrane permeability, 149
Area postrema, 119
Arteriography, 272
  dexamethasone after, 409
  glucocorticoids and, 348
  sagittal sinus occlusion on, 199
  surgery and, 393
L-asparaginase, 152
Astrocytoma
  cell surface antigen studies with, 176–179
  metastases to, 8
Ataxia, 195, 382

ATPase activity, 356
Automobile accident syndrome, 201
Autopsy studies, of brain metastases, 16–18

Basal cisterns, 220
Basal lamina of tumor vessels, 125
BCG, and immunotherapy, 182
BCNU
  bronchogenic carcinoma and, 331
  malignant melanoma and, 331–332
  permeability of blood-brain barrier and, 150
  Radiation Therapy Oncology Group (RTOG) studies and, 284
Behavior
  brain metastases and, 196
  glucocorticoids and, 349
Bladder cancer, 68, 294
Blood
  arrest of cells and, 41
  brain-CSF interfaces with, 146
  within brain metastases, 11
  brain microcirculatory units in, 90–92
  brain tumor microvasculature and, 115–133
  cell detachment and, 35–36
  cerebral, on positron-emission tomography, 249–250
  cytotoxic factors in, 39
  distribution of brain metastases and, 11
  drug permeability studies with, 160–163
  experimental metastatic patterns and, 50–51
  microinjury hypothesis and, 86–89
  migration of tumor cells and, 92–96
  site of single brain metastasis and, 21
  spread of brain metastases and, 18
  trauma to cancer cells in, 38–39
  tumor emboli in, 84–86
  See also Microvasculature
Blood-brain barrier
  adrenocorticosteroid hormones and, 341
  brain changes and osmotic opening in, 103–105
  in center of brain tumors, 328
  chemotherapy and, 144

dexamethasone and, 344
edema control and, 25
expression of permeability in, 148
malignant cells in central nervous system and, 23
mannitol and methotrexate and, 139–140
methotrexate and, 109–110, 111–112
murine sarcoma virus 3 and absence of, 126
physiologic evidence for osmotic barrier opening in, 101–103
physiology of movement of drugs across, 146–149
on positron-emission tomography, 251
prophylaxis with chemotherapy and, 329
quantification of barrier permeability in, 106–109
regional differences in, 149
simplified model of drug transport across, 149–152
structure and function of, 101
tracer studies of, 141–142
unique aspects of brain metastases and, 24–25
Bone graft marrow, 262
Bone tumors, 73–76, 294
Brain
　blood-CSF interfaces with, 146
　microcirculatory units of, 90–92
　osmotic opening in blood-brain barrier and changes in, 103–105
　See also Blood-brain barrier
Brain metastases
　central necrosis in, 4
　classification of, 4, 11–13
　clinical manifestations of, 189–191
　definition of, 4
　focal symptoms of, 189–191
　frequency of, 14–18
　generalized symptoms of, 191
　histologic types of tumors in, 82–84
　incidence of, 14
　microscopic appearance of, 11
　model for, 134–145
　number of, 20–21
　presenting signs of, 195–196
　presenting symptoms of, 191–195
　reasons for special attention to, 2
　unique aspects of, 24–25
　unusual clinical syndromes in, 199–203
　varieties of, 4–8
Brain stem cancer, 92
Brain stem metastases, 8
　on CT scan, 238

hydrocephalus and, 25
site of single metastasis and blood supply in, 21
Breast cancer
　brain metastases and, 81
　cascade process and, 72, 73–76
　CCNU therapy for, 335
　chemotherapy for, 387
　circulation of tumor cells and, 85, 92, 96
　CT scan for, 214, 216
　meningeal carcinomatosis with, 338
　Ontario Cancer Institute studies on, 291, 292, 294
　as primary cancer, 18
　prophylactic chemotherapy for, 329
　radiation therapy for, 387
　Radiation Therapy Oncology Group (RTOG) studies of, 280–281
　single metastasis from, 20–21
　Southern California Permanent Medical Group studies of, 306–307
　subdural effusions and, 200
　surgical treatment of metastases from, 382, 392
　survival times for, 275, 292, 294, 387, 395
Bronchogenic carcinoma, and BCNU therapy, 331, 332, 335
Brown-Pearce carcinoma
　circulation of tumor cells and, 87
　patterns of metastatic development and, 50–51
B16 melanoma cells
　cell periphery characteristics of, 32
　circulation of, 94
　development of experimental models for, 51–52
　properties of brain-colonizing variants of, 61–62

Calcified metastases, 216
Calcium and cell adhesion, 37–38
Calvarial metastases, 212
Cancer cells. *See* Cells
Cancer coagulative factor, 41
Cancer mortality rates, 2
Carboxypeptidase, 152
Carcinoembryonic antigen (CEA), 44
Cascade process, 66–80
　brain metastases and, 76–78
　breast and prostate cancer and, 73–76
　nature of, 67–72
　organ-specific subpopulations of cancer cells and, 33
　pulmonary metastases and, 72–73
　schematic diagrams for, 68–72, 73–75

statistical analysis for, 67
CCNU
  malignant melanoma and, 332
  metastatic brain tumor model and,
    136–138
  permeability of blood-brain barrier
    and, 150
  radiation therapy combined with, 364–
    379
Cecum tumors, 294
Cells
  adhesion of, 35, 37–38
  arrest cycle in, 39–42
  circulation of, 38–40
  deformability of, 40
  detachment of, 35–36, 39–40
  development of metastasis and, 42–44
  differences between cancer and nor-
    mal periphery in, 30
  dormancy of, 43
  movement of, 36–38
  nonadherence of, 37–38
  periphery studies of, 30–49
  surface proteins of, and organ specific-
    ity, 60–61
Cell-surface antigens
  classes of, 173–176
  escape mechanisms and, 181
  immunotherapy and, 182
  renal cancer and astrocytoma serologic
    analysis in, 176–179
  tumor-specific, 165–167
Central nervous system (CNS)
  blood-brain barrier and malignant cells
    in, 23
  cascade process and, 68
  chemotherapy and, 144, 328–339
  metastases to tumors within, 8
  radiation effects on, 314–327
  unique aspects of brain metastases
    and, 24
Cerebellar metastases, 8
  blood supply and site of, 21
  CT scan and, 238
  gait ataxia and, 202
  hydrocephalus and, 25
  tumor distribution in, 135
Cerebrospinal fluid (CSF)
  blood-brain interfaces with, 146
  CT contrast and, 211
  in diagnosis, 205
  glucocorticoids and, 345
  methotrexate therapy and, 140
  onset of neurologic dysfunction and,
    197
  unique aspects of brain metastasis
    and, 24, 25

Cerebrum
  B16 melanoma metastases to, 54
  glucocorticoids and, 348
  microcirculatory units in, 91–92
  positron-emission tomography on,
    248–251
  site of single metastases and blood
    supply in, 21
  tumor distribution in, 135
Cervical cancer, 68, 294
Chemotherapy
  blood-brain barrier and, 100, 144
  bone marrow graft after, 262
  brain tumor microvasculature and, 115
  cascade process and choice of, 78
  central nervous system metastases
    and, 144, 328–339
  CT scan and, 224
  edema and, 328
  intraarterial drugs in, 156–158
  irradiation combined with, 364–379
  malignant cells in central nervous sys-
    tem and blood-brain barrier and,
    23
  meningeal carcinomatosis and, 336–
    338
  metastatic brain tumor model and,
    135–138
  organ-preferring melanoma variants
    and sensitivities to, 61–62
  physiology of blood-brain barrier and,
    146–149
  progressive multifocal leukoen-
    cephalopathy from, 223
  prophylactic use of, 329–330
  rate of drug inactivation, metabolism,
    and excretion in, 156
  rescue techniques and, 151–152
  simplified model of blood-brain trans-
    port in, 149–155
  site of drug administration and, 156
  after surgery, 389
  survival times and, 328–329
  time course of drug activity in, 158–160
Choriocarcinomas, 197, 210
Choroid plexus
  circulation of tumor cells and, 94
  endothelial defects and, 131
  metastases to, 8
  steroids and, 344, 356, 357
  tumor distribution in, 135
Chromophobe adenomas, 231
Cimetidine, 350
Circulation. *See* Blood
Citrovorum factor (CF), 152, 336
Classification of brain metastases, 4, 11–
    13

Cloudman S91 melanoma, 51
Coagulation, and circulation of tumor cells, 42, 85
Cognitive behavior, and brain metastases, 196
Colon cancer, 214, 216, 294
Computed tomography (CT), 208–241, 272
  accuracy of detection on, 224
  cascade process and, 77
  combined chemotherapy and radiation therapy on, 224, 378
  complications in, 238–239
  contrast enhancement in, 210–211, 239
  in diagnosis of brain metastases, 203–205
  in differential diagnosis, 205, 223
  equipment in, 209–210
  errors in use of, 238
  interpretation of, 212–223
  onset of neurologic dysfunction and, 197
  progressive multifocal leukoencephalopathy and, 223
  radiation dosage in, 238
  radionuclide scans as complementary to, 243–244
  radionuclide scan compared with, 203–204, 205
  as screening process, 228–238
  steroids and, 347–348
  surgery and, 227–228, 380, 384, 391, 399, 407, 409
  technical considerations in, 209–211
  treatment and, 224–228
Confusional states, 200–201
Convulsions. *See* Seizures
Corticosteroids
  anti-inflammatory effects of, 356
  CT scan and, 224
  massive doses of, 384
  radiation therapy with, 266, 267
  Radiation Therapy Oncology Group (RTOG) studies and, 281
  surgery and, 383, 384
  systemic effects of, 357
Cortisol, 357
Cortisone, 341
Cost-effectiveness of treatment, 300–301
Craniopharyngiomas, 131
Craniotomy. *See* Surgery
Creatinine, 239
CSF. *See* Cerebrospinal fluid (CSF)
Cyclic adenosine monophosphate (AMP), 352
Cyclophosphamide, 387

metastatic brain tumor model and, 134–135, 136–138
  for oat-cell carcinoma, 365
Cystic brain metastases, 4
Cytosine arabinoside
  blood-brain barrier and, 100, 107, 109, 110–111
  circulation of, 153
  meningeal carcinomatosis treatment with, 335, 336

Delta activity on EEG, 345, 346
Depression
  glucocorticoids and, 349
  as symptom, 194
Dexamethasone
  administration of, 344
  CT scans and, 347–348
  edema treatment with, 343
  glioblastoma treatment with, 352
  lung cancer improvement on EEG with, 345
  metastatic brain tumor model and, 136–138
  Ontario Cancer Institute studies with, 291
  radionuclide brain scans and, 347
  side effect of, 350
  surgery and, 391, 407
  systemic effect of, 357
Diagnosis of brain metastases, 186–253
  computed tomography (CT) in, 203–205
  surgical treatment and, 384–386
Dianhydrogalactitol, 150
Diazepam, 344
Differential diagnosis, and CT scan, 205, 223
Diphenylhydantoin, 384
Disseminated intravascular coagulation (DIC), 41
Doxorubicin hydrochloride, 364–379
Drugs. *See* Chemotherapy
Dural metastases
  breast or lung cancer and, 92
  on CT scan, 218
  frequency of, 17
  intracranial metastasis in, 2
  malignant melanoma and, 20

Edema
  blood-brain barrier and, 25, 105
  cerebral metastases surrounded by, 8
  chemotherapy and, 328
  clearance of, 356–357
  on CT scan, 212, 224, 228, 347

on EEG, 345–346
production of, 334–356
sodium metabolism and, 354–356
steroids for, 274, 341, 342, 343, 353–357
after surgery, 410
as symptom, 191
vascular permeability and, 354
Electroencephalography (EEG)
  diagnosis with, 205
  glucocorticoids and, 345–346
  steroids and, 353
  surgery and, 385
Electron microscopy, 123–128
Encephalitic brain tumor, 201
Endocrine gland cancer, 68
Endothelial cells
  in brain microvasculature, 117
  electron microscopy of, 123–128
  fenestrations in, 119, 128, 130
  gaps in, 128
  light microscopy of brain tumor micro-
    vasculature and, 122
  permeability in brain tumors and, 130–
    131
  pinocytotic vesicles in, 117
  tight junctions of, 117
Enzyme activity, and cell detachment, 36
Ependymoblastoma, 344, 352
Ependymoma, 8
Epidemiologic studies of brain metasta-
    ses, 14
Epidermoid carcinoma, 82, 88
Epidural metastases, 199
Epipodophyllotoxin, 150
Esophageal cancer, 68, 294
Experimental brain metastases, 50–65
  cell-surface proteins and organ prefer-
    ence of, 60–61
  development of models for malignant
    melanoma with, 51–52
  drug sensitivities and organ preference
    in, 61–62
  patterns of, 50–51
^{18}F-2-fluoro-2-deoxy-D-glucose (^{18}F-
    FDG), 249
Falx metastases, 218
Fenestrated endothelium, 119, 128, 130
Fertile soil theory, 18
Fibrin system, 42, 85
Fibroblasts, 36
Fibrosarcoma, 94
5-fluorouracil, 150, 389
Forebrain metastases, 54, 56
Frequency of brain metastases, 14–18,
    22–23
Frontal pole metastases, 8

Gait ataxia, 195, 202
Gallium brain scans, 251, 347
Gamma-ray emission tomography, 247–
    248
Gastrointestinal bleeding, and steroids,
    350
Gastrointestinal cancer, 68, 384
Genetic analysis, of cell surface antigen,
    180–181
Germimoma, 329
Gingiva tumors, 294
Glioblastomas, 130, 352
Gliomas
  blood-brain barrier and, 126
  on CT scan, 220, 223, 228
Glucocorticoids
  arteriography and, 348
  clinical response to, 343–344
  edema and, 353–357
  effects of, 345–348
  mechanisms of action of, 351–357
  radionuclide brain scans and, 347
  See also Steroids
Glucoheptonate, 242, 244
Glucose metabolic rate, 248–249
Graft, bone marrow, 262
Granulomas, 220, 234
Gray matter
  brain metastases at junction of white
    matter with, 4
  microcirculatory units in, 90
  permeability of blood-brain barrier in,
    149

Hahnemann Medical College and Hospi-
    tal, 269–278
Headache
  steroids for, 342
  as symptom, 192–193, 282, 394
Head cancers, 68, 315
Hemangioblastomas, 131
Hematomas, subdural, 395, 407, 408
Hemiparesis
  steroids for, 341, 342
  subdural effusions and, 200
  as symptom, 191, 193–194
Hemorrhage, cerebral, 233
Hemorrhagic brain metastases, 4
Hepatoma, 87
Host defense mechanism, 43
Hydrocephalus
  brain metastases and CSF absorption
    and, 25
  on CT scan, 211, 220
  gait ataxia and, 195

Immune adherence (IA) studies, 167–169
Immunology, 165–185
    absorption tests in, 170–176
    central nervous system and, 382
    dormancy of metastatic cells and, 43–44
    escape mechanism for antigenic tumors and, 181
    malignant melanoma studies in, 167–176
    tumor-cell arrest and, 42
    tumor-specific cell surface components in, 165–167
Immunosuppression, and leukoencephalopathy, 223
Immunotherapy
    misonidazole with, 385
    tumor-specific cell surface antigens and, 182
Incidence of brain metastases, 14, 22–23, 270
Infarction, on CT scan, 223, 231–232
Intracerebral metastases, on CT scan, 212–220
Intracranial metastases
    anatomic classification of, 2–4
    on CT scan, 238
    definition of, 2–4
    frequency of, 17
    site of, 18

Karyotypes of cancer cells, 31
Kidney cancer. *See* Renal cancer

Large-cell carcinomas, 82, 84
Latent period, and metastatic development, 81–82
Leptomeningeal metastases, 82
    breast or lung cancer and, 92, 96
    frequency of, 17
    intracranial metastases invading, 2
    lymphoblastic leukemia and, 23
    meningeal carcinomatosis and, 337
Leukemia
    on CT scan, 220
    as primary cancer, 18
    prophylactic chemotherapy for, 329
    prophylactic irradiation for, 261
Leukoencephalopathy, 223, 236
Lewis sarcoma, 41
Liver metastases, 68
Lumbar puncture, 345
Lung cancer
    brain-colonizing variants of B16 melanoma and, 54, 61
    brain metastases and, 81
    cascade process and, 68, 72–73
    CCNU for, 380
    chemotherapy in treatment of, 332
    combined chemotherapy and irradiation for, 364–379
    CT scan for, 214, 216
    dormancy of metastatic cells and. 43
    EEG improvement with dexmethasone for, 345
    meningeal carcinomatosis with, 338
    multiple metastases from, 21
    in Ontario Cancer Institute studies, 291, 292, 294
    organ specificity by tumor metastases and, 51, 52
    as primary site, 18
    prophylactic chemotherapy for, 329
    Radiation Therapy Oncology Group (RTOG) studies of, 280–281, 282
    Southern California Permanent Medical Group studies of, 305–306
    surgical treatment of, 381, 391
    survival rate and, 275, 292, 294, 395
    treatment of, 261
Lungs, and arrest cycle of cancer cells, 39–40
Lymph node tumors, 294
Lymphoblastic leukemia, 23
Lymphomas
    CT scans for, 214, 216
    endothelial defects and, 131
    meningeal carcinomatosis with, 338
    as primary cancer, 18
    prophylactic chemotherapy for, 329
    radiation therapy for, 325
    survival rate for, 275
Lysosomal enzymes
    arrest of tumor cells and, 42
    cell detachment and, 36
    deformability of cancer cells and, 40
Lytic metastases, 212

Mania, 194
Mannitol, 139–140, 409
Medulloblastoma defects, 130
Melanoma
    BCNU therapy for, 331
    blood-borne tumor emboli from, 84, 85
    brain metastases and, 81
    cell-surface antigen studies with, 178–179
    cell-surface proteins and, 60–61
    chemotherapy for, 331–332, 335
    confusional states from multiple metastases in, 200
    CT contrast for, 210, 218
    drug sensitivities and organ preference of, 61–62

experimental metastases models for,
51–52
immunologic studies with, 167–175
multiple metastases from, 21
onset of neurologic dysfunction in, 197
Ontario Cancer Institute experience
with, 291, 292
patterns of metastatic development
and, 51
as primary cancer, 18, 20
properties of brain-colonizing variants
of, 52–60
steroids and, 352
surgical treatment of, 381, 382, 392
See also B16 melanoma cells
Memorial Hospital, 265–268
Meningeal carcinomas, 220, 330
Meningeal carcinomatosis
chemotherapy and, 331, 332, 335
treatment of, 336–338
Meningiomas
on CT scans, 218, 223, 228–231
metastases to, 8
Mental disturbances, as symptom, 194
Metastasis, definition, 2
Methotrexate (MTX)
blood-brain barrier and, 100, 107, 109–
110, 111–112
after breast cancer surgery, 387
citrovorum factor rescue and, 152
intracarotid mannitol and, 139–140
for meningeal carcinomatosis, 335, 336
metastatic brain tumor model and,
136–138, 139–140
Methyl-CCNU, 136–138
Methylprednisolone, 386
Metrizamide, 210–211
Microcirculation units of brain, 90–92
Microinjury thesis, 86–89
Micrometastasis, 86, 88
Microvasculature
brain tumor, 115–133
electron microscopy of, 123–128
light microscopy of, 120–123
in normal brain, 117–119
Misonidazole, 385
Mixed hemadsorption (MHA) studies,
167–169, 182
Model for brain metastases, 167–169, 182
Monoparesis, as symptom, 193–194
Mortality rates, 2
Motor loss, as symptom, 282
Motor strip, 200–201
Multiple metastases
confusional states from, 200–201
CT scan and, 220
frequency of, 20–21

incidence of, 272
Multiple sclerosis, 236
Murine sarcoma virus 3, 126
Muscle tumors, 294
Muscle weakness, and steroids, 349–350
Myelitis, radiation, 314–327

Neck cancers, 68, 315
Necrosis
in brain metastases, 4
cell detachment and, 36
circulation of tumor cells and, 85
radiation, 234–235
Needle biopsy, 386
Neovascularization, 23
Neurilemoma, 130
Neuroblastomas, 130
Neurologic dysfunction
course of, 198–199
mode of onset of, 197–198
pseudovascular forms in, 199
Neurological function
Radiation Therapy Oncology Group
(RTOG) studies of, 281
steroids and, 341–343
surgical treatment and, 383–384
Nitrosoureas
metastatic brain tumor model and,
136–138
prophylaxis with, 329
radiation therapy with, 385
response rate for, 335
Nominal standard dose (NSD) of radiation, 288, 316

Oat-cell carcinomas
chemotherapy for, 333
confusional states from multiple metastases in, 200
cyclophosphamide for, 365
prophylactic irradiation for, 261
Occipital metastases, 8, 201
Ontario Cancer Institute, 286
Organ specificity
cell-surface proteins and, 60–61
drug-sensitivities of melanoma variants and, 61–62
Osmotic therapy, 259
Osteochondrosarcomas, 68
Osteogenic sarcoma, 216
Ovarian cancer, 294
brain-colonizing variants of B16 malignant melanoma and, 58–59, 61
cascade process and, 68
frequency of brain metastases with, 22
as primary cancer, 18
Oxygen extraction fraction, in PET, 250

PALA therapy, 153
Pancreatic tumors, 294
Papilledema
  sagittal sinus occlusion with, 199
  as symptom of brain metastases, 193
  withdrawal from steroids and, 351
Parietal metastases, 8, 201
Penile cancer, 294
Pentylenetetrazol, 348
Phenobarbital, 344, 387
Phenytoin, 275, 344
N-(phosphonacetyl)-L-aspartate, 153
Pineal gland, 8, 135, 383
Pituitary gland, 130, 135, 341
Platelet aggregating activity, 94
Plial network, brain, 90
Pneumoencephalography, 205, 208–209
Pneumonitis, radiation, 261
Positron-emission tomography (PET),
      244, 246–253
  application of, 248–251
  blood-brain barrier on, 251
  cerebral hemodynamics and, 249–250
  cerebral metabolism on, 248–249
  CT scan use and, 205
  theoretical basis for, 247–248
  tissue chemical composition on, 251
Postcentral gyrus, 21
Prednisolone, 341, 344, 352
Prednisone, 357
Primary cancer
  cancer cells in metastases different
      from, 31–34
  cascade process and location of, 77
  classification of brain metastases by, 11
  single or multiple metastases and na-
      ture of, 20–21
  site of, and brain metastases, 18–20
  surgical treatment of metastases and,
      381–382
Procarbazine, 136–138
Prostate cancer, 294
  cascade process and, 72, 73–76
  as primary cancer, 18
  subdural effusions and, 200
Protein A assay (PA), 167
Proteins, cell-surface, 60–61
Pseudorheumatism, 351
Pseudovascular forms, 199
Pulmonary cancer. *See* Lung cancer

Quality of life, and treatment, 311–312

Radiation necrosis, 234–235
Radiation pneumonitis, 261
Radiation therapy
  cascade process and choice of, 78

chemotherapy combined with, 364–
      379
complications in, 399
craniotomy prior to, 274
CT scan use and, 224
deaths from, 298
Hahnemann Medical College and Hos-
      pital experience with, 269–278
Memorial Hospital experience with,
      265–268
meningeal carcinomatosis treatment
      with, 336
metastatic brain tumor model and,
      138–139
misonidazole with, 385
myelitis from, 314–317
nervous system and, 314–317
nominal single dose (NSD) concept in,
      288, 316
in Ontario Cancer Institute, 287–288
prophylactic use of, 261
Radiation Therapy Oncology Group
      (RTOG) and, 279–285
retreatment with, 274
Southern California Permanente Medi-
      cal Group experience with, 304
steroids and, 343
after surgery, 392, 406–407
surgery compared with, 399–406
survival and, 298
time-benefit ratio for, 259
time-dose fractionation schemes for,
      267, 316–325
Radiation Therapy Oncology Group
      (RTOG), 279–285
Radiography, 208
Radionuclide scans, 242–245
  accuracy of detection on, 224
  combined chemotherapy and radi-
      otherapy on, 367, 378
  cost of, 243
  CT scan as complementary to, 243–244
  CT scan compared with, 203–204, 205
  glucorticoids and, 347
  instrumentation in, 242–243
  localization of metastases with, 243
  as screening technique, 244
  surgery and, 383
Rectal tumors, 68, 294
Renal cancer, 294
  brain metastases and, 81
  cascade process and, 68
  cell-surface antigens and, 176–179
  CT scan and, 214
  endothelial defects and, 131
  single metastases from, 21
  surgery for metastases from, 382, 394

Renal failure, from CT contrast material, 239

Rescue techniques, and drug circulation, 151–152

Reticulum-cell sarcoma, 51, 200–201

Retinoic acid, 62

Retreatment, 261, 274

Sagittal sinus occlusion, 199

Sarcomas
  blood-brain barrier and, 126
  cell arrest and, 41
  cell movement in, 36
  circulation of tumor cells and, 85
  frequency of brain metastases with, 22
  as primary cancer, 18
  surgical treatment of, 392–393

Screening programs
  with CT scans, 228–238
  with radionuclide scans, 244

Seizures
  from CT contrast material, 239
  phenytoin for, 344
  steroids and, 348–349
  surgery and, 384
  as symptom, 194–195, 394

Sex differences, in distribution of metastases, 92

Signs of brain metastases
  presenting, 195–196
  surgical treatment and, 394

Single brain metastasis, 4, 8
  frequency of, 20
  location of, 8
  site of, 8, 21
  surgery for, 338, 390–414

Site of cancer
  cascade process and, 68–72, 76
  characteristics of cancer cells and, 31
  within intracranial cavity, 18
  microcirculation of tumor cells and, 92
  of primary cancer, 18–20
  of single metastasis, 21
  survival rates and, 275

Skin tumors, 68, 294

Skull metastases, 2–4, 211

Skull radiography, 208, 385

Small-cell carcinomas, 82, 84

Solid tumors, 37–38

Southern California Permanent Medical Group, 303–313

Spirohydantoin mustard, 151, 158

Squamous-cell carcinomas, 84

Steroids
  anti-inflammatory effects of, 356
  CT scans and, 224, 347–348
  edema and, 353–357

effects of, 341–351

Ontario Cancer Institute use of, 291

radiation therapy with, 274, 290, 367, 368

re-operations and, 407–408

systemic effects of, 357

time-benefit ratio for, 259

untoward effects of, 348–350

withdrawal from, 329, 350–351

See also Adrenocorticosteroid hormones

Stomach tumors, 294

Subdural effusions, 200

Surgery, 380–414
  clinical presentations and, 381–382
  complications after, 395
  CT scan use and, 227–228
  diagnostic workup for, 382–384
  factors in selection for, 395–397, 411–413
  negative explorations in, 408–409
  neurological evaluation in, 383–384
  prior to radiation therapy, 274
  radiation therapy after, 406–407
  radiation therapy compared with, 399–406
  re-operations in, 407–408
  survival and, 386–387, 394–395, 404–405
  time-benefit ratio for, 258–259

Survival times
  breast cancer and, 292, 294
  chemotherapy evaluation with, 328–329
  combined chemotherapy and radiation and, 367
  degree of systemic disease and, 409–410
  lung cancer and, 292, 294
  meningeal carcinomatosis and, 337, 338
  in Ontario Cancer Institute studies, 292, 294
  quality of life and, 311–312
  radiation therapy and, 298
  in Radiation Therapy Oncology Group (RTOG) studies, 282
  site of primary tumor and, 275
  Southern California Permanent Medical Group and, 303–313
  surgery and, 386–387

Symptoms
  focal, 189–191
  generalized, 191
  presenting, 191–195, 270
  in Radiation Therapy Oncology Group (RTOG) studies, 282
  surgical treatment and, 394

Technetium glucoheptonate scans, 347
Testicle tumors, 68, 294
Thorax cancer, 315
Thrombosis, and cell arrest, 41–42
Thymidine, 153
Thymus leukemia (TL) antigen, 166
Thyroid tumors, 294
Time-benefit ratio, 258–259
T-lymphocytes, 43
Tongue tumors, 294
Treatment of metastases, 255–416
   adrenocorticosteroid hormones in,
      340–363
   in advance of expected metastases, 261
   analysis of benefits of, 257–264
   cascade process and choice of, 78
   concomitant primary tumor and brain
      metastases in, 261
   cost-effectiveness of, 300–301
   CT scans in, 224–228
   Memorial Hospital experience with,
      265–268
   of meningeal carcinomatosis, 336–338
   new techniques of management in,
      261–262
   Ontario Cancer Institute experience
      with, 286–302
   patient's view of, 257–258
   physician's role in, 259–260
   quality of life and, 311–312
   retreatment and, 261
   social factors in, 262
   Southern California Permanente Medi-
      cal Group experience with, 303–
      313
   time-benefit ratio in, 258–259
   treatment alternatives in, 260–262
   See also Chemotherapy; Radiation
      therapy
Tumor-specific transplantation antigens
   (TSA), 166

Urea levels, 239
Uridine, 153
Uterine tumors, 68, 294

Vertebral metastases, 73
Vitamin A, 36, 62
V2 carcinomas
   circulation of tumor cells and, 87
   patterns of metastatic development
      and, 50–51

Walker 256 carcinomas
   circulation of tumor cells and, 85, 86
   drug permeability studies with, 160
   migration of tumor cells from, 92, 94

   model for brain metastases and, 134,
      135, 138
Water content of brain, 348
White matter
   brain metastases at junction of gray
      matter with, 4
   microcirculatory units in, 90
   permeability of blood-brain barrier in,
      149
Withdrawal from steroids, 329, 350–351

Zonulae occludentes, brain, 117

Author Index

Abbatucci, J. S., 314, 316, 318, 324
Abbo, A. W., 299
Abercombie, M., 36, 37
Agostino, D., 86
Aita, J. F., 236
Alberti, E., 345
Alderson, P. O., 243
Alexander, J. W., 86, 87
Alexander, M., 329
Alexander, P., 43
Allen, J. C., 139, 236
Allen, M. B., Jr., 270
Alpers, B. J., 201
Alpert, N. M., 250
Altemeier, W. A., 86, 87
Amatruda, T. T., 351
Ambrus, J. L., 2
Anuigbo, W. I. B., 84
Appenzeller, O., 195
Aronson, S. M., 16, 18, 21
Arseni, C., 14, 15
Athens, J. W., 39
Atkins, H. L., 318, 320, 321, 322, 324
Axelrod, L., 349
Azmitia, E. C., 352, 358

Baethmann, A., 352, 356
Bahn, A. K., 316
Bajpai, D., 269–278
Baker, H. I., 236
Baldwin, R. W., 32, 44
Ballinger, W. E., 94
Bardfeld, P. A., 210, 216, 224
Barnes, D. W. H., 43
Baserga, R., 86
Batson, O. V., 11
Becker, H., 212
Bedikian, A. Y., 263
Beggs, J. L., 115, 124, 130, 131
Bennett, H. S., 91
Benua, R. S., 242–245
Berenblum, I., 84
Beresford, H. R., 53
Bergstrom, M., 233
Berkovich, M. L., 87
Berkowitz, R. S., 22
Bernard-Weil, E., 343
Berry, H. C., 406
Bhavilai, D., 322, 324
Bigner, D. D., 11, 115, 116, 134
Black, T. W., 195, 196
Blasberg, R. G., 23, 141, 142, 144, 146–164, 148, 149, 151, 160
Blumenson, L. E., 73
Boden, G., 317, 318, 319, 324

Bond, W., 349
Boone, C. W., 184
Borgelt, B., 279, 280, 282
Bosch, E. P., 223
Bouzarth, W. E., 357
Boyse, E. A., 165
Brady, L. W., 269–278, 286
Brewis, M., 14
Brightman, M. W., 102, 115, 117, 146
Brizzee, K. R., 119
Brooks, S. M., 344
Bross, I. D. J., 33, 66–80, 66, 73, 77, 79, 352
Brown, J. W., 194
Brown, W. J., 314
Brownell, G. L., 248
Bruning, J. L., 316
Brunson, K. W., 50–65, 52, 53, 54, 56, 58, 59, 60, 61
Budinger, T. F., 248
Buell, U., 224
Buell, V., 243
Bunn, P. A., Jr., 261
Burger, M. M., 32, 45
Buss, J. M., 50, 87
Butler, A. R., 210
Butler, T. P., 45
Byfield, J. E., 320, 324, 364–379

Cain, M. L., 347
Cairncross, 406
Cala, L. A., 236
Campbell, T., 364–379
Capon, A., 344, 348
Carella, R. J., 385
Carey, T. E., 167, 176, 178
Carr, I., 84
Carter, L. P., 131
Catane, R., 18
Chabner, B. A., 153
Chan, P. Y. M., 314–327, 364–379
Chang, C. H., 210, 218
Chang, P., 22
Chao, J. H., 265, 283, 367
Charney, A. N., 356
Chason, J. L., 16, 20, 21
Chernik, N. L., 11, 16, 20
Chernukh, A. M., 87
Chesler, D. A., 248
Chew, E. C., 41, 94
Chiueh, C. C., 103, 104
Cho, Z. H., 248
Christensen, E., 15
Christie, J. H., 243
Christopherson, W. M., 85, 86

Chu, F. C. H., 259, 265–268, 266, 267, 311
Clifton, E. E., 86
Cobb, L. M., 158
Collander, R., 102
Collier, J., 191
Coman, D. R., 35
Constant, P., 218, 220
Cook, P., 218, 220
Copeland, D. D., 117
Cortes, E. P., 378
Cotran, R., 131
Cowles, A. L., 110, 156
Cox, D. J., 115
Coy, P., 322, 324
Crocker, E. F., 224, 347
Crone, C., 101, 107, 149, 156
Cushing, H., 14, 15
Czerwinski, A. W., 349, 350

Dafny, N., 352
Dalessio, D. J., 193
Danziger, A., 234
Davis, R. L., 324
Davis, W., 158
Dayes, L. A., 390
Deck, M. D. F., 208–241, 214, 216, 236
Deeley, T. J., 367, 406
Dellen, J. R., van, 234
Den Hood-Sijtsema, S., 322, 324
Dische, S., 385
Donald, K. J., 39
Doring, L., 8
Dresden, M. H., 50
Driscoll, J., 151
Dubois, P. J., 220
Dunn, T. B., 51
Dutreix, J., 299
Dynes, J. B., 317, 318, 321, 322, 324

Earle, K. M., 16
Eaves, G., 50
Eccles, S. A., 43
Edwards, J. M. R., 367, 406
Ehrenkranz, J. R. L., 340–363
Ehrlich, P., 340
Eisenberg, H., 354
Eisenhardt, L., 15
Ekbom, K., 193
Elkington, J. S. C., 15, 196
Ellis, F., 288, 316
El-Shaboury, A. H., 357
Engell, H. C., 85
Enzmann, D. R., 216, 218, 220
Escourolle, R., 81, 82
Espana, P., 20, 22
Evens, R. G., 244

Eyster, E. F., 317, 321, 324

Feldman, R. A., 390
Feldman, S., 352
Fenstermacher, J. D., 100, 110, 156
Fewer, D., 378
Fidler, I. J., 32, 45, 50, 51, 52, 56, 58, 61, 94, 349
Fisher, B., 43, 86
Fisher, B. A., 73
Fishman, R. A., 340, 341, 345
Fitzpatrick, P. J., 286–302, 300
Fletcher, J. W., 347
Florey, H. W., 84
Fogelholm, R., 317, 324
Folger, R., 38
Folkman, J., 131
Foote, W. E., 352
Fordham, E. W., 243, 245
Foulds, L., 31
Frank, A. L., 41
Frasher, W. G., 88
Frei, E., 153, 343
French, L. A., 341, 342, 343
Friedell, G. H., 37
Fuchs, K., 303–313

Galicich, J. H., 341, 343, 390–414, 391
Gallagher, B. B., 356
Gamache, F. W., 191, 195, 390–414
Garde, A., 196
Gasic, G. J., 94
Gassel, M. M., 191
Gawler, J., 224, 236
Gelber, R., 258
Gercovich, R. G., 22
Gilbert, H., 303–313, 314–327
Gilbert, R. W., 26
Gildersleeve, N., 216
Glaser, G. H., 356
Glass, J. P., 336
Glaves, D., 38, 40, 42
Goldblatt, S. A., 85
Goldman, E. E., 340
Good, R. A., 351
Gottlieb, J. A., 22, 343
Grasso, R. J., 352
Green, J., 4, 332
Greene, H. S. N., 31, 46
Griffiths, C. T., 22
Griffiths, J. D., 85
Gruener, R., 352
Gudman-Hoyer, E., 350
Gulati, D. R., 341
Güldner, F. -H., 87
Gullberg, G. T., 248
Gullino, P. M., 45

Guner, M., 352
Guomundsson, K. R., 14
Gurcay, O., 352
Gutin, P. H., 343, 344

Haar, F., 390, 398, 399, 407, 410
Hadjidimos, A., 348
Hagan, R., 354
Hakulinen, T., 2
Hall, T. C., 342
Hama, K., 119
Hansen, H. H., 367
Hanson, J. C., 195
Haque, N., 195, 344
Hardman, J., 90
Harlos, J. P., 41
Harwood, A. R., 294, 298, 299, 310
Hasegawa, H., 100, 109, 135, 136
Hashimoto, P. H., 119
Hawkins, N. V., 301
Hazra, T., 343
Heidorn, G. H., 357
Hendley, E. D., 356
Hendrickson, F. R., 258, 259, 261, 262,
    279–285, 279, 299, 310, 364, 367
Henkin, R. I., 352
Henry, P., 318, 324
Hilal, S. K., 210, 218
Hilaris, B. S., 259, 265, 266, 311
Hildebrand, J., 16, 195
Hindo, W. A., 299
Hirano, A., 11, 90, 91, 115, 130, 131
Ho, D. H., 153
Hoffman, E. J., 248
Hollenberg, N. K., 86, 94
Holyoke, E. D., 41, 42, 44
Hoppe, E., 86
Hoppe, J. O., 109
Horenstein, S., 194
Horton, J., 259, 343
Hounsfield, G. N., 208
Houser, O. W., 236
Huber, D., 35
Huckman, M., 210
Hustu, J., 261
Hutchinson, D. J., 140
Hyman, R. A., 224

Ido, T., 249
Inagaki, J., 2
Ingraham, F. D., 341
Irie, K., 167

Jack, H., 350, 360
Jack, W., 344
Jackson, D. V., 329
Jacobs, L., 84, 203, 228, 232

Jellinger, K., 317, 318, 319, 324
Johannson, B., 354
Johns, D. G., 100, 153
Johnson, C. E., 352
Johnson, R. K., 153
Jones, T., 250
Jonnson, O., 105
Josephson, R. L., 92, 93
Jost, R. G., 244

Kagan, A. R., 303–327, 314, 315, 316
Kane, W., 92, 96
Karnovsky, M. J., 101
Kato, Y., 333
Katz, F. H., 344
Kaufmann, J. C. E., 95
Kawaguchi, T., 87, 88
Kazner, E., 220
Keen, C. W., 286–302
Kennedy, C., 149
Kernohan, J. W., 191, 342
Kido, D. K., 212
Kim, J.-H., 138, 267
Kindt, G. W., 270
Kinkel, W. R., 232
Kinsey, D. L., 51
Klara, P. M., 119
Klastersky, J., 2
Klatzo, I., 354
Klein, E., 167
Klintz, B. L., 316
Kobayashi, T., 151
Kofman, S., 340, 341, 342. 352
Kotsilimbas, D. G., 352
Kramer, R. A., 210
Kramer, S., 279
Kremer, M., 193
Kretzchmar, K., 224
Kricheff, I. I., 210
Krishnamurthy, G. T., 242
Kuhl, D. E., 243, 249
Kullberg, G., 345, 353
Kung, P. C., 84

Lachmann, P. J., 184
Lambert, P. M., 319, 321, 322, 324
Lane, B., 223
Lang, E. F., 198, 258
Lang, E. J., 381, 386, 403, 410
Lanksch, W., 347, 348
Larson, E. B., 208
Lasse, S., 16, 21, 23
Lassen, N. A., 2, 107
Lawrence, D. J. R., 43
Latchaw, L. E., 210
Laws, E. R., 356
Le Blanc, R. A., 8

Leighton, J., 31
Leveille, J., 242
Levin, V. A., 100, 144, 149, 151, 152, 328
Levy, M., 193
Lichtman, M. A., 40
Lieber, S., 349
Lieberman, A., 343, 384
Lindgren, M., 314
Liotta, L. A., 45
Livingston, K. E., 15, 412
Locksmith, J. B., 321, 322, 324
Long, D. M., 8, 11, 127, 130, 341, 348, 354, 356
Lotan, R., 62
Luce, J. K., 343
Luna, M. A., 22
Lundberg, N., 193, 345

McCann, W. P., 353
McEwen, B., 344, 352, 356
McKissock, W., 14, 15, 81, 82, 191, 383, 388
McLelland, J., 344
Madow, L., 201
Maier, J. G., 320, 321, 324
Malamud, N., 194, 319, 324
Mandybur, T. I., 197
Marchalonis, J. J., 60
Marchesi, V. T., 84
Marshall, L. R., 343
Martin, J. H., 91
Marty, R., 347
Marynick, S. P., 344
Masdeu, J. C., 232
Maslow, D. E., 41
Mastaglia, F. L., 236
Matsui, T., 11, 90, 91, 115
Matsuoka, S., 345, 353
Matthews, M. J., 82, 91
Maurice-Williams, R. S., 195
Mayer, R. J., 22
Mayhew, E., 40
Meagher, R., 15
Mealey, J., 352
Mehta, B. M., 140, 336
Meikle, A. W., 343
Menig, G., 341, 348, 361
Messeter, K., 251
Messina, A. V., 238
Metzgar, R. S., 167
Meyer, P. C., 20, 21, 84
Meyza, J., 158
Michel, D., 199
Mikhael, M. A., 234
Miller, J. D., 356, 357
Mitchison, N. A., 184
Modesti, L. M., 390

Montana, G. S., 281, 390, 403
Mori, K., 197
Morrison, G. M., 301
Murphy, B. E. P., 344
Muss, H. B., 244

Nadel, E. M., 85
Nakamura, K., 87, 88
Netsky, M. G., 16, 21, 23
New, P. F. J., 210, 213, 224, 243
Newell, J., 387
Newman, S. J., 367
Nickson, J. J., 265
Nicolson, G. L., 32, 33, 45, 50–65, 53, 54, 58, 59, 60, 61, 62
Nisce, L. Z., 266, 267, 281, 311, 367
Novak, E., 349
Nulsen, F. E., 356
Nussbaum, H., 303–313, 314–327
Nystrom, S., 128

O'Connor, J. S., 356
Odom, G. L., 383, 412
Oettgen, H. F., 165–185
Ohno, K., 107, 109, 110
Old, L. J., 165–185, 165, 167
Oldendorf, W. H., 107
Olenick, S. R., 167
Olson, M. E., 336
O'Meara, R. A. Q., 41
Onuigbo, W. I. B., 11
Order, S. E., 257–264, 263, 281, 283, 310, 311, 364, 367, 390
Ortega, B. O., 356
Ortega, P., 8
Overton, E., 102

Paillas, J. E., 14, 15, 21, 193, 194, 195, 196, 197, 198
Pallis, C. A., 317, 319, 321, 324
Palmer, J. J., 317, 321, 324
Papo, L., 15
Pappius, H. M., 105, 353, 357
Parks, R. C., 51
Parsons, L., 37
Patlak, C. S., 100
Patterson, R. H., 390, 398, 399, 407, 410
Pay, N. T., 224
Pellet, W., 14, 15, 21, 193, 194, 195, 196, 197, 198
Pendergras, H., 224
Peng, G. W., 151
Percy, A. K., 14
Perret, G. E., 342
Peters, A., 117
Peterson, H.-I., 85
Petit-Dutaillis, D., 15

Peylan-Ramu, N., 236
Pfreundschuh, M., 165–185, 167, 177
Phelps, M. E., 247, 248, 250
Phillips, R., 265
Pickren, J. W., 66, 67
Pilgrim, H. I., 51
Pimm, M. V., 32
Plowman, J., 158
Poirier, J., 81, 82
Pontecorvu, G., 184
Porter, J., 350
Posner, J. B., 2–29, 11, 15, 20, 52, 189–207, 191, 193, 195, 197, 267, 281, 283, 341, 342, 352, 381, 385, 386, 390–414, 390, 404, 405, 406
Poste, G., 30
Potter, M., 51
Powers, W. E., 321, 322, 324
Prados, M., 341
Prato, F. S., 261
Price, H. I., 234
Price, M. R., 234

Rabotti, G., 31, 47
Raichle, M. E., 107, 246–253, 246, 248, 249, 251
Rall, D. P., 328
Ransohoff, J., 343, 354, 356, 381–389, 407, 410
Rao, A. R., 303–313, 314–327, 364–379
Rapoport, S. I., 100–114, 100, 101, 102, 103, 104, 106, 107, 108, 109, 110, 117, 127, 140, 151, 341
Rapp, H. J., 33
Raskind, R., 381, 386, 405, 410
Rassmussen, T., 341
Reagen, T. J., 317, 318, 319, 321, 323, 324
Reah, T. G., 20, 21
Rech, T. C., 84
Redvanly, C. S., 246, 249
Reese, T. S., 101, 117
Reinhold, H. S., 322, 323, 324
Reivich, M., 105, 249
Renaudin, J., 343, 384, 408
Resnick, L., 167
Reulen, H. J., 191, 340, 341, 354
Richards, P., 14, 15, 81, 82, 381, 386, 410
Rider, W. D., 287
Ritchie, A. C., 85
Robbins, J. C., 60
Roberts, S. S., 85
Robinson, K. P., 86
Romanul, F. C. A., 90
Rosenblatt, M. B., 2
Ross, W. C., 158
Rotstein, J., 351
Rottenberg, D. A., 234, 314

Rovit, R., 354
Rubin, P., 4, 332
Rubinstein, L. J., 4, 11, 81, 82, 314
Ruderman, N. B., 342
Russell, D. S., 4, 11

Sadoff, L., 364–379
Saffiotti, U., 86
Sakurada, O., 149, 160
Salsbury, A. J., 85
Sandberg, A. A., 31
Sato, H., 38, 40
Schaul, N., 345, 346
Schechter, J., 131
Schermm, F. R., 357
Schimpff, R. D., 94
Schmiedek, 343
Schwartz, M. L., 344, 356, 357
Sears, E. S., 236
Seligman, A. M., 158
Shapiro, W. R., 52, 109, 134–145, 160, 328–329, 335, 336, 341, 352
Shehata, W. M., 259, 299, 367
Shiku, H., 165–185, 167, 169, 170, 171, 172, 174, 176, 178, 183
Shubik, P., 85
Siesjo, B. K., 251
Sikora, K., 184
Silen, N. H., 352
Silverberg, E., 2
Simionescu, M. D., 192, 195
Simionescu, M. E., 14, 15
Simpson, W. J., 294, 298, 299, 310
Skipper, H. E., 158
Slack, N. H., 73, 79, 352
Slater, J., 198, 258, 383, 388, 403, 412
Sligar, P., 342
Smedal, M. I., 317, 318, 321, 322, 324
Sokoloff, L., 105, 149, 249
Solis, O. J., 216, 218, 220
Sporn, M. B., 62
Stastny, F. H., 356
Stern, L., 352
Sterrett, P. T., 102
Steudel, W. I., 346, 347
Stevens, E. A., 234
Stevenson, G. T., 43
Stewart, H. L., 92
Stjernholm, M. R., 344
Stoker, M. G. P., 39
Stormont, J. M., 357, 363
Stortebecker, T. P., 14, 15, 192, 259, 383, 385, 412
Sträuli, P., 38
Strub, R. L., 195, 196
Studer, R. K., 354
Sturm, K. W., 317, 318, 319, 324

Subjeck, J. R., 41
Sugarbaker, E. D., 51
Suzuki, M., 38, 40
Swenberg, J. A., 134
Symonds, C., 193

Tachibana, T., 167
Takahashi, T., 165–185, 167, 178
Talalla, A., 191
Tani, E., 131
Tao, T. W., 32, 45
Tarnoff, J. F., 392
Tator, C. H., 100
Teppo, L., 2
Ter-Pogossian, M. M., 248
Thomas, J. P., 357
Thompson, H. K., 103
Todd, M., 287
Tretter, P., 318, 320, 321, 322, 324
Tritapepe, R. C., 15
Tyler, F. H., 343

Ueda, R., 165–185, 167, 177
Urtasun, R. C., 387
Ushio, Y., 134, 138, 140, 160

Vales, O., 87
Van Eck, J. H. M., 15, 192, 197
Van Harreveld, A., 352, 356
Viadana, E., 2, 23, 66, 67, 72
Vick, N. A., 11, 115–133, 115, 116, 117, 144, 152, 328
Vider, M., 11
Vieth, R. G., 381, 412
Vincent, F. M., 344
Volkman, A., 39

Waggener, J. D., 115, 124, 130, 131
Wagner, J., 303–313
Walker, M.D., 115
Wallace, A. C., 86, 94
Wallack, M. K., 184
Wara, W. M., 279–285, 316, 317, 321, 322, 323, 324
Warren, B. A., 4, 81–99, 84, 85, 87, 94, 95
Waxman, A. D., 347
Wayland, H. A., 88
Webster, D. R., 85
Weed, R. J., 40
Weinstein, J. D., 345, 348
Weinstein, M. A., 208
Weiss, L., 30–49, 30, 31, 35, 36, 38, 39, 40, 41, 42, 43, 50, 85
Weiss, S. R., 407
Wiess, M. H., 356
Werk, E. E., 344

West, K. A., 345, 353
Westergaard, E., 117, 127
Wharam, M. D., 262
Wheelock, E. F., 43, 44
White, D. R., 244
Whiteside, J. A., 100
Wiernik, P. H., 22
Wilfong, R. F., 117
Williams, C., 329
Willis, R. A., 2, 16, 18, 85
Wilson, C. B., 317, 321, 324, 335
Wolf, A. P., 246, 249
Wolff, E., 37, 193
Wolk, R. W., 23
Wollin, M., 314–327, 315, 316
Wollman, H. W., 191
Woodbury, D. M., 348, 351, 352
Woods, S., Jr., 89
Wright, R. L., 352

Yamada, K., 37
Young, D. F., 191, 193, 195, 267, 335, 336, 399
Yung, W. K., 115, 116

Zharko, D. S., 158
Zeidman, I., 31, 50, 87
Zimmerman, H. M., 11, 131
Zubrod, C. C., 328
Zulch, K. J., 15, 191
Zweifach, B. W., 88